TRANSFORMING COGNITIVE REHABILITATION

Also Available

Cognitive Rehabilitation:
An Integrative Neuropsychological Approach
McKay Moore Sohlberg and Catherine A. Mateer

TRANSFORMING COGNITIVE REHABILITATION

Effective Instructional Methods

McKay Moore Sohlberg
Justine Hamilton
Lyn S. Turkstra

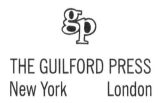

THE GUILFORD PRESS
New York   London

The authors have checked with sources believed to be reliable in their efforts to provide
information that is complete and generally in accord with the standards of practice that are
accepted at the time of publication. However, in view of the possibility of human error or
changes in behavioral, mental health, or medical sciences, neither the authors, nor the editors
and publisher, nor any other party who has been involved in the preparation or publication
of this work warrants that the information contained herein is in every respect accurate or
complete, and they are not responsible for any errors or omissions or the results obtained from
the use of such information. Readers are encouraged to confirm the information contained in
this book with other sources.

Library of Congress Cataloging-in-Publication Data

Names: Sohlberg, McKay Moore, author. | Hamilton, Justine, author. |
  Turkstra, Lyn, author.
Title: Transforming cognitive rehabilitation : effective instructional
  methods / McKay Moore Sohlberg, Justine Hamilton, Lyn S. Turkstra.
Description: New York, NY : The Guilford Press, [2023] | Includes
  bibliographical references and index.
Identifiers: LCCN 2022019588 | ISBN 9781462550876 (cloth)
Subjects: LCSH: Cognitive therapy. | Brain
  damage—Patients—Rehabilitation.
Classification: LCC RC489.C63 S657 2023 | DDC
  616.89/1425—dc23/eng/20220716
LC record available at https://lccn.loc.gov/2022019588

About the Authors

McKay Moore Sohlberg, PhD, CCC-SLP, is Professor of Communication Disorders and Sciences at the University of Oregon, where she has been teaching, conducting research, and providing clinical training since 1994. Dr. Sohlberg is known internationally for her pioneering work in the field of cognitive rehabilitation. She has published widely on the development and evaluation of treatments to assist people with acquired brain injury in managing cognitive impairments in order to function optimally in their communities. Dr. Sohlberg has contributed to a number of evidence-based practice guidelines supported by the Academy of Neurologic Communication Disorders and Sciences.

Justine Hamilton, MClSc, MBA, is Assistant Professor and Director of Clinical Education in the Speech–Language Pathology Program at the School of Rehabilitation Science, McMaster University, Hamilton, Ontario, Canada. Ms. Hamilton joined McMaster to help develop the first problem-based learning program in speech–language pathology in North America. Her teaching responsibilities include problem-based tutorial and clinical skills lab courses. Prior to joining McMaster, Ms. Hamilton was the cofounder of a speech–language pathology practice with three locations across southern Ontario. Her interests include assessment and treatment of aphasia and cognitive–communication disorders as well as objective measurement of meaningful, real-world outcomes.

Lyn S. Turkstra, PhD, is Assistant Dean and Professor in the Speech–Language Pathology Program at the School of Rehabilitation Science, McMaster University, Hamilton, Ontario, Canada. She is a clinical speech–language pathologist by training and senior scholar in the field of acquired cognitive–communication disorders. Dr. Turkstra's research aims to advance our understanding of cognitive mechanisms underlying communication disorders, and to translate research findings into assessment and intervention methods that improve life participation for adolescents and adults with acquired brain injury. Dr. Turkstra has coauthored national and international practice guidelines in cognitive rehabilitation for both civilian and military populations.

Contributors

Rose Dunn*, PhD, Neuropsychologist, Neuropsychology and Behavioral Health Consultants, Dallas, Texas

Mary K. Ferraro, PhD, Occupational Therapist, Moss Rehabilitation Research Institute, Einstein Medical Center, Elkins Park, Pennsylvania

Tessa Hart, PhD, Neuropsychologist, Moss Rehabilitation Research Institute, Einstein Medical Center, Elkins Park, Pennsylvania; Department of Rehabilitation Medicine, Sidney Kimmel Medical College, Thomas Jefferson University, Philadelphia, Pennsylvania

Pauline Mashima*, PhD, Speech–Language Pathologist, Communication Sciences and Disorders, John A. Burns School of Medicine, University of Hawai'i at Mānoa, Honolulu, Hawaii

Diane Paul*, PhD, Speech–Language Pathologist and Senior Director, Clinical Issues in Speech–Language Pathology, American Speech–Language–Hearing Association, Rockville, Maryland

Kelly Ann Peña*, MS, Speech–Language Pathologist, Department of Rehabilitation and Movement Sciences, School of Health Professions, Rutgers, The State University of New Jersey, Newark, New Jersey

Amanda R. Rabinowitz, PhD, Director, Brain Injury Neuropsychology Lab, Moss Rehabilitation Research Institute, Einstein Medical Center, Elkins Park, Pennsylvania; Department of Rehabilitation Medicine, Sidney Kimmel Medical College, Thomas Jefferson University, Philadelphia, Pennsylvania

Katharine Seagly*, PhD, Neuropsychologist and Rehabilitation Psychologist, Traumatic Brain Injury Rehabilitation Program; Department of Physical Medicine and Rehabilitation, University of Michigan, Ann Arbor, Michigan

Brigid Waldron-Perrine*, PhD, Neuropsychologist and Rehabilitation Psychologist, Department of Physical Medicine and Rehabilitation, University of Michigan, Ann Arbor, Michigan

---

*Members of the Joint Committee on Interprofessional Relations Between the American Psychological Association and the American Speech–Language–Hearing Association.

Preface

It has been over a decade since the publication of our last textbook on cognitive rehabilitation, *Optimizing Cognitive Rehabilitation* (Sohlberg & Turkstra, 2011). There has been so much progress and evolution in the field since then, and what started out as a revision has ended up as a new volume. In particular, this text reflects the changing contexts of cognitive rehabilitation practice, increased recognition of the multitude of psychological and somatic factors that affect cognitive function, and the emergence of novel theories that inform and guide clinical practice.

This new textbook, *Transforming Cognitive Rehabilitation*, begins with five chapters that set the stage for the remainder of the volume. Chapter 1 introduces five paradigms that serve as the context for cognitive rehabilitation today. In Chapter 2, we review key cognitive functions typically affected by acquired brain damage. Chapter 3, a new chapter, introduces the concept of "psychological mindedness" and provides counseling frameworks and strategies that can be incorporated in cognitive rehabilitation sessions to promote client engagement and motivation. Chapter 4 is also a new chapter and provides an overview of the Rehabilitation Treatment Specification System (RTSS; Hart et al., 2019), a framework to describe and classify our treatments. The RTSS encourages clinicians and researchers to specify their intervention methods and desired outcomes, and is applied throughout the remainder of the text. Chapter 5 further builds on the Planning, Implementation, and Evaluation (PIE) framework, first introduced in *Optimizing Cognitive Rehabilitation*.

The remaining chapters apply the principles and frameworks to instruction in the use of cognitive strategies (Chapter 7) and external cognitive aids (Chapter 8), teaching discrete facts and routines (Chapter 6), and methods to support social competence after brain injury (Chapter 9). Topics new to this text are rehabilitation in the inpatient setting (Chapter 10); a review of the current state of computer-based, drill-focused cognitive rehabilitation (Chapter 11), necessitated by the intensified marketing and media promotion targeting cognitive rehabilitation providers; and cognitive rehabilitation for clients with functional cognitive symptoms (Chapter 12).

We describe cognitive rehabilitation principles and frameworks, intervention options, and types of evaluation that are broadly applicable across etiologies of cognitive impairment. Many disorders and diseases can affect cognitive functioning, including acute-onset disorders such as stroke and traumatic brain injury; degenerative diseases such as multiple sclerosis, Parkinson disease, and Alzheimer's disease; and viruses and infections such as COVID-19, meningitis, and encephalitis. Each has unique features that will inform assessment and treatment, and requires that practitioners be informed about the specific etiology, symptomatology, recovery trajectories, and comorbidities. Knowing which techniques and treatment approaches fit with particular client profiles requires that clinicians are familiar with the populations that they serve.

Finally, this book has been designed to support the reader in translating knowledge into practice. Each intervention chapter follows a similar format, beginning with a summary of current knowledge and supporting evidence. We provide practical examples to illustrate the concepts as well as blank treatment planning forms to help clinicians structure their therapy sessions according to the framework outlined in each chapter. Case Applications are then provided in a stepwise manner whereby readers are encouraged to take the narrative information provided in the chapter and map it onto a session planning or progress monitoring form, and then compare their work to completed Case Application: Sample Answer forms at the end of the chapter. Blank forms are provided at the end of each intervention chapter and are also available for downloading at the book's companion website. As discussed in Chapter 4, to develop a new skill, clients must have lots of opportunities for hands-on practice, and this is no less true for clinicians seeking to improve their skills. It is our hope that this level of structure and supported practice will allow clinicians to easily put their new learning into action!

Acknowledgments

This book was written during a pandemic, a backdrop that created a sense of urgency and hope, mirroring our disposition toward the field of cognitive rehabilitation. For most of the writing and editing, the three of us were quarantined in our homes, meeting electronically every several weeks. We experienced in new ways what our clients, their significant others, and caregivers had already taught us: our greatest powers are rooted in connection, and our most effective actions are collective. We channeled our collective clinical community. Our clients, those whom we have served directly and those treated by our students and mentees, guided the creation of this book. We humbly and gratefully acknowledge every client who has embarked on the journey of recovering from brain injury, and every person who has supported them. You have not only helped us become better practitioners, researchers, and instructors, you have helped us become better citizens, family members, and friends. You have deepened our professional and personal selves.

We also wish to thank our respective colleagues. This book rests upon decades of research and vast clinical expertise. Each of us has been mentored and inspired by many people in the field of neurorehabilitation. We so hope that this volume reflects your lessons.

Students, you too have shaped this text. We know that in learning we will teach, and that in teaching we will learn. Thank you. We have learned much from every student who has crossed our paths. You have provided a vision and optimism that our practices will evolve to serve our clients optimally.

Every demanding and worthwhile endeavor benefits from the support of those individuals who provide encouragement and resources that help the project come to fruition. We thank those who gave us the space and reinforcement to write this book. We hope it will help "transform" the field of cognitive rehabilitation and the lives of people living with cognitive and communication challenges after brain injury.

Contents

List of Reproducibles

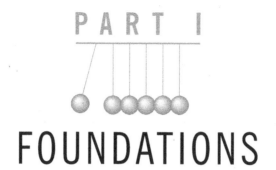

PART I

FOUNDATIONS

CHAPTER 1

Introduction

THE PURPOSE OF COGNITIVE REHABILITATION

Cognitive rehabilitation refers to a diverse assortment of approaches aimed at optimizing function in people experiencing cognitive changes after brain injury. In contrast to other branches of medicine that seek to cure or eliminate disease, rehabilitation recognizes that brain injury often results in conditions that cannot be cured. The recognition that cognitive impairments can be persistent beyond physical recovery led to the development of the cognitive rehabilitation field, which focuses on helping people with acquired cognitive impairments optimize their daily functioning and quality of life.

Cognitive rehabilitation requires an array of knowledge and skills related to understanding the intersections among cognitive processing, physical states, and psychosocial functioning, as well as behavior change and adaptation. As such, successful cognitive rehabilitation takes a professional and community "village" in which, ideally, practitioners from a number of clinical disciplines partner with clients and their natural supports to deliver rehabilitation. While the implementation of clinical practices will vary based on client profiles and practice contexts, *the goal is to encourage functional change and an increased sense of well-being in every client who seeks our expertise.* Holding this goal as the beacon guiding our rehabilitation efforts will enhance our clinical outcomes. Describing cognitive rehabilitation practices that have the potential to enhance individual function and quality of life is the foundational purpose of this book.[1]

HISTORY LESSONS

An examination of past and current practices is essential for guiding our research and clinical endeavors. Based on careful examination, we can leverage the knowledge gained

---

[1] For consistency, we use the term *client* throughout the text, to refer to those who are receiving cognitive rehabilitation. We also use the gender-neutral pronoun *they* except when the individual in a case example has self-identified as male or female.

through experimental and clinical research and apply it to our therapies. In so doing, we can discontinue practices that are not effective and modify existing practices to optimize outcomes. Perhaps one of the most striking examples of the utility of scrutinizing historical practice patterns can be found by considering early cognitive rehabilitation efforts that focused on *process-oriented drill and practice.*

In the late 1970s and early 80s, video games, educational software, and eventually specially designed brain-training drills became a mainstream cognitive rehabilitation approach in the brain injury field. The paper-and-pencil drills were hypothesized to stimulate the rewiring of brain networks and generalize to changes in cognitive processing (Bracy, 1983; Lynch, 2002; Sohlberg & Mateer, 1987). Common tasks included list memorization, practice recalling stories, and puzzles and games designed to improve attentional focus and problem solving. Over time, research studies showed no robust evidence that nonspecific practice drills restored general cognitive processes, let alone improved functional abilities (e.g., Park & Ingles, 2001). An unfortunate legacy of the drill approach, however, was a proliferation of cognitive rehabilitation workbooks and computer programs with decontextualized, nonadaptive, general cognitive exercises. Of concern, these tools continue to be part of mainstream practice today (see Chapter 11 for a discussion of "brain training" methods and associated research).

A positive outcome of early cognitive rehabilitation approaches is that they furthered our knowledge about what *does* work in rehabilitation and provided several key lessons. For example, research showed that specific aspects of attention may be amenable to improvement in certain client populations; however, the changes were restricted to highly similar tasks (Serino et al., 2007; Sohlberg, Harn, MacPherson, & Wade, 2014; van Heugten, Ponds, & Kessels, 2016). The early process-focused drill work also helped define the range of factors that together are necessary to enhance the neuroplasticity that is the hypothesized mechanism underlying functional changes (see Chapter 4 for a discussion of those factors and Chapter 11 for further discussion of neuroplasticity as it relates to cognitive rehabilitation).

The limitations of process-oriented approaches led to a shift away from dichotomizing therapy interventions into those that promote process-oriented changes (i.e., "restorative" approaches) versus those that train adaptive techniques ("compensatory" approaches). Any intervention that produces enduring changes in thinking and behavior has changed how the brain operates, and clients can be using strategies unconsciously even early in recovery, so the distinction of compensatory versus restorative is an artificial one. This dichotomy is also inconsistent with evidence that strategy use can improve performance on impairment-based measures. As examples, when children with disabilities used augmentative communication devices, they also verbalized more (Millar, Light, & Schlosser, 2006); children who learned mindfulness strategies improved their scores on executive function tests (Zelazo, Forston, Masten, & Carlson, 2018); and adults with aphasia who used conversation strategies also produced more words (Cunningham & Ward, 2003). In clinic, telling a client that their therapy is compensatory rather than restorative also can convey a message that their brain can no longer change and that we have abandoned hope for improvement in basic cognitive functions.

As a field dedicated to helping our clients manage acquired cognitive impairments, our challenge and responsibility are the ongoing evaluation and analysis of our clinical practices to build lines of inquiry that clarify which client profiles have the most potential to benefit from which treatment components. This is how we ensure our clinical practice reflects the current state of knowledge. We hope that this book will move us forward in such an effort.

We seek to facilitate the evolution of effective neurorehabilitation that results in functional changes by describing evidence-based practices and practice-based evidence pertinent to rehabilitation providers who treat clients with acquired cognitive impairments. In addition to translating current knowledge into practice recommendations, we hope to clarify key questions that remain unanswered and deserve more examination. In the decade since the publication of *Optimizing Cognitive Rehabilitation: Effective Instructional Methods* (Sohlberg & Turkstra, 2011), there have been key advancements in our knowledge and service delivery with the potential to positively impact our clinical outcomes. Below we describe five paradigms that are beginning to gain clinical traction, and that we believe should be harnessed to optimize the delivery of cognitive rehabilitation.

FIVE EVOLVING PARADIGMS
WITH POTENTIAL FOR POSITIVE INFLUENCE IN COGNITIVE REHABILITATION

International Classification of Functioning, Disability, and Health

Most readers will be familiar with the World Health Organization's International Classification of Functioning, Disability and Health (ICF; World Health Organization [WHO], 2021), a biopsychosocial model of disability that was developed to classify health and outcomes from health conditions. The ICF for adults was first published in 2001, and a companion for children and youth was published in 2007. While the ICF is not new and has been foundational in cognitive rehabilitation research, we include it here, as there is a need to apply it more robustly to our clinical practice.

The ICF classifies functioning into the following categories:

- *Body structures and functions*, including brain and cognitive functions
- *Activities,* including everyday thinking tasks like remembering instructions or having a conversation
- *Participation* in all aspects of life, including family, school, social, and other life roles
- *Environmental factors* that can be facilitators or barriers

Health and outcomes from health conditions also are influenced by *personal factors*, which are not formally classified in the ICF but are critical contributors to health outcomes. Personal factors include psychological factors such as mood, beliefs, and motivation, which are discussed in Chapter 3, as well as factors such as a person's preinjury knowledge and skills. A person's level of function is the product of dynamic interactions among all of the factors in the model.

Readers are encouraged to access materials at the main ICF website (*www.who.int/ standards/classifications/international-classification-of-functioning-disability-and-health*), and a fillable ICF diagram is provided as Form 1.1 at the end of this chapter and also in the digital files accompanying this book. In this text, we use the ICF to select targets of cognitive rehabilitation—the *what* and *why* of treatment—and the Rehabilitation Treatment Specification System (RTSS; Hart et al., 2019), described in Chapter 4, to specify *how* that treatment is implemented.

Interprofessional Collaboration and Communication in the Delivery of Cognitive Rehabilitation

Support for interdisciplinary care in the treatment of brain injury is not new. Unfortunately, however, integrated care based on interprofessional collaboration and communication remains elusive, with much of our medical rehabilitation being delivered in silos. A primary barrier to interdisciplinary care is reimbursement mandates that are not set up to encourage collaboration. Furthermore, the practice of interprofessional collaboration is still in the early stages of integration into rehabilitation training programs.

Cognitive rehabilitation is delivered by rehabilitation professionals from varying disciplines, including but not limited to neuropsychologists, rehabilitation psychologists, speech-language pathologists, occupational therapists, and physical therapists. Conceptual and practice frameworks differ among these professions, which can result in duplicative, disjointed care and a missed opportunity to integrate knowledge. A recent paper written by an interprofessional collaborative group of speech-language pathologists, rehabilitation psychologists, and neuropsychologists (Mashima et al., 2021) identified challenges in the interprofessional rehabilitation of clients with acquired cognitive impairments after brain injury and offered suggestions for mitigating the problem of siloed care. The authors discussed the specific challenge of defining and operationalizing cognitive rehabilitation and suggested recommendations for interprofessional training, development of a shared perspective and language, and the establishment of interprofessional communication systems. The evolution of systems that promote interprofessional collaboration is key for optimizing our treatment of clients with acquired cognitive impairments.

In this text, we do not discuss roles and qualifications for administering cognitive rehabilitation. There are a number of licensed rehabilitation professionals well suited for delivering cognitive rehabilitation. As in all areas of specialization, regardless of the discipline, it is imperative to receive training specific to brain injury to be qualified to deliver this therapy. Different disciplines will also have distinct areas of expertise critical to successful cognitive rehabilitation. For example, speech-language pathologists are uniquely positioned to understand and treat social communication issues following brain injury; clinical psychologists have expertise in treating comorbid or resulting mental health issues arising from injury and trauma; and occupational therapists have particular knowledge in managing visuospatial challenges related to brain injury. Each of these disciplines may be addressing problems in the cognitive domains of attention, memory, and executive functions. What is needed is interprofessional collaboration using common language, a shared perspective, and clear communication processes.

Emphasis on Empowerment and Self-Efficacy as Integral to Cognitive Rehabilitation

The recognition that psychological functions should be targets in rehabilitation is slowly changing how we practice cognitive rehabilitation. It is accepted that optimal rehabilitation outcomes, including cognitive outcomes, depend on factors such as client motivation and self-efficacy (Kreutzer et al., 2018). Furthermore, nascent research suggests that actively cultivating resilience as a therapy target can lead to improved clinical outcomes for people with brain injury (Neils-Strunjas et al., 2017). Behavioral health science offers a range of evidence-backed behavioral change interventions that can facilitate the uptake and use of clinical interventions and promote adjustment (Michie, van Stralen, & West, 2011). Relevant to cognitive rehabilitation are interventions relating to psychoeducation, persuasion (e.g., motivational interviewing), and enablement through establishing environmental supports. While the gap between recognition and practice remains large, the shift toward person-centered care in rehabilitation is progressing and there is now a foundation for addressing these psychological factors in rehabilitation (DiLollo & Favreau, 2010). Health providers delivering cognitive rehabilitation across disciplines are beginning to use techniques such as motivational interviewing, as they recognize the benefits of collaborating with clients in decisions about rehabilitation goals and therapy approaches (Medley & Powell, 2010). There is a shift away from historic practices where clinicians selected therapy activities believed to match specific areas of cognitive impairments and toward engagement of the client in decision making around goals and targets. Furthermore, while the research remains sparse, there is increasing recognition of the power of establishing a strong therapeutic alliance in neurorehabilitation that can promote engagement, adherence, and client satisfaction (Shelton & Shryock, 2007).

Throughout this book, practices that target and promote client understanding of their condition, engagement, enablement, and self-efficacy are embedded in the recommended therapy (Michie et al., 2011). Chapter 3 is devoted to describing models and concepts of psychological mindedness that are feasible for clinicians to implement as part of their cognitive rehabilitation practice.

Development of the RTSS (Hart et al., 2019)

In Chapter 4 of this text, we introduce the RTSS, a system for describing and classifying rehabilitation treatments. The RTSS was developed by a multidisciplinary group of rehabilitation specialists who observed that rehabilitation was often viewed as a "black box": clients enter with problems and are discharged when they're better, but what happens in the middle is a mystery to most people other than the individual clinician (Hart et al., 2014). In cognitive rehabilitation clinical practice and research, treatments are often described only by variables like duration (e.g., number of sessions), type of impairment or population (e.g., memory therapy, brain injury rehabilitation), or provider (e.g., occupational therapy, speech therapy). These variables do not tell us what the clinician actually *does* during a session. The lack of information about rehabilitation treatments has implications for rehabilitation research, as it makes it difficult to aggregate results across studies, replicate studies, or identify active ingredients. It also creates challenges for aspects of clinical practice, such as transfer of care from one clinician to another and communication among team members. The RTSS is used throughout the remainder of this text to specify treatment targets (goals) and ingredients (clinician actions and the objects they provide).

Adoption of Implementation Science in Research Practices

Implementation science is the study of methods that influence the integration of evidence-based interventions into practice settings. It is a game-changer for the neurorehabilitation field as it addresses the prohibitive lag time inherent in the traditional research pipeline, where the progression from research efficacy to research effectiveness often takes more than a decade (Douglas, Campbell, & Hinckley, 2015). Implementation science also addresses the challenge of limited adoption of tested therapy techniques, as it emphasizes researchers partnering with stakeholders—including clients, clinicians, and administrators—from the beginning of the research process (Sohlberg, Kucheria, Fickas, & Wade, 2015). Interventions developed without consideration of key implementation variables may not be adaptable to meet practice needs. Addressing this challenge is a primary goal of implementation science.

Implementation science has also helped to systematize practice-based evidence (PBE) as a way of closing the evidence gap in neurorehabilitation. PBE uses careful observation methods and detailed case descriptions with frontline clinicians involved in the design and delivery of therapy, which contributes to best practices by allowing the study of a diversity of client and practice variables (Horn, DeJong, & Deutscher, 2012; Lemoncello & Ness, 2013). Chapter 5 includes an example of PBE: the application of single-subject design methodology to clinical practice, to objectively evaluate client outcomes.

The field of cognitive rehabilitation is evolving. We recognize, and hope, that the recommendations and practices offered in this text will change and progress in the years to come. With grounded models, a clear purpose to facilitate functional change and quality of life in our clients with acquired cognitive impairments, and a commitment to ongoing systematic evaluation of our practices, together, we will continue to advance the field of cognitive rehabilitation.

International Classification of Functioning, Disability and Health (ICF)

Health Condition

Body Functions and Structure

Activity

Participation

Environmental Factors

Personal Factors

CHAPTER 2

Cognition

What Clinicians Need to Know

Historically, the focus of cognitive rehabilitation for people with acquired brain injury (ABI) was to remediate ABI-related cognitive impairments, typically focusing on attention, memory, and executive functions. Over time, our understanding of the cognitive effects of ABI has expanded. We've learned how cognitive functions interact in complex and dynamic ways and have identified new cognitive domains affected by ABI, such as social cognition and empathy. We've also developed a keen appreciation of the myriad of contextual, somatic, and psychosocial factors that influence cognition irrespective of direct brain damage. While it has long been accepted that these factors affect cognitive functioning, this knowledge is now front and center when we develop rehabilitation treatments.

Our rehabilitation history is rooted in, and still heavily influenced by, the medical model, which assumes that the remediation of a cognitive impairment should serve as the primary rehabilitation goal (White-Chu, Graves, Godfrey, Bonner, & Sloane, 2009). This means that treatment selection often still relies on matching therapy activities to areas of cognitive impairment identified on standardized tests. As emphasized in our introductory chapter, however, design and delivery of treatment must focus on functional outcomes, which might or might not improve as a result of treatment of specific cognitive functions. Indeed, current mainstream definitions of cognitive rehabilitation, including those written by the Brain Injury Association of America, the Brain Injury Interdisciplinary Special Interest Group of the American Congress of Rehabilitative Medicine, and the Veterans Health Administration emphasize functional change as central to the purpose of cognitive rehabilitation (Koehler, Willhelm, Shoulson, et al., 2012).

COGNITIVE MODELS AND FRAMEWORKS

Our understanding of neural mechanisms underlying human beings' unparalleled cognitive abilities has vastly increased over the past few decades, in part due to advances in noninvasive imaging techniques and the evolution of statistical techniques for analyzing large and complex datasets. At the same time, the field of cognitive rehabilitation has deepened its commitment to develop techniques that foster meaningful, relevant functional changes in the everyday lives of individuals with ABI. One might argue that knowledge of cognitive models and framework is unnecessary given the focus on function. We propose that these models and frameworks guide our clinical observations, helping us interpret test results and select intervention options. For example, understanding models of attention and memory can help a clinician identify strategies for a client who has stopped a previously pleasurable reading activity because they say they can't retain what they read. The clinician might try to sort out whether deficits are related to (1) reduced working memory and not being able to hold onto information as it is read, so they do not form schemas as they read; (2) inability to consolidate and store new concepts; (3) poor retrieval or access to information that was read and stored and can be recognized when asked; or (4) some combination of these. Based on client responses to interview questions, the clinician could select cognitive tests to help sort out the source of the problem and identify a reading strategy that matches the identified problem. For a problem with working memory, the clinician and client may create a strategy that emphasizes setting up the environment to minimize distractions, uses information chunking, and includes active periodic review using the client's own words. For a client whose primary issue is retrieving what they read, the most helpful approach might be a prereading strategy that activates background knowledge and creates an organizing schema for the reading content. Theoretical models might not always explain what we see clinically, but they provide a foundation for identifying aspects of cognition that can be disrupted by injury or disease and inform our treatment decisions.

REMINDER OF FUNDAMENTALS

This chapter is not intended to provide comprehensive background on cognition and cognitive theory. Rather, it focuses on fundamental concepts critical to practicing cognitive rehabilitation. We begin with three key considerations for linking theory to practice:

1. **Cognitive domains are complex and multifactorial.** Domains such as attention, memory, executive functions, and social cognition have a number of subcomponents with important clinical significance.

2. **Cognitive domains interact and have significant overlap with one another.** In this chapter, we describe cognitive functions as if they were independent from each other. These descriptions will help us generate hypotheses about cognitive contributors to a client's behavior and generate ideas for treatment. In everyday functioning, however, it is not possible to isolate cognitive domains and, as discussed in Chapter 11, targeting treatment at a specific cognitive function may not improve everyday performance.

3. **Cognition is affected by a myriad of contextual factors.** The models discussed in this chapter present cognition in isolation for heuristic purposes; however, we know that cognition is affected by many other factors. For example, psychological factors such as motivation and engagement can affect an individual's level of attention and executive function. Somatic factors such as pain or fatigue can decrease cognitive functioning across cognitive domains. Environmental factors such as noise, lighting, or space can influence cognition. These factors are discussed in detail in other chapters. Chapter 3 reviews methods to promote motivation and engagement, and the Plan, Implement, and Evaluate (PIE) model reviewed in Chapter 5 reminds the clinician to consider somatic and environmental factors in the planning and implementation phase of treatment.

In this chapter, we focus on three interrelated cognitive functions that are commonly impaired by ABI: attention, memory, and executive functions. Related to executive functions, we also discuss self-awareness. We describe these functions using models that have been well validated by research and have heuristic value for clinical intervention. We also discuss social cognition, a more recent addition to the cognitive rehabilitation literature, and provide relevant background in this area. We do not discuss language or visuospatial functions and refer readers to other rehabilitation volumes dedicated to these processes.

Attention

Attention encompasses a broad range of skills, processes, and cognitive states. There is considerable overlap among anatomical (Posner & Petersen, 1990); factor-analytic (e.g., Spikman, Boelen, Lamberts, Brouwer, & Fasotti, 2010); cognitive processing (Baddeley & Hitch, 1974); and clinical models of attention (e.g., Mirsky, Anthony, Duncan, Ahearn, & Kellam, 1991). Most attention models, regardless of their theoretical orientation, include four core concepts: the speed with which incoming information is processed, the capacity or amount of incoming information that can be processed, controlling attention and allocating it to specific mental operations, and sustaining attention over time (vigilance). Driving provides a good example of the different types of attention as it requires that an individual must be quick enough to read and understand written signs while driving by them; have the capacity to simultaneously process how cars are moving in their own and nearby lanes while operating the car and attending to traffic signals; be able to suddenly allocate attention to a siren and safely pull over; and keep paying attention throughout the driving process without lapses in vigilance. Each of these four attention functions is vulnerable to brain injury (Sohlberg & Mateer, 2001).

Clinically, it is useful to distinguish between attention functions that are *bottom up* versus *top down*. Bottom-up processes are reflexive and stimulus-bound attentional functions, such as speed of processing, automatic orientation to novel stimuli, and overall attentional capacity. Top-down processes refer to internally generated, task-independent processes used to allocate or control attention processes (Fish, 2017). A common clinical model of top-down attentional processes (e.g., Sohlberg & Mateer, 2001) includes the following subcomponents:

• Sustained attention, also referred to as vigilance: maintaining attention on an internal or external stimulus over time. An example is being able to complete a continuous task such as reading an article without your mind wandering.

• Attentional control: voluntary attentional control processes that affect attention allocation to specific tasks, including selective, divided, and alternating attention. An example of using these types of processes would be during the activity of driving when the driver divides their attention between different oncoming sources of information, for example, motorically operating the car while paying attention to the visual information on the road. The driver allocates or alternates attention when they listen to or glance at navigation guidance and then return their primary attention to the road.

Different types of strategies and interventions can be used to affect the bottom-up versus top-down processes. For example, a bottom-up intervention might be to structure tasks to be repetitive so working memory demands are decreased. Chapter 11 reviews some instances when drill-based therapy might be used in conjunction with top-down activities, such as a person repeating a self-selected phrase like "focus" when they feel like their attention is wavering on a drill-based task.

Attention processes must be inferred and can be part of clinicians' hypothesis testing as they observe clients, listen to their concerns, and discern if a particular subcomponent or set of subcomponents of attention might be managed by a cognitive strategy designed to support that component.

Memory

There are two general types of memory models: structural models, which describe different types of memory; and process models, which describe how information is learned, stored, and recalled over time. We begin by describing structural models, as these are a common starting point when discussing clients with ABI.

Structural Models

A critical clinical distinction in structural models is between the two main time-dependent forms of memory: *short-term* versus *long-term memory*, which are primarily distinguished by (1) duration of memory storage and (2) capacity of the memory storage. Long-term memory is thought to hold information permanently and in unlimited capacity. Short-term memory is what is "on your mind" at any moment in time, your "mental workspace" (Baddeley, Eysenck, & Anderson, 2009). It is what a person can hold in conscious thought (if they are not interrupted) and thus has a short duration and limited capacity (about seven items or chunks of information). The original notion of short-term memory has been subsumed into the current term, *working memory*, and we use that term here.

WORKING MEMORY

Working memory refers to both the short-term storage of information and also the active process of manipulating that information for either storage or retrieval (Baddeley et al., 2009). Working memory allows us to temporarily hold information in mind while applying strategies such as elaboration during learning (Markowitsch, 1998), or while searching long-term memory for an idea or word we are trying to retrieve. Capacity for short-term storage of information is typically measured via tests of *simple span*, like asking a client to repeat a series of numbers or words. The active manipulation of information in working memory, sometimes called *operational span*, is typically measured by asking the client to perform a series of mental operations on information, such as presenting a mixed string of numbers and letters and asking the client to repeat it with numbers in numerical order and letters in alphabetical order.

To get a sense of simple and operational working memory span, imagine planning your workday: you might hold a number of different tasks in mind and mentally sort through and rearrange them according to constraints such as priority, available time, and schedules of other people involved. This exercise shows how working memory requires active control processes, such as rehearsal and retrieval strategies that encourage information to be held in temporary storage or to be encoded (Baddeley & Hitch, 1974). It also shows how working memory requires control of attention, as once attention is shifted, the contents of working memory can no longer be consciously recalled (Baddeley & Hitch, 1974). These examples demonstrate the interrelation of attention and memory, and also interrelations among both of these and executive functions (discussed in the next section).

Working memory plays a critical role in communication, a factor that can be overlooked in clinical practice. Consider the following sentence, from *The Identicals* by E. Hilderbrand (2017, p. 360):

> Eleanor hears about Tabitha's love affair with the builder and that the builder's sister is the woman Harper betrayed with Billy's doctor.

This three-clause sentence is written in active voice and has relatively simple concepts (sister, love, builder, doctor), but it is a mentally exhausting sentence to understand. The reason is the large number of different people to keep in mind (seven) and the number of words or phrases that need to be reordered to understand the meaning (six), that is, the simple and operational working memory load. Although this is an extreme example, clinicians should keep working memory in mind (pun intended) when interacting with clients, and also when evaluating clients' comprehension of spoken and written information in everyday interactions.

Working memory is important for rehabilitation specialists to understand because it is often disrupted following brain injury. It provides the mental workspace for us to perform complex activities such as reasoning, learning, and comprehension. It also is the mental workspace for *executive functions*—the cognitive processes that underlie goal-directed behavior—and *metacognition*—the process of thinking about one's own thinking and making adjustments accordingly (see below). A person with a working memory impairment might appear to have an executive function impairment because they cannot hold information in mind long enough to plan, organize, or sequence it. What appears to be a deficit in metacognition (i.e., lack of awareness of one's deficits) also can be due to working memory impairments, as it is difficult to reflect on one's own performance when working memory resources are already consumed by task performance (Kennedy et al., 2008).

LONG-TERM MEMORY

Long-term memory encompasses a number of different types of memory that are distinguished by the types of information stored and how that information is learned and retrieved. Table 2.1 provides definitions of key types of long-term memory. The most basic distinction is between explicit or *declarative* learning and memory and implicit or

TABLE 2.1. Definition of Different Types of Content-Dependent Forms of Memory

Types of long-term memory	Description
Declarative memory	Explicit knowledge base
Episodic memory	Storage of events that are tagged in time and place
Semantic memory	Storage of facts and concepts
Metamemory (subset of metacognition)	Awareness about one's own memory functioning
Prospective memory	Remembering to initiate future intentions
Nondeclarative memory	Implicit memory; doesn't require conscious awareness of learning
Procedural memory	Acquisition of rules, sequences, perceptual motor skills
Emotional associations	Association of feelings with people and events
Priming	Increased probability of producing a response because of having previously produced it

nondeclarative learning and memory (see review by Baron & Arbel, 2022). These two memory types are distinguished not only by how they are learned and retrieved, but also by their trajectory of development and decline over the lifespan, the neural mechanisms thought to underlie each and, related to those mechanisms, the likelihood that each learning and memory type will be impaired versus spared in clients with acquired cognitive impairments.

Declarative learning is the conscious process of acquiring new memories. Declarative memories are the knowledge base of information about which we have conscious awareness. This is the type of learning and memory most laypeople mean when they use the term *memory*. Two distinct categories of declarative memory are *semantic* and *episodic* memory. Semantic memory is our "mental encyclopedia" and comprises our knowledge base. Knowing that spiders have eight legs and Jupiter is the largest planet are examples of semantic memory. Episodic memory is memory for temporally related events and comprises our autobiographical memory. Recall of the spider you saw this morning and your trip to the planetarium are examples of episodic memory. Although semantic and episodic memories differ in some characteristics, they are highly interdependent at both encoding and retrieval phases of learning. For example, existing semantic knowledge affects the learning of new episodic memories in both healthy and impaired learners (Greenberg & Verfaellie, 2010). There also is some debate about whether they are truly different memory types, or if they are different instantiations of a unitary memory representation (Irish & Vatansever, 2020).

Declarative learning and memory improve throughout the first two decades of life, in both the amount of information we accumulate and our ability to form and retrieve those memories. The rate of new declarative learning slows down after the sixth or seventh decade of life, and retrieval slows down as well, but there is great individual variability. Declarative learning is highly dependent on brain structures such as the hippocampus that are vulnerable to loss of oxygen. As loss of oxygen to the brain (hypoxia or anoxia) is a common feature of brain injury, impaired declarative learning is relatively common among individuals with ABI.

Declarative learning is enhanced by conscious strategies such as elaboration, trial-and-error, or discovery methods. It is not tied to the learning context, so it can be generalized to other situations. For example, you can probably recall a family holiday event from your childhood without physically being in the setting in which it occurred, although that setting might provide useful cues to help retrieve specific memories. Retrieval of long-term declarative memory is helped by meaning cues and prompts, as well as by an effortful search of long-term memory (e.g., thinking of relatives who might have been at that family event, or eliciting hints from family members). Because declarative memory is conscious, it is encoded and retrieved using working memory. This is another case in which a working memory impairment can masquerade as a long-term declarative memory impairment: if the client cannot hold information in their mind long enough to use an encoding strategy, they might appear to have a declarative memory impairment. If the information is divided into smaller chunks or made simpler, however, or if distractions are reduced, the client might perform normally.

Nondeclarative learning is the process of acquiring memories through automatic association or repeated practice, without conscious awareness of the learning process. Nondeclarative memory includes memory for procedures (*procedural memory*) as well as emotional associations that we form unconsciously throughout our lives, like connecting exams with anxiety, or the smell of a certain perfume with love. A key feature of procedural learning is that it is *probabilistic*: that is, what is learned is the information or behavior that is repeated most often, regardless of the importance of the stimulus. Stated another way, "Practice makes habits." When a person fails to retrieve information from nondeclarative memory, attempts to consciously retrieve it are unhelpful. For example, to remember the number of days in a month, many people have learned the "30 days has September . . ." rhyme. To recall a particular month, it is often necessary to start at the beginning of the rhyme. Hints, cues, and encouragement to "try harder" (all of which rely on declarative memory processes) are likely to be less effective. Priming is another example of nondeclarative memory. It occurs when the introduction of one stimulus influences the memory or reaction to a subsequent stimulus, due to the activation of an association just before that second stimulus is introduced. For example, briefly showing someone a photo of a person they know may increase the likelihood they would give that name when asked to think of a name for a random person in a new photo, even if they have no recollection of being shown the original photo.

Unlike declarative learning and memory, nondeclarative learning and memory are highly context dependent. You might be able to recall a childhood family event by thinking consciously about it, but you are unlikely to remember procedural information such as how you learned the social skills you used on that day or how you learned to hold your fork at dinner. Because of this context dependence, nondeclarative memories do not automatically generalize except to situations with highly similar surface features. This *hyperspecificity* of learning is a challenge in rehabilitation and likely underlies much of the failure to generalize treatment gains outside of the clinic. Strategies to promote generalization of nondeclarative learning are discussed in subsequent chapters.

Also unlike declarative memory, nondeclarative learning and memory are virtually adultlike at birth and largely preserved throughout life. Phenomena such as language and social skill learning depend on this type of memory, and evidence to date suggests that it is highly resistant to disease. The robustness and persistence of nondeclarative learning underlie the effectiveness of error-controlled instructional methods such as spaced retrieval training, discussed in Chapters 4 and 6. Nondeclarative learning and memory are thought to rely on structures such as the cerebellum, basal ganglia, and amygdala, although debate continues about which neural systems are essential for different types of nondeclarative learning.

Memory Process Models

While structural models describe memory types, process models describe how information is transformed over time, including how we detect, learn, store, retrieve, recognize, extinguish, and forget information, and what helps or hinders each of these processes. A classic process model is that developed by Baddeley, Wilson, and Watts (see Baddeley, 1995). This model begins with an *attention* stage, which is the initial registration of information and incorporates the range of bottom-up and top-down attention functions described above. It is a logical component of memory as it is this capacity that initially allows the system to gain access to and ultimately use incoming information. The *encoding* stage is the level of analysis performed on material to be remembered. It relies on working memory and the ability to hold information in mind so it can be further processed. A person must be able to process and interpret incoming information if it is to be remembered and later recalled. For example, a language comprehension deficit will prohibit the encoding of associated verbal information and thus prevent the formation of memory traces. The *consolidation* stage is the process of stabilizing a memory trace after the initial activation of information, and contrasts with *storage*, which is thought to be a passive process of retaining information. *Retrieval* refers to the act of consciously recalling or reaccessing events or information that has been previously encoded or stored.

A key component of process models is *time*. Studies have shown that memories are consolidated over times that extend from milliseconds, for consolidation in working memory (Ricker, Nieuwenstein, Bayliss, & Barrouillet, 2018), to months or even years, for long-term and lifelong memories (McGaugh, 2000), and that different brain regions and cellular mechanisms are engaged at different stages of this process (Gallistel & Balsam, 2014; McGaugh, 2000). Process models also attempt to explain why some types of information are remembered better than others, for example, why emotional memories are more enduring and why some teaching strategies are effective for specific types of information, like elaborative encoding strategies for declarative learning or high-dose repetition for nondeclarative learning. Process models also help explain memory phenomena in dementia, when distant, well-consolidated events are recalled but not those encoded after memory storage mechanisms had degenerated.

The concept of *prospective memory* illustrates the utility of considering time when discussing memory. Prospective memory is the ability to remember to carry out intended actions in the absence of an explicit direction to perform the action. Remembering to hand in completed homework or return a phone call at a particular time are examples of prospective memory. It is perhaps one of the most functional constructs of memory and may be disrupted due to memory consolidation impairments, that is, incompletely encoding the to-be-remembered information. Prospective memory also can be disrupted by attention or executive function deficits—for example, not noticing cues to future actions or not initiating an intended action, even if it is remembered. Determining whether prospective memory is disrupting everyday functioning, and if so, pinpointing the source of the disruption in the attention, memory, and executive function systems, will lead to the identification of strategies that allow people to manage prospective memory deficits.

As a resource for this manual and for clinicians working in the field of neurorehabilitation, Appendix A at the end of the book provides a list of terms relevant to learning and memory processes.

Common Memory Impairments

People with memory impairment may experience preservation of some types of memory and not others, which is why it is critical that rehabilitation professionals understand these distinctions. The process of choosing an intervention—including those in this text—requires careful consideration of the type of learning required for each treatment target, and selection of ingredients matched to the target and the client's memory profile (see Chapter 4 for definitions of *target* and *ingredient*). With that caveat, common impairments in ABI are summarized next.

As noted above, declarative learning is dependent on brain structures that commonly are affected by acquired brain damage and so is commonly impaired in clients with ABI. If the impairment affects new declarative learning after injury, it is referred to as *anterograde*, and if it affects recall of facts and events that occurred prior to injury, it is referred to as *retrograde*. Thus, if a client is not making any new declarative memories, their condition is called *anterograde amnesia*, and inability to access previously learned declarative memories is *retrograde amnesia*. Complete and persistent anterograde or retrograde amnesia is very rare. More often, the client has a period of time surrounding the injury for which they have no recall, a reverse gradient of preinjury recall so that events more remote from the injury were better consolidated and thus are remembered better, and impairments in new declarative learning.

A special case of anterograde amnesia is *posttraumatic amnesia* (PTA). PTA is a period of anterograde amnesia and other behavioral disturbances that can occur after a traumatic brain injury (TBI). PTA can be brief, as in mild TBI (concussion), where it can be diagnosed as "confusion" or last for days or weeks after more severe injuries. In medical settings, PTA is typically assessed using tools such as the Orientation Log (O-Log; Jackson, Novack, & Dowler, 1998) or Galveston Orientation and Amnesia Test (Levin, O'Donnell, & Grossman, 1979), administered daily until the client meets a criterion for emergence from PTA. While a full discussion of PTA is beyond the scope of this book, it is worth noting that management of clients in PTA shares principles with management of other client groups with impaired declarative learning and recall and relatively spared nondeclarative learning (e.g., minimizing use of trial-and-error methods and other opportunities for learning errors, maximizing positive emotional associations). Readers are referred to the PTA protocol described by Hart and colleagues (2020) as an example (see Chapter 10).

In contrast to the prevalence of impairments in declarative learning and memory, clients with ABI commonly have spared *nondeclarative* learning. As noted earlier, nondeclarative learning also is relatively adultlike from early in life and is preserved into older age. Thus, interventions for individuals with ABI often emphasize learning new procedures (including strategies) that can become automatic for the client. Some of the techniques discussed in this book, such as spaced retrieval and errorless learning, take advantage of intact nondeclarative learning and memory.

Executive Functions

Executive functions (EFs) are cognitive functions that allow us to control our thoughts, feelings, and actions. We call them "top-down" processes because, as Diamond stated in her excellent review of EFs (Diamond, 2013), they are needed "when you have to concentrate and pay attention, when going on automatic or relying on instinct or intuition would be ill-advised, insufficient, or impossible" (p. 136). In other words, they shape our response to bottom-up stimuli that elicit reflexive actions. Figure 2.1, from Diamond's review, shows the three core functions that comprise EFs: *inhibition, cognitive flexibility*, and *working memory*. Each of these is discussed in the next sections, along with higher-order EFs that are built on these functions, such as reasoning, problem solving, and planning, shown in Figure 2.1, and each also functions like organization and metacognition.[1]

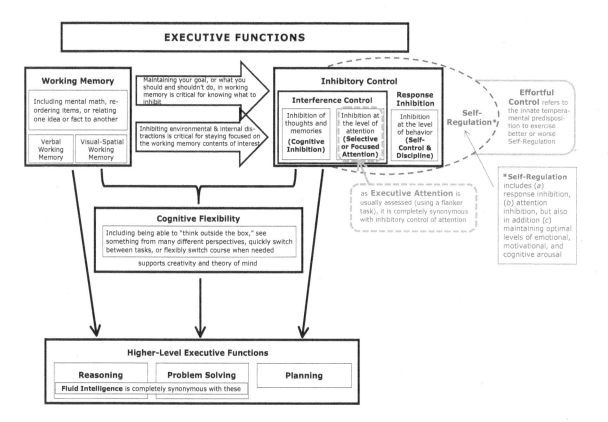

FIGURE 2.1. Executive functions and related terms. From Diamond (2013). Reprinted with permission of Annual Reviews, Inc.; permission conveyed through Copyright Clearance Center, Inc.

---

[1]There is still considerable scholarly and clinical debate about the nature of EFs and how they interact or overlap. This debate is described in detail in Diamond's review (2013), and readers are encouraged to consult that source for more information.

Inhibition

Inhibition is our ability to "override a strong internal predisposition or external lure, and instead do what's more appropriate or needed" (Diamond, 2013, p. 137). It is required for *self-control*, the cognitive function that allows us to resist temptation and delay gratification [illustrated by the Marshmallow Test, which is widely studied in fields such as health psychology (Prinsen, Evers, & de Ridder, 2016; Shmueli & Prochaska, 2009)], and also underlies control of other cognitive functions, like the ability to focus on a target, resist distractions, and stay on task, in order to achieve a goal. Inhibitory control, also known as *self-regulation*, allows you to do physical tasks, like sticking to an exercise regimen or quitting smoking, and also cognitive tasks, like controlling negative thoughts or weighing all arguments before coming to a conclusion.

Two aspects of inhibitory control are particularly important for TBI rehabilitation. First, delaying a response often helps achieve a better outcome. This delay benefit underlies many problem-solving and self-regulation rehabilitation strategies, like the Stop-Relax-Refocus strategy used by Novakovic-Agopian and colleagues (2019) to help veterans with TBI. Second, self-regulation resources can be depleted. Self-regulation depletion has been well studied in the social psychology and marketing fields (Baumeister, Tice, & Vohs, 2018; Muraven & Baumeister, 2000). It is well known that people are less likely to persist on a task if their preceding activity depleted self-regulatory resources (e.g., be patient with a partner in the evening after being on their best behavior all day at work) (Baumeister et al., 2018). When clients say they have "mental fatigue" or "hit a mental wall" at some point during the day, they may be talking about self-regulation depletion. Self-regulation depletion crosses modalities and contexts (Baumeister et al., 2018), so a cognitively demanding work environment, for example, can reduce self-control for alcohol consumption in the evening.

The good news is that self-regulation capacity can increase with practice [at least in people without TBI (Oaten & Cheng, 2006), especially children (Blair & Raver, 2014)], and self-regulation resources are replenishable (or *repletable*). *Repletion* activities used in experimental tasks include self-talk with affirmations (e.g., reflecting on successful performance, positive self-talk like "I can do it!") as well as physical activity or activities like meditation (Vinney, van Mersbergen, Connor, & Turkstra, 2016). Activities that replenish self-regulation vary from person to person, however, so it may be useful to ask that person what they like to do to take a "mental break" or "recharge."

A client's attitude about their self-regulation capacity also might play a role in performance. In one study, participants who believed self-regulation was limitless performed better on a sustained learning task (Miller et al., 2012), so it may be helpful to consider both a client's signs of self-regulation fatigue and also their beliefs about their own cognitive resources.

Cognitive Flexibility

Cognitive flexibility develops in childhood after working memory and inhibitory control and builds on those functions (Diamond, 2013). Cognitive flexibility includes spatial flexibility—literally imagining how something would appear from another perspective—and also the ability to shift one's response to a stimulus, as on tests like the Stroop Test, where the examinee must switch from reading a color word to naming the color of the word. In everyday adult life, cognitive flexibility includes figurative shifts in perspective that allow you to "see" how others see things (theory of mind), understand nonliteral meanings such as sarcasm and abstract language, change our thinking and actions to adapt to ongoing conditions, and generate new ways of doing things when current methods aren't successful. Neuropsychological tests of cognitive flexibility include tests such as verbal fluency (How many words can you think of starting with the letter *F*?) and alternation tasks like the Trailmaking Test (switching between letters and numbers).

Cognitive flexibility requires inhibitory control, as we need to stop doing or thinking about something to start doing something else, and working memory, the workspace in which to maintain whatever perspective we choose. Sorting out which of these EFs is the problem for a given client can be a challenge, even with neuropsychological tests (e.g., Does the client name only *F* names for animals because they got stuck in the animal category, couldn't keep the instructions in working memory, or thought the examiner would approve of that strategy?).

Working Memory

As discussed earlier in this chapter, working memory is the type of memory that underlies our ability to hold information in mind and manipulate it for either storage or retrieval (Baddeley et al., 2009). It is included in Figure 2.1 because it is the *workspace for EFs*. If you cannot hold information in mind and manipulate it, you cannot perform tasks requiring reasoning, learning, and understanding complex information. Working memory has a bidirectional relationship with inhibitory control and cognitive flexibility. We need control to block information from taking up space in working memory, and we need flexibility to manipulate information in working memory to solve problems. Conversely, we need to have enough working memory space and processing capacity to keep information in mind long enough to decide what is extraneous or compare alternative solutions.

We mention relations among working memory, inhibitory control, and flexibility because it can be a challenge clinically to sort out which of these is driving the client's performance, and sorting that out is important for intervention. As noted earlier in this chapter, a client with a limited working memory span might not be able to hold enough information in their mind to make a plan, in which case having them write a list might be helpful. Alternatively, the client might have trouble holding information in working memory because they have poor inhibitory control, in which case the task of writing a list might introduce even more distractions; or they could have limited flexibility, in which case they might not be able to generate list items. Likewise, a behavior that appears to reflect a deficit in metacognition might occur because the person is perseverating on old information (lack of inhibition), can't shift perspectives to consider that the injury might be the reason for their challenges (flexibility), or can't hold current task performance in mind long enough to evaluate it (working memory). Sorting out these factors is a key task for the rehabilitation of clients with cognitive impairments.

Higher-Order EFs

Higher-order EFs include *reasoning*—that is, using logic and rational thinking to arrive at a conclusion; *planning* and its close relative, *organization*; and *problem solving*, the process of identifying a problem, generating solutions, and implementing those solutions. Reasoning and problem solving are synonymous with fluid intelligence (Diamond, 2013). Another higher-order EF is *metacognition* (thinking about one's thinking). A widely used model of metacognition was proposed by Nelson and Narens (1990) and includes two processes: monitoring, which is thinking about one's own thoughts or behavior; and control, which is changing actions as a result of data acquired via monitoring. This model does not imply that our evaluation of our own thoughts and behavior is accurate, only that we collect those data on an ongoing basis and adjust our actions accordingly. Deficits in metacognition are commonly reported in adults with ABI, typically as impairments in *insight* or *awareness* about cognitive problems, and can reflect impairments in either monitoring or control of thoughts and behavior (or both). The concept of self-awareness and its deficits are discussed later in this chapter.

As shown in Figure 2.1, higher-order functions require combinations of the core EFs along with other cognitive functions as needed. For example, planning and organization may involve holding information in one's mind while reorganizing it according to priority or time (working memory), considering different ways of grouping or sequencing elements (flexibility), and focusing on relevant variables while ignoring others (inhibition). In addition, organization could require declarative knowledge about the nature of items to be organized, sustained attention, and language or visuospatial skills (if the to-be-organized items are verbal or visuospatial); and metacognition may require a combination of control, to focus thoughts on specific aspects of behavior; working memory, to hold monitored data in mind; and flexibility, to generate ways to modify and make those modifications as needed; as well as other cognitive functions like social cognition so that others' thoughts and feelings can be added to metacognitive "data."

As an example, consider the thought processes involved when a person with ABI is deciding whether to order a specific beverage in a restaurant. The reasoning steps might include:

- Flexibility to think of consequences associated with different beverage choices
- Working memory to hold information about different consequences in mind while weighing pros and cons
- Inhibitory control to stay on task, not be distracted by noise in the environment and others' comments, and refrain from choosing without thinking

If the client makes a maladaptive decision, identifying the cognitive contributors to that decision will guide the selection of a strategy (e.g., a "stop-and-think" strategy to support impulse control, avoidance of that context if distractions cannot be controlled, training in a scripted response to reduce working memory load while making decisions). Another example is provided later in this chapter, in the context of social cognition and social behavior.

In summary, Diamond (2013) described three core EFs: inhibition, cognitive flexibility, and working memory. These core functions combine with other cognitive and sensorimotor functions to achieve higher-level EFs such as reasoning, problem solving, planning, organizing, and metacognition. Perhaps because EFs require dynamic coordination among multiple cognitive functions and thus multiple brain systems, they are vulnerable to any type of brain dysfunction and thus are commonly impaired in clients with ABI.

A Few Words about Standardized EF Tests

There has been a longstanding debate about whether standardized EF tests capture everyday EF problems (e.g., Chaytor & Schmitter-Edgecombe, 2003), especially in clients with non-TBI reasons for EF impairments, such as comorbid mental health problems or functional cognitive symptoms (see Chapter 12). Comorbid conditions might explain both the lack of congruence between objective and subjective EF measures in populations like military personnel with mild TBI (Schiehser et al., 2011), where the prevalence of comorbid depression and anxiety is high, and also the overall lack of concordance between objective data and self-reported problems in this clinical population (Armistead-Jehle, 2010; Cooper et al., 2018). Typical EF tests also provide instructions and structure and are administered in controlled settings, so they are unlikely to capture the demands for inhibition and flexibility in everyday life. In rehabilitation, we are treating the person who has beliefs about their own cognitive functioning, so selection of targets is based on self-reported and observed problems, informed by test data.

Self-Awareness

Self-awareness or insight into one's own abilities and challenges is a key consideration in cognitive rehabilitation. Some frameworks include it as part of EFs. For example, self-awareness can be viewed within the construct of metacognition discussed above as a higher-level EF. We have elected to review self-awareness as a distinct cognitive domain due to the prevalence of self-awareness challenges following brain injury and their impact on the therapy process and outcomes.

Self-awareness is the ability to view ourselves somewhat objectively and perceive our actions from the perspective of other people. It allows us to incorporate feedback and modify our behavior accordingly. Impairments in self-awareness can result in unsafe or inappropriate behavior, as well as nonadherence to therapy recommendations. A number of different models have described types and stages of self-awareness, as well as the cognitive, emotional, and contextual factors that influence a person's self-awareness (e.g., Toglia & Kirk, 2000). These models can help direct hypothesis testing about the sources and influences of unawareness and reveal whether the development of targets and associated treatment ingredients that address self-awareness are warranted (Fleming, Strong, & Ashton, 1998).

Most models of self-awareness after brain injury differentiate between two major awareness constructs: *intellectual awareness*, or knowing that a challenge or deficit exists, and *online awareness*, or the ability to recognize a challenge as it is occurring during task performance (Crosson et al., 1989; Schmidt, Fleming, Ownsworth, & Lannin, 2013; Schmidt, Lannin, Fleming, & Ownsworth, 2011; Toglia & Kirk, 2000). In neurologically healthy individuals, the two types of awareness interact: We have preexisting knowledge and beliefs about our abilities based on our experiences, and these beliefs are partly shaped—and sometimes challenged—by results of a process of self-monitoring and attending to internal and external feedback while actively performing tasks or activities. A host of factors will influence both intellectual and online awareness following brain injury, including situational factors such as the type of task and context, as well as personal factors such as motivation, self-efficacy, and cognitive abilities (Toglia & Kirk, 2000). For example, some individuals may have challenges with intellectual awareness and endorse a physical impairment, but not perceive having cognitive impairments. For example, they might not "know" that they have a memory impairment. Some individuals may be able to accurately describe their strengths and challenges but, during real-time task completion, be unable to self-monitor and modify their performance in response to feedback. They may not "respond in the situation." The first individual may benefit from initial psychoeducation and brain injury education and time, while the second individual may benefit from structured and supportive self-reflection exercises during functional and meaningful tasks. Often, cognitive rehabilitation will require addressing self-awareness either concurrently with or prior to treating other rehabilitation targets.

Diminished self-awareness can result from damage to brain structures and networks that support self-awareness, psychological responses to injury, or a combination of both. Understanding the source of self-awareness deficits is important to match appropriate management and intervention (Langer & Padrone, 1992). Two conditions that result in impaired self-awareness due to brain damage to structures and networks that support self-awareness are *apathy syndromes* and *anosognosia*. *Apathy* refers to a syndrome of disinterest, disengagement, inertia, lack of motivation, and absence of emotional responsivity. A cardinal feature of apathy after brain injury is diminished goal-directed behavior (Worthington & Wood, 2018). Apathy may result from damage to the mesial frontal lobes and might respond to medication, specifically psychostimulants (Rao & Lyketsos, 2000). Cognitive rehabilitation, with its focus on behavior and skill, is not likely to change apathy. *Anosognosia* is a neurological condition in which the person is cognitively unaware of their disability. Three key factors define anosognosia: (1) underreporting of striking symptoms or disability, (2) a tendency toward positive self-evaluation, and (3) avoidance of adverse information that reveals difficulty accompanied by an increased likelihood of a failure to recognize errors (Gasquoine, 2016). Typically, anosognosia is caused by damage in the fronto-temporal-parietal region in the right hemisphere (Moro, Pernigo, Zapparoli, Cordioli, & Aglioti, 2011). It is important to remember that, when brain networks allowing accurate self-appraisal are damaged, anosognosia is similar to other cognitive deficits such as changes in attention or memory (i.e., it is a deficit, not a coping mechanism). Anosognosia often lessens over time and, for clients who are able to participate in rehabilitation, is typically addressed by psychoeducation and structured supportive feedback programs in a milieu where there is high therapeutic alliance (see Chapter 3).

Denial is a psychologically mediated condition that results in a distortion of self-awareness. Typically, denial serves to protect a person from despair (Prigatano & Sherer, 2020). A person's psyche may lead them to deny the existence or degree of a disability in order to spare themselves the pain of loss. Denial is not just a psychological phenomenon that can occur in people after brain injury; it may be present in any individual struggling to accept painful circumstances, including the family and friends of clients. Denial may manifest as resistance to information and a tendency to blame external sources for problems, and might result in hostility when problems are pointed out. A characteristic distinguishing denial from anosognosia is how the client responds to feedback. A client with anosognosia may show indifference to being told that test results suggest they have cognitive impairments, whereas a client with denial may reject this information (Langer & Padrone, 1992). Importantly, however, individuals can have both unawareness and denial, and these cognitive and psychological processes can interact (Toglia &

Kirk, 2000). Depending on the client's profile, issues stemming from denial are often addressed using the counseling techniques described in Chapter 3.

Social Cognition

Social cognition refers to the ability to identify and interpret social signals (Schulkin, 2000). It includes, at minimum, processes such as the ability to recognize others' emotions from affective and vocal displays, the ability to demonstrate empathy, and *theory of mind*, defined as the understanding that others have thoughts separate from one's own and these thoughts can influence behaviors (Premack & Woodruff, 1978). Some definitions of social cognition also include embodied social simulation (feeling the emotions of others), the ability to identify and express one's own feelings, and social knowledge (Beer & Ochsner, 2006).

Development of social cognition begins very early in life, evidenced by the findings that infants at around age 6 months can differentiate animate versus inanimate objects (Brune & Brune-Cohrs, 2006). By age 3 or 4 years, children can separate their own versus others' thoughts, and by adolescence they can easily take the perspective of others and recognize complex social emotions like disgust and shame (Blakemore & Choudhury, 2006). Some aspects of social cognition appear to cross cultures, such as understanding intents (Tomasello, Carpenter, Call, Behne, & Moll, 2005), and thus are universal; but development of social cognition is also influenced by environmental factors (e.g., parents who talk about feelings) and language development, as we know about others' internal states mostly through their words (Brune & Brune-Cohrs, 2006), so there may be individual differences even in adults. Sex and gender differences may also exist, though those differences appear to be small and their everyday significance is unclear (Turkstra et al., 2020).

There are very few standardized tools for assessment of social cognition for adults with acquired brain damage, in part because most research and clinical work has been done in children with autism and in part because it is difficult to create tools that fully capture social cognition in everyday life. Assessment of social cognition also is challenging because it interacts with other cognitive functions, not only language as noted above, but also EFs and memory.

PUTTING IT ALL TOGETHER

The cognitive functions summarized here interact in complex and dynamic ways in the real life of a person with ABI. To illustrate these interactions, consider the earlier beverage-selection example in the broader context of a social interaction. Cognitive functions involved in the person's decision about ordering a beverage could include the three listed earlier and additional items from all five cognitive functions summarized in this chapter:

- *Attention:* sustained attention to complete the task
- *Memory:* declarative recall of previous semantic and episodic information, including the physician's recommendations regarding alcohol consumption, past consequences of beverage consumption, social rules for alcohol consumption in

that particular context, and amount consumed in the past few hours; nondeclarative knowledge of automatic social behaviors, such as implicit politeness rules for
ordering from a food server
- *Executive functions:* flexibility to think of different outcomes associated with
  different beverage choices; working memory to hold information about different
  outcomes in mind while weighing pros and cons; inhibitory control to stay on
  task, not be distracted by noise in the environment and others' comments, and
  refrain from choosing without thinking; higher-level EFs such as metacognition
  to gauge one's own capacity to make a good decision, and organization to generate the actions needed to achieve the goal
- *Self-awareness:* in addition to metacognition, awareness of variables such as relationship to others in the social environment and physical capacity to execute the
  target behavior
- *Social cognition:* theory of mind, to determine if the social gathering is continuing or ending, beverage consumption is appropriate, and possibly if others also
  would like a beverage; recognition of others' affect cues that might provide evaluative cues to appropriate behavior in that context

These cognitive functions are in addition to functions not discussed in this chapter,
including language comprehension and expression, visuospatial functions (e.g., to navigate the physical space), and calculation, to determine if the person has adequate funds
for a beverage purchase. As described in the example above, selection of an appropriate
strategy will depend on which of these functions is the main contributor to the maladaptive behavior. If the main cause is poor declarative recall or metacognition, memorized
rules for behavior might be helpful; if it is social cognition, then the client might learn
to ask others for guidance about appropriate behavior; and a stop-and-think strategy
might be helpful if the problem is lack of inhibitory control.

CONCLUSION

This chapter provided an overview of cognitive concepts that are fundamental to the
practice of cognitive rehabilitation. We proposed that understanding relevant cognitive
theories and frameworks helps us tailor intervention to meet a client's individual needs.
Chapter 3 describes clinical techniques to promote client engagement in therapy, including clients with diminished self-awareness. Chapter 4 describes instructional methods
that align with different cognitive strengths and challenges, and Chapter 5 introduces
hypothesis testing as a method to help determine which underlying cognitive process(es)
may be contributing to a client's performance on any given functional task. The concepts described here also are the foundation for subsequent chapters on specific intervention techniques and populations.

CHAPTER 3

Practicing Psychological Mindedness in Cognitive Rehabilitation

Katharine Seagly, Brigid Waldron-Perrine, McKay Moore Sohlberg, Rose Dunn, Pauline Mashima, Diane Paul, and Kelly Ann Peña[1]

A person-centered, biopsychosocial–cultural approach to cognitive rehabilitation requires clinicians on an interdisciplinary team to recognize and account for psychological, social, and cultural factors in their assessment and treatment of clients. While not all clinicians on an interdisciplinary cognitive rehabilitation team formally treat psychological factors, psychological mindedness (PM) is an advantageous skill and perspective for all team members, to optimize clients' outcomes. Broadly speaking, PM refers to a person's capacity for examination, reflection, and insight regarding their thoughts, feelings, and behaviors and those of others. While addressing PM directly may sound challenging without formal psychological training, there are several accessible approaches to foster clients' PM and, in so doing, increase motivation and engagement in the cognitive rehabilitation process. Being able to foster PM in our clients also requires that we clinicians examine our own feelings and biases and bring a high degree of self-awareness to our clinical sessions.

This chapter offers a practical guide for incorporating psychologically based strategies into assessment and treatment practices for individuals with cognitive challenges. Specific evidence-based approaches, including cognitive-behavioral therapy (CBT), motivational interviewing (MI), and acceptance and commitment therapy (ACT), are discussed and used to identify treatment ingredients to help improve outcomes of cognitive rehabilitation.

---

[1]On behalf of the Joint Committee on Interprofessional Relations Between the American Psychological Association and the American Speech–Language–Hearing Association.

THE BIOPSYCHOSOCIAL–CULTURAL FRAMEWORK

The biopsychosocial–cultural framework includes attention to biological, psychological, and social aspects of illness and functioning, including cognition and recovery (Engel, 1977). The framework is consistent with the International Classification of Functioning, Disability and Health (ICF) framework discussed in Chapter 1 and includes the following factors:

Biological
- Medical diagnoses and extent of brain involvement
- Genetic predispositions and risks
- Medication effects

Psychological
- Adaptive and maladaptive coping mechanisms
- Sense of self
- Emotional states

Social
- Family circumstances and relationships
- Peers
- Stress or safety of the environment

Although the cultural aspects of illness, function, and recovery have sometimes been incorporated under the *social* umbrella, we are choosing to highlight these in their own right, as cultural factors have been underemphasized for many years, despite their significant impact on a client's progress and recovery (Nazroo, 1998; White et al., 2018). Cultural factors can include aspects of identity, including but not limited to racial or ethnic heritage, gender identity, disability identity, degree of acculturation, and importantly, how the dominant culture values or devalues various identities.

When fostering PM in cognitive rehabilitation, we must conceptualize both ourselves and our clients through biopsychosocial and cultural lenses, and approach factors or identities relevant to our clients, including those we may not yet understand, with a sense of humility and curiosity, to increase our understanding and decrease potential bias. In this way, we can address the whole person in our rehabilitation rather than just the cognitive symptoms, thereby optimizing outcomes.

PM should be integrated into all three of the PIE phases described in Chapter 5—Planning, Implementation, and Evaluation—and should provide the intervention framework for cognitive rehabilitation. In particular, the implementation phase will be delivered in the context of a therapeutic relationship between the client and clinician, which requires the clinician to develop a collaborative working alliance that helps the client engage in the rehabilitation process. In this chapter, we describe active ingredients that clinicians can employ within a cognitive rehabilitation session to enhance therapeutic alliance and increase client engagement.

The therapeutic relationship between the client and clinician is not the only relationship critical to optimizing cognitive rehabilitation outcomes. Communication and interaction among all team members treating and caring for the client are also important. The traditional rehabilitation model, while multidisciplinary, has not always been *inter*disciplinary, meaning that the various disciplines often take a siloed approach to client care, meeting once or twice a week to touch base, but for the most part pursuing separate treatments within their own disciplines. In this traditional model, mental health professionals are typically the team members who evaluate and treat social, emotional, and behavioral problems and communicate their findings and progress to the team. We expand this traditional model to include every practitioner as well as the client and their everyday people, to optimize cognitive rehabilitation and therapeutic progress by acknowledging the whole client, the whole clinician, and their interaction.

WHY FOCUS ON PM?

Why is PM important when addressing targets and aims associated with cognitive challenges? It is well documented that clients with cognitive challenges after brain injury struggle with loss, identity, and motivation, which can affect their ability to participate in all life activities—including rehabilitation (Carroll & Coetzer, 2011; Kusec, Panday, Froese, Albright, & Harris, 2020). Our cognitive rehabilitation protocols will be more effective if practitioners are skilled in person-centered practices, which requires clinicians to embrace PM. It is not effective to deliver a siloed cognitive rehabilitation program that does not incorporate and acknowledge client values, needs, preferences, and emotional states. As the person-centered movement has begun to be infused into rehabilitation, clinicians are increasingly attending to client values and preferences but may be less mindful of clients' emotional states, which are also key factors in responsivity to rehabilitation. Fortunately, PM has begun to be instilled in the practices of all disciplines on a rehabilitation team, and we are seeing the evolution of person-centered rehabilitation to include methods to attend to emotional states.

PM includes the clinician's ability to identify emotions, both their own and those of others, and a willingness to reflect on their own and others' thoughts, feelings, and actions in a nonjudgmental manner, with an interest in the meaning and values behind their own and others' behaviors. Recognizing that it is impossible, even in the clinical practice of psychology, to master a purely nonjudgmental and aware stance, the goal is to be open and willing to explore the connections among thoughts, emotions, sensations, and behaviors as a means of being attuned to what may be driving symptoms or reinforcing barriers, or conversely, what might drive progress, provide stepping-stones, or whittle away at roadblocks.

There are two foundational clinical orientations that depend on PM and help to ensure person-centered practice. The first is the *cultivation of a therapeutic alliance*, and the second is the *cultivation of a productive client mindset* that allows full engagement in the therapy process. Below we describe the required principles and clinical values necessary for each orientation and propose supporting clinical treatment ingredients.

Cultivating Therapeutic Alliance

Therapeutic alliance, also called working alliance, is a mainstay of person-centered practice. It can be conceptualized as the degree to which a client and practitioner are collaboratively engaged in a rehabilitation process that is beneficial to the client's recovery. Figure 3.1 depicts the three core values that clinicians must embrace to build a collaborative, client-focused working relationship (Horvath & Luborsky, 1993; Raskin & Rogers, 2005):

- *Congruence:* The clinician is real, authentic, and genuine with their clients.
- *Unconditional positive regard:* The clinician genuinely cares for their clients and does not evaluate or judge clients' thoughts, feelings, or behaviors as good or bad.
- *Empathic understanding:* The clinician understands their clients' experience and feelings in an accurate and compassionate way.

As discussed later in the chapter, embracing these three core values requires that clinicians are aware of their own biases, judgments, and feelings. To build therapeutic alliance, the three core values are mapped onto three essential activities: (1) agreement on the goals of the treatment, (2) agreement on the therapy tasks, and (3) development of a personal bond (Horvath & Luborsky, 1993). As described in Chapter 5, the PIE planning phase includes an assessment process with a clinical interview that involves collaborative goal setting and target selection, which facilitates joint decision making about goals and treatment components. Development of a personal bond results when clinicians are present and engage in reflective listening throughout this process. The section on MI later in this chapter describes methods that promote connection between clinicians and clients.

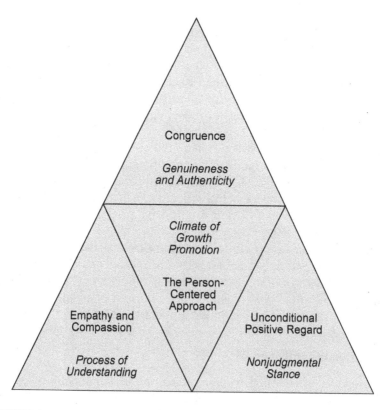

FIGURE 3.1. Components of therapeutic alliance (Horvath & Luborsky, 1993).

While there is limited research on factors affecting working alliance in neurorehabilitation, a scoping review of research examining working alliance in acquired brain injury (ABI) rehabilitation concluded that enhancement of working alliance improved rehabilitation outcomes (Stagg, Douglas, & Iacono, 2019). Studies reviewed showed that participation outcomes, including return to work, school, and driving, were associated with stronger working alliance. Also reported in individual studies were positive subjective outcomes, such as client perceptions of lessened somatic symptoms and increased social communication functioning.

Clients with diminished self-awareness due to either anosognosia or denial, as described in Chapter 2, present a challenge to developing a working alliance, as they may not have the cognitive function to understand their limitations due to brain injury (anosognosia) or may have a psychological condition that does not recognize limitations, to protect themselves from pain of loss (denial). While limited self-awareness is a challenge to developing alliance, it is also critical in order to support the client and help them manage their impairments. Without a strong therapeutic alliance, clients with limited self-awareness may not benefit from therapy.

Building therapeutic alliance with clients participating in cognitive rehabilitation depends on being intentional about our interactions. Perhaps the most basic action is to take the time to get to know our clients and build rapport. We can ask questions about their lives and follow up in future sessions with questions related to their responses, showing that we are listening and care about them as whole people. Knowing how to listen reflexively and respond to their disclosed feelings and concerns is key for therapeutic alliance. If a clinician notes a client's response to a query on how they feel about their progress, and also notes how they responded to words of encouragement, the clinician can use that information to guide progress conversations in later sessions. In summary, approaching the clinical session with values that align with person-centered practice, working collaboratively to set goals and agree on treatment approaches, and taking time to develop rapport with clients will cultivate a therapeutic alliance that will provide a fruitful rehabilitation environment.

Cultivating a Productive Client Mindset for Engaging in Rehabilitation

Perhaps the most important factor in any rehabilitation is the client's willingness to engage in the treatment process. Motivation and engagement are critical, regardless of the severity of cognitive impairments. Moderate to severe brain injury can affect every aspect of a client's functioning and understandably can lead to affective states that impede therapy progress, including low motivation and self-efficacy. As discussed in Chapter 12, mild traumatic brain injury or concussion can result in a complicated interaction of psychological, somatic, and cognitive symptoms, which likewise can affect clients' ability to engage in therapy. In the context of rehabilitation and recovery, motivation is commonly identified as a precursor to engagement (Lequerica & Kortte, 2010). Thus, when delivering cognitive rehabilitation interventions, it is imperative that we use evidence-supported strategies and ingredients that optimize client engagement and motivation.

A number of well-validated counseling frameworks offer principles and strategies to maximize motivation and engagement that can be embedded within cognitive rehabilitation sessions and used by clinicians who are not trained as psychologists (Holland

& Ryan, 2020; Rothbart & Sohlberg, 2021). In the sections that follow, we discuss three influential and effective counseling frameworks and apply them to the practice of cognitive rehabilitation: CBT (Beck, 2011), MI (Miller & Rollnick, 2012), and ACT (Harris, 2009; Hayes, Strosahl, & Wilson, 2016). For each, we provide a brief background and description and then give examples of how they may offer treatment ingredients that can maximize a productive mindset for a range of skill and knowledge targets and also be used to address specific targets to increase motivation, engagement, and hope.

COGNITIVE-BEHAVIORAL THERAPY

Cognitive-behavioral interventions have a strong evidence base in the clinical psychology literature (Hofmann, Asnaani, Vonk, Sawyer, & Fang, 2012). These are interventions that consider thoughts, behaviors, and emotions and represent an approach that has been found to be effective across health populations (Dobson & Dobson, 2018). CBT is a formal psychological modality delivered by licensed psychologists and other mental health practitioners and is intended to help clients identify and change unhelpful ways of thinking that can negatively affect their mental health or behavior (Beck & Weishaar, 2005). CBT is a psychotherapy approach and thus is distinct from cognitive rehabilitation; however, rehabilitation professionals have successfully integrated some of the tenets of CBT into cognitive rehabilitation to optimize treatment outcomes (Cooper et al., 2015; Mateer, Sira, & O'Connell, 2005). Next, we describe the application of these tenets to rehabilitation.

We know that empowerment and self-efficacy are critical factors for successful rehabilitation (Jones & Riazi, 2011; Sit et al., 2016; Tschopp, Frain, & Bishop, 2009). As clients are confronted with multiple challenges after brain injury, they can develop unhelpful thought patterns that can undermine their self-efficacy and negatively impact engagement and motivation in cognitive rehabilitation. This cycle is depicted in Figure 3.2, which is a simplified rubric of the cognitive-behavioral model that is the core of CBT. Assisting clients in recognizing and replacing these negative thought patterns can help increase their engagement in therapy.

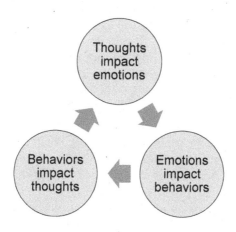

FIGURE 3.2. A simplified cognitive-behavioral model.

Applying Cognitive-Behavioral Principles to Cognitive Rehabilitation

During cognitive rehabilitation sessions, clinicians may notice some of the thought patterns that are preventing clients from fully benefiting from therapy. Clinicians can describe how false patterns arise and how the client might benefit from replacing counterproductive thoughts with different, more productive thoughts. The clinician could share a version of the cognitive-behavioral cycle shown in Figure 3.1 to help illustrate the relationships among thoughts, feelings, and behaviors. Below we contrast an unhelpful versus more helpful thought process that might be used when working with a client who has *learned helplessness and associated amotivation.*

Example of the Unhelpful Cycle

Client-identified thought: "I want to be like I was before my stroke, but I don't know if or when that can happen."

Client-identified emotions: Worried, uncertain, glum, "less than."

Client-identified behavior: Avoids doing cognitive rehabilitation homework because it is uncomfortable to face feelings of uncertainty and not being "good enough." As a result, progress is less than expected.

Clinician response: Listens but does not address thoughts, feelings, or emotions.

Example of a More Helpful Cycle

Client-identified thought: "I want to be like I was before my stroke, but I don't know if or when that can happen."

Client-identified emotions: Worried, uncertain, glum, "less than."

Client-identified behavior: Avoids doing cognitive rehabilitation homework because it is uncomfortable to face feelings of uncertainty and not being "good enough." As a result, progress is less than expected.

Clinician response: Helps client identify the cycle of learned helplessness and its association with avoidance of uncomfortable emotions and activities that evoke difficult emotions and counterproductive behavior.

Table 3.1 lists some common negative thought patterns that clinicians can help clients recognize and replace to optimize motivation for cognitive rehabilitation.

MOTIVATIONAL INTERVIEWING

Motivational interviewing (MI) is a person-centered and directive counseling approach. MI increases readiness for change by helping clients to examine and possibly even resolve their ambivalence about change (Rollnick & Miller, 1995). Effective use of MI can cultivate readiness for change, overcome resistance or resolve ambivalence, build intrinsic motivation and commitment to using therapeutic strategies, foster resilience and psychosocial adjustment with coping strategies, and promote self-efficacy by increasing clients' insight into their own limitations and reinforcing their belief in having the capabilities to self-monitor and self-regulate behavior (Medley & Powell, 2010). MI comprises a set of principles and communication techniques that are grounded in the following concepts:

- *Compassion:* The clinician always keeps the client's best interests in mind and tries to see things from the client's point of view.
- *Partnership:* The clinician and client work collaboratively, and the clinician avoids playing the role of the "expert."
- *Acceptance:* The clinician respects the client's autonomy, potential, strengths, and perspective.

TABLE 3.1. Unhelpful Thought Patterns

Unhelpful thought pattern	Client examples	Clinician-guided response
Fortune telling: predicting that things will turn out badly. But, in reality, we cannot predict the future because we don't have a crystal ball!	• "I know I'll mess this up." • "I will never be able to manage my memory problems."	"We may feel things will not go our way, but in reality no one can predict the future. What if we focus on what can be done right now?"
Black-and-white thinking: looking at situations in terms of extremes (e.g., things are either good or bad, a success or a failure). But, in reality, most events call for a more "moderate" explanation. For example, making an error does not mean you have failed completely; you had a small setback, and you can get back on track.	• "Anything less than perfect is a failure." • "I left my grocery list at home, and I forgot some items at the store. My whole day was ruined. Why should I even bother making lists?"	"Making mistakes can feel terrible, but they are bound to happen. As long as we keep moving forward, one setback cannot define us. We can always get back on track."
Mind reading: believing that we know what others are thinking and assuming that they are thinking the worst of us. In reality, no one can read minds, so we don't really know what others are thinking!	• "Others think I'm stupid." • "My friends think I'm a burden to hang out with."	"It's easy to feel as though we are being judged, but in reality, we don't know what others are thinking. If you're concerned that your friends feel burdened, why not talk with them about it?"
Overgeneralization: using words like "always" or "never" to describe situations or events. This type of thinking is not helpful because it does not take all situations or events into account. For example, sometimes we make mistakes, but we don't always make mistakes.	• "I always make mistakes." • "I am never able to concentrate."	"We all make mistakes sometimes and have difficulties achieving our goals, but this isn't always true. Tell me about a time when things went well."
Labeling: talking to ourselves in mean ways and using a single negative word to describe ourselves or others. This kind of thinking is unhelpful and unfair. We are too complex to be summed up in a single word!	• "I'm stupid." • "I'm a loser."	"We all may feel stupid sometimes, but feelings are not facts. And anyway, feelings are much too complex to be summed up in one or two words."

The principles of MI help to reinforce the basic concepts of compassion, partnership, and acceptance, and may be remembered using the acronym RULE:

- *Resist* the righting reflex.
- *Understand* the client's motivation.
- *Listen* to and *empower* your client.

The righting reflex in MI is the tendency to want to solve a client's problems for them. It can be particularly hard for clinicians to resist trying to fix problems when delivering cognitive rehabilitation. Clinicians have specialized training in the field of brain injury and knowledge of the strategies that can be employed by people with brain injury to facilitate functional everyday skills. With this background, it is easy for clinicians to believe that they know the "best" therapies and strategies to help their clients. It may be very difficult when, in the context of a collaborative approach to therapy, the client identifies a goal or strategy that seems to be "wrong"—that is, not what the clinician would suggest as the best strategy. In this situation, clinicians might experience an overwhelming urge to "correct" clients, point out the flaws in their choices, and help them select the "best" course of treatment (Hoepner, Sievert, & Guenther, 2021). Instead, MI provides communication strategies to guide the client in selecting targets that will help them achieve their desired aim.

MI communication strategies include *open-ended questions, affirmations, reflections,* and *summaries* (often collectively referred to as OARS). Open-ended questions do not constrain the responses and allow clients to freely share their concerns. Open-ended questions may be broad and generic (e.g., "What would you like to be doing that you are not doing right now?") or more specific (e.g., "What happens when you try to read?"). Affirmations are statements that recognize clients' strengths and acknowledge behaviors that lead to positive change. Affirmations are effective when they are specific and used sparingly. For example, a frequent "good job" is less potent than an affirmation in response to a client's description of their home program, such as "It seems like you had a more satisfying interaction when you used your question-asking strategy." Reflections can be a useful strategy to draw more discussion from a client related to a specific question. Reflections are statements relevant to what the client has said, and they let the client know that you are listening and hear what they are saying. Importantly, reflections are more than just repeating what the client has said; they may be used to frame hypotheses about what the client really means to say. For example, a clinician might reflect, "As I'm listening, it sounds like a big concern is that people will find out that you have a memory issue and not want to be your friend. Is that right?" Summaries are used to gather and connect related information within an interview or conversation. They convey to clients that the clinician has been listening and understands what the client has said. Summaries can be used to highlight and focus on specific information that can set the stage for informing clients about available strategies and developing specific goals associated with the strategies they select.

MI is backed by robust research support. Recent meta-analyses found MI to be particularly helpful in optimizing outcomes in health care settings, even for those with multimorbidity, and in optimizing treatment adherence and behavioral health outcomes (Lundahl et al., 2013; McKenzie, Pierce, & Gunn, 2015; Morton et al., 2015). A meta-analytic study on MI showed a large initial effect and moderate long-term effect on treatment outcomes, particularly for ethnic minorities and when practiced without a manual (Hettema, Steele, & Miller, 2005). Of note, many of the clinicians in these studies were non-psychologist health care providers who successfully implemented MI principles, indicating that formal psychotherapy training is not required to incorporate psychology-based strategies into cognitive rehabilitation. Although MI principles and components can (and should) be implemented by any practitioner involved in goal setting and cognitive rehabilitation, certain MI applications require specific training. For example, the use of open-ended questions in discussions about the client's aims is a straightforward interview technique and can be used intentionally by any practitioner engaged in collaborative goal setting. By contrast, understanding the best ratio of simple to complex reflections or knowing how to engage clients who are highly resistant to therapy in change talk requires specific MI training.

Applying MI to Cognitive Rehabilitation

The goal of MI is for the clinician to set the stage for treatment by allowing the client to sort out ambivalence about making any specific behavior change (such as using a memory strategy or pacing for activities) while helping the client to reflect on desires and encouraging them to engage in "change talk" that opens the door for using strategies. The clinician asks the client's permission to give information on how the client is doing, and if the client agrees, the clinician offers feedback. The clinician then requests the client's response to the feedback and follows with open-ended questions, affirmations, reflections, and summaries. The use of MI is particularly helpful in reviewing assessment results, setting goals, and managing lack of adherence.

At times, the goals of the client and family may be unrealistic in the context of a finite care encounter. MI skills—including asking open-ended questions, using reflective listening, and summarizing statements—can help the clinician understand the client and family's goals as well as logical steps to achieve those goals from a nondefensive and nonconfrontational perspective. These MI ingredients may help identify immediate tasks that can be achieved within the therapy encounter and that are steps toward larger or longer-term aims that will also require other interventions. For example, a family might have the aim of the client living independently, and the use of MI ingredients can help the clinician show how cognitive rehabilitation might contribute to that aim, for example, by addressing safety targets.

There may also be incongruence between the client's present aims for cognitive rehabilitation, as defined by the system of care, and their own values. For instance, a supported residential facility may value organization, cleanliness, and planning, but an individual client may not necessarily identify these areas as of high value. MI can help facilitate a discussion and awareness of this incongruence, which is essential, as it may be a notable barrier to progress. Table 3.2 provides examples of using MI language.

Use of MI with Clients Who Have Diminished Self-Awareness

MI is particularly useful for clients with poor self-awareness due to either anosognosia or denial (Medley & Powell, 2010). Some clients with reduced self-awareness may not be ready to participate in cognitive rehabilitation. Engaging in change talk that explores ambivalence about therapy or neutrally sharing discrepancies between their perceptions

TABLE 3.2. Example Statements for MI Processes in a Cognitive Rehabilitation Client Session

Permission	• "Can I share with you what the data tell us about how you're doing?" • "May I have permission to discuss this with you?"
Request feedback response	• "So how are you taking that in?" • "Can you tell me what you're hearing in your own words?"
Open-ended questions	• "Tell me more about what you're thinking." • "What happened during your day?" • "What do you think you'll do about this problem?"
Affirmations	• "That sounds like a step in the right direction." • "You've accomplished a lot this week." • "Your intentions were good even if they didn't work out."
Reflections	• "I'm hearing you say that you know you need this, but it's hard to face how different things are since your injury." • [Client: "I've had a really tough day."] • "This is hard, and you're understandably frustrated." or • [Client: "I don't think I'm having as much trouble with my memory as you say I am."] • "You are definitely the expert on your own experience. I'm here to help optimize your memory, regardless of the starting point."
Summaries	• "You realize that you are making progress in rehab, but you wish it were faster, and it is hard to be patient with the process." • "So, let me see if I have this right. You know you need to do your homework in order to improve, but it's hard to stick to a schedule. I noticed you mentioned that you might be ready to try something different this time. Can you tell me more about what you're thinking?"
Empathic statement	• "I can imagine that this is really hard." • "It is natural to have many different feelings about this process." • "Our feelings may not be facts, but they are always valid and should be given the attention they deserve."

Note. Adapted from Milman et al. (2019) and Working Group to Develop a Clinician's Guide to Cognitive Rehabilitation in Mild Traumatic Brain Injury (2017; *www.asha.org/siteassets/practice-portal/traumatic-brain-injury-adult/clinicians-guide-to-cognitive-rehabilitation-in-mild-traumatic-brain-injury.pdf*).

and those of others and asking for the client's thoughts may lay the groundwork for a gradual increase in insight or acceptance. It is important that therapists develop a solid therapeutic alliance with clients in order to work on readiness for therapy.

The undergirding clinical principle when working with clients who have diminished awareness is to resist the urge to tell or convince them of their needs or impairment (i.e., resist the righting reflex). Instead, the clinician's objective is to help the client understand their challenges and strengths and personal priorities. Ultimately, the clinician's role is to facilitate client motivation and engagement by helping the client identify meaningful activities and acceptable therapeutic processes for accomplishing these activities. An MI technique that can be useful for clients with diminished self-awareness is to use *scaling questions* and ask them to rate (1) the importance of working on a target and (2) their confidence in performing the particular target or activity. Clients with diminished self-awareness may show a pattern where they rate the importance for change in a particular area as low, but their confidence in their ability to perform a particular task as high. Clients with this profile may benefit from initial sessions with MI. However, prolonged discussion in which the clinician explains why change is beneficial is often unproductive.

Some clients may benefit from experiential learning, where they are supported in completing activities that showcase strengths and difficulties, followed by MI sessions. For example, consider a client who is videotaped doing an activity of daily living or engaged in a communication exchange, as in TBI Express (Togher et al., 2010), the communication partner training described in Chapter 9. The client could be asked to point out strengths as well as evidence of the target problem. If the client is able to recognize problems, a follow-up MI discussion that elicits change talk may be useful. This change talk might contain the following types of questions to help guide a client toward selection of productive therapy goals:

Desire

"What do you want to happen?"
"Why might you want to improve your ability to _____?"

Ability

"What could you do to _____?"
"What have you done before to _____?"

Reasons

"If you were able to _____ better, how would that help?"
"Why would you want to _____?"

Need

"How important is it for you to _____?"
"How much do you need to _____?"

Use of MI on an Interprofessional Team

MI has been described as a helpful intervention for interprofessional collaborative management of ABI symptoms (Milman et al., 2019). A shared MI communication style bolsters therapeutic alliance and provides consistent messaging from all rehabilitation team clinicians because it uses empathic listening and collaborative decision making. Mashima and colleagues (2019) provided the example of a client who expressed resistance to using a written planner to track appointments because it involved "extra steps that weren't necessary" prior to injury. The speech-language pathologist employed MI principles to help the client identify benefits of using a strategy to compensate for memory lapses, such as not missing appointments. The client stated that they preferred the planner over other options because it did not involve technology or the assistance of others, so the team recognized and reinforced the increased independence the planner would offer. The psychologist on the team reinforced use of the planner to increase the client's follow-through by noting events that triggered anxiety in the client's daily routine. These MI practices helped the client achieve their treatment targets and move forward through rehabilitation in a person-centered and collaborative manner, consistent with a PM approach of addressing the whole person and recognizing each client's needs.

ACCEPTANCE AND COMMITMENT THERAPY

Acceptance and commitment therapy is a psychotherapeutic intervention that draws heavily from behavior therapy, particularly relational frame theory (RFT) and mindfulness (Powers, Vording, & Emmelkamp, 2009). As in MI, ACT integrates PM. ACT was developed by clinical psychologist Steven Hayes as one of the "third wave" cognitive-behavioral therapies (Hayes, Strosahl, & Wilson, 2009; Hayes et al., 2016) and has been adapted for many life situations and unhelpful behaviors (Gloster, Walder, Levin, Twohig, & Karekla, 2020). The goal of ACT is to guide clients to a values-based, mindful existence and help them live a fulfilling and enriched life by using ACT principles, regardless of their cognitive status.

> ### Among the Key ACT Concepts (Harris, 2009)
> - Take effective action guided by one's deepest values.
> - Be fully present and engaged.
> - Use mindfulness to handle "unpleasant" and "unwanted" experiences.

A key component of ACT that sets it apart from other behavior therapies is its emphasis on values-guided, mindful action. For example, when a client is thinking about who they want to become and what changes they want to make, the clinician asks values-guided questions, such as "What really matters to you?" For clients at any level of cognitive or communication ability, the client then works with the clinician to determine if they are acting in accordance with their personal values and "making room" for unwanted thoughts and feelings that are difficult to extinguish (Ylvisaker, Mcpherson, Kayes, & Pellett, 2008). If the client is not engaging in values-consistent behavior, the clinician assists the client in moving toward alignment through values-guided action with ACT-based skills and principles to achieve an enriched and fulfilling life (Harris, 2009).

Over the past decade, studies have shown manualized ACT to be efficacious in clients with ABI, although more research is needed (Kangas & McDonald, 2011). ACT must be adapted for clients with cognitive impairments, particularly in executive function and processing speed, as clients with cognitive impairments have been shown to have poorer ACT outcomes if ACT procedures are not adapted (Herbert et al., 2018). Two adaptations are the degree to which the clinician is directive in values-guided processes and the extent to which the clinician engages the client's support system. It is particularly important for the clinician to engage the support system in conversations about values to ensure that the client has the structure at home to consistently engage in values-guided action.

Another way in which ACT differs from other behavioral approaches is that it does not focus directly on symptom alleviation, which makes it especially well suited for cognitive symptoms that might not entirely resolve. ACT provides the perspective that all people can live fulfilling and enriched lives by using ACT principles, regardless of symptom experience or cognitive status. ACT assumes, first, that quality of life is primarily dependent on purposeful, values-guided action and, second, that this is possible regardless of one's symptoms, provided that the individual responds to symptoms in as mindful a way as they are capable (Harris, 2009). While the goal of ACT is not to alleviate symptoms, symptom reduction has been reported as a "side effect" in randomized controlled trials using this therapy approach, often over and above the results of traditional CBT (Jiménez, 2012). Paradoxically, if one is focusing on alleviating symptoms, then one is, by definition, focusing on the symptoms (i.e., "spotlighting"), which can exacerbate the degree to which the symptom negatively affects the client's quality of life. When the spotlight is shifted away from the symptoms and toward values-based action, symptom-based barriers can be reduced. If cognitive rehabilitation focuses on a client's values by interweaving strength-based work and values-guided action, then deficits will likely play a smaller part in the client's self-concept, thus reducing their impact on treatment and quality of life. Such an approach is consistent with the holistic and client-centered focus of PM.

In rehabilitation interventions, the psychologist can initiate more intensive therapeutic strategies based on the principles of ACT and consult with those providing cognitive rehabilitation to infuse the use of values and acceptance language to reinforce concepts of ACT. However, even in the absence of psychologist consultation, clinicians providing cognitive rehabilitation can independently incorporate the tenets of ACT into sessions without exceeding their scope of practice. For example, the cognitive rehabilitation clinician might say, "Is asking your professor for additional time to complete your work in line with your goals and what you think is appropriate?" or "It's normal to feel apprehensive about doing this. See if you can explore or reflect on this feeling, or even just sit with it for a minute or two, then do what you know is important."

Applying ACT to Cognitive Rehabilitation

The application of ACT to cognitive rehabilitation can take many forms. Some of the easiest and most effective are the incorporation of client values into goal setting and basic mindfulness training to improve a client's ability to be present and engage in cognitive rehabilitation. Mindfulness training can also increase tolerance for unpleasant experiences and emotions, which are bound to arise at points during rehabilitation.

The provider or client may access a list of values online or from an ACT-based text, as it is often helpful to have a list of values from which the client can choose, rather than asking the the client to identify values without a reference. The values that are most important to the client can then be applied to the goal-setting process to ensure that goals have deep personal meaning to the client, thus increasing client engagement and motivation. For example, a client may identify independence as a top value. As in the previous example, this value could then be incorporated into memory-aid training by highlighting that using an aid, rather than relying solely on others, is consistent with the client's value of independence.

A simple mindfulness exercise that can be incorporated into cognitive rehabilitation is to ask the client to engage their five senses (or select senses depending on preference or sensory limitations) by noticing what they see, hear, smell, taste, and feel (tactile) in the present moment. The clinician can explain that noticing their experience right now can keep the client's mind from drifting to the past, which cannot be changed, or to the future, which cannot be predicted. This can highlight for clients that we only have a say in right now, which can help increase engagement and motivation in the present rehabilitation activities. When helping clients use mindfulness to increase their tolerance of unpleasant experiences and emotions, a simple deep-breathing exercise can be helpful. For example, if a client expresses grief over their loss of cognitive abilities, it can be acknowledged that grief is an uncomfortable emotional experience and that the best way to navigate that feeling is to accept and make room for it, rather than trying to deny or avoid it. Clients can be encouraged to breathe in deeply and allow the grief to fill them up, then breathe out slowly for as long as they can and allow the grief to recede. Visualization may also be a helpful mindfulness tool when making room for unpleasant experiences. For example, a client can be encouraged to imagine their grief as a tide washing over them. It can be difficult to tolerate when we are awash with it, but we know it will recede, as the tide always does. Thinking of uncomfortable emotions and unwanted experiences as ebbing and flowing, like the tide, can help clients let go of the unhelpful notion that we can control the past or future and can also foster resilience, as we know we can tolerate uncomfortable emotions until they eventually pass.

There are many excellent mindfulness texts, apps, websites, and research organizations aimed at educating beginners (suggestions are listed in Appendix B). The use of mindfulness exercises, like all rehabilitation practices, requires that clinicians have received some training in their application.

CULTURALLY INFORMED COGNITIVE REHABILITATION

Culturally informed practice means that clinicians use assessment and treatment methods that have been evaluated and/or adapted for groups with differing perspectives, experiences, beliefs, and values. This is particularly important for the field of brain injury rehabilitation, when the demographics of people recovering from ABI, at least in North America, include a large percentage of people who are not represented in the dominant culture (Centers for Disease Control and Prevention, 2015). Unfortunately, the field of brain injury does not have many cognitive rehabilitation tools that have been adapted for different populations; hence, the person-centered practices described throughout this text are critical to ensuring our rehabilitation methods align with the values and needs of clients from diverse backgrounds. A clinician can avoid making "ethnocentric" assumptions by asking the client questions about their preferences and values, ensuring that goals will be meaningful to that client.

An example of a traditional rehabilitation assumption is that therapy should be directed at making clients as independent as possible, often helping them prepare to live on their own. Some cultures, however, value interdependence or providing care for persons with disabilities and thus might prefer to set up a home and community that provide ongoing external support. Soliciting input from clients and their everyday people about preferences for how therapy is delivered can also be important for working with clients who come from different cultures. Most often, clinicians work one-on-one with clients, but many cultures value having families attend therapy and be in the room even if the therapy is individually directed. Likewise, group interactions might be valued in some cultures but be unacceptable in others because of public sharing of information. Culturally informed practice requires the clinician to take the time to ask questions about preferences, values, and needs at all stages of the therapy process. Asnaani and Hofmann (2012) offer the following suggestions to help establish cross cultural therapeutic alliance that can be adopted in a cognitive rehabilitation session:

- Conduct a thorough culturally informed but person-specific assessment of the presenting problem.
- Identify and incorporate client's cultural strengths and resources into treatment.
- Explore the client's perspective on seeking treatment and the therapeutic relationship.

FIRST, KNOW THYSELF

The core of PM is to be culturally, biopsychosocially sensitive clinicians, recognize that we bring our own culture and biopsychosocial factors to every treatment session, and optimize the treatment process by recognizing how our own factors interact with those of the client. In the interprofessional rehabilitation literature, it is well documented that members of different professional groups often come to the team with professional biases, and we all need to be aware of this potential and differences in thinking and perceiving others from different professional and cultural backgrounds (American Speech–Language–Hearing Association, 2021). We all also bring to the therapeutic relationship our own personal biases and beliefs, of which we may be more or less aware. Similarly, every client we see will have their own biases based on their past experiences, including experiences with other professionals. Our recognition of all these potential influences will help us to treat clients with sensitivity and optimize progress in cognitive rehabilitation and be able to facilitate behavior change.

In any human interaction, both parties bring beliefs, thoughts, feelings, and actions. We must be prepared to acknowledge these, even without formal training in PM and self-reflection. Clinicians who practice self-reflection and mindfulness will be best equipped to explore and understand possible biases and influences. A very helpful resource is the counseling text by Holland and Ryan (2020) written for the nonpsychologist, which draws heavily from positive psychology and contains self-reflection exercises.

CONCLUSIONS

While some clinicians may be concerned about scope of practice, and justifiably may hesitate to venture into psychotherapy territory, PM via MI-, CBT-, and ACT-based strategies are techniques that all skilled clinicians can integrate into their cognitive rehabilitation work with clients. In this chapter, we proposed a framework and specific strategies that are meant in part to "give permission" to non-psychologist clinicians to integrate PM into their client care in a manner that is within their comfort zone, knowledge, skills, and scope of practice. To clarify the difference between being psychologically minded and doing formal psychotherapy, we conceptualized these strategies on a continuum ranging from the practices of psychologists who are licensed and trained to treat psychological disorders to the practices of clinicians such as occupational therapists, physical therapists, and speech-language pathologists who specialize in other areas but understand how to recognize psychosocial-cultural factors and optimize therapy outcomes by increasing self-reflection and resilience, in both clients and themselves. The training of most rehabilitation clinicians includes coursework that reviews counseling and client communication techniques, and training will be enhanced by including foundational skills and values grounded in PM.

CHAPTER 4

Applying RTSS and Systematic Instruction to Cognitive Rehabilitation

In Chapter 1, we discussed the International Classification of Functioning, Disability and Health (ICF) as a framework for identifying *what* to focus on in intervention. In this chapter, we focus on the *how* of intervention: What methods can clinicians use to help clients make meaningful changes in their everyday cognitive performance? The chapter begins with a description of the Rehabilitation Treatment Specification System (RTSS; Hart et al., 2019), a system designed to specify the client functions we are attempting to change and how to change them. We then describe *systematic instruction*, a general approach to intervention that is particularly helpful for clients with declarative learning and memory impairments. The chapter ends with a summary of principles of neuroplasticity, which guide critical components of our treatment, such as dose. The information presented here is the basis for all of the subsequent chapters in this text.

THE REHABILITATION TREATMENT SPECIFICATION SYSTEM

The RTSS (Hart et al., 2019) is a system for describing and classifying rehabilitation treatments. It was developed by a multidisciplinary group of rehabilitation specialists, motivated by the lack of information about rehabilitation treatment methods, not only in research studies, but also in clinical practice. While there are several systems for describing client and study characteristics (e.g., CONSORT; Boutron et al., 2017) and systems for classifying goals of treatment (e.g., the ICF; WHO, 2021), these systems describe the *who* and *what* of rehabilitation. The treatments themselves, however, often are described only in terms of duration of a particular service (e.g., hours of speech therapy) or by the problems they are intended to treat (e.g., cognitive rehabilitation). What these systems do not tell us is the *how* of rehabilitation: what the clinician does or provides to a client in a therapy session. The RTSS is intended to organize treatments according to these clinician actions, specifically clinician actions that are known or hypothesized to account for changes in client functioning.

The RTSS is a "top-down" approach, based on *treatment theory* (Hart et al., 2019). Treatment theories specify how changes occur—that is, what actions by a clinician lead to changes in client function, and by what underlying mechanisms (Keith & Lipsey, 1993). In the RTSS, *treatment is specified according to the clinician's theories about actions or objects that will improve the client's functioning.* This stands in contrast to "bottom-up" approaches like practice-based evidence that collect data from clinical practice and seek to identify practices that improve functioning (Horn, DeJong, & Deutscher, 2012). *The RTSS is concerned only with direct interactions with clients or other treatment recipients* (e.g., family members); that is, it is concerned with what happens during a treatment session. It is not concerned with other aspects of rehabilitation that can influence client outcome, including assessments that precede treatment (e.g., neuropsychological testing), health care system features (e.g., access to services), institutional practices (e.g., team meetings), or environmental features that support client functioning in general (e.g., closed captioning or curb cuts). These aspects of rehabilitation are the province of *enablement theory* (Whyte, 2014), which addresses the broader context of intervention and the many factors that contribute to successful outcomes. For example, return to work might require not only treatment of specific skills, but also nontreatment factors such as transportation, employment opportunities, and family support. Thus, training of specific skills would be the province of treatment theory, but the many factors contributing to employment would be the province of enablement theory.

The RTSS has a tripartite structure: ingredients, targets, and mechanisms of action, as shown in Figure 4.1. *Ingredients* are what the clinician says, does, or provides to improve client functioning. *Targets* are the aspect of client functioning that the clinician desires to change, and *mechanisms of action* are mechanisms by which the clinician believes change occurs. A note about the word *target*. Clinicians may be accustomed to using terms such as *long- and short-term objectives* or *goals*. The meaning and use of

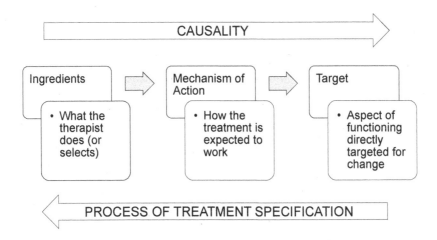

FIGURE 4.1. Tripartite structure of the Rehabilitation Treatment Specification System.

those terms vary across settings: sometimes they refer to what is expected to improve in a session or across sessions, sometimes it's what is expected as an outcome of a rehabilitation stay or after a fixed time interval (e.g., 1 week), and sometimes it is what we hope for in the client's life after discharge. The RTSS authors chose to use the word "target" to be clear that it is the specific aspect of client functioning that the clinician hopes to improve by *direct* interactions with clients or other treatment recipients, and that is what the clinician chooses to address within a treatment session.

Targets are contrasted with *aims*, which are aspects of functioning that might or might not change in response to the treatment of a single target. Aims often are what clinicians refer to as long-term goals or objectives, that is, aspects of functioning that will require more than just achievement of a single target. For example, the client may have the aim of *remembering appointments at work*, and that might require a series of targets: increasing knowledge about different calendar apps, developing skill in using a particular app, and developing the habit of using that app in specific contexts.

Ingredients are always observable, and targets are always measurable, at least in principle. By contrast, mechanisms of action often are invisible to us, particularly for treatments like cognitive rehabilitation, where the mechanism of action might be "changes in the brain" (see further discussion in Chapter 11). As shown in Figure 4.1, clinical reasoning typically proceeds from the target to the ingredients; that is, the clinician identifies the aspect of function (target) that should be improved and then chooses ingredients that they theorize will improve that target.

Targets can be divided into three different groups: *organ functions* (O), *mental representations* (R) (i.e., knowledge, beliefs, and attitudes), and *skills and habits* (S) (see Table 4.1). O targets are relatively rare in cognitive rehabilitation, as we are not typically treating the brain directly. A possible exception is treatments in which energy is applied directly to the brain, such as in transcranial direct current stimulation, although even that is often paired with behavioral treatments, so it is not clear that the electrical current alone accounts for behavioral changes.

Most targets in cognitive rehabilitation are about knowledge and attitudes (R targets) or skills and habits (S targets), and most therapy involves a mix of both. For example, for the remembering appointments aim described above, the target types would be increasing knowledge about different technology options (R target), developing skill in using a particular app (S target), and developing the habit of using that app in specific contexts (S target).

Some ingredients are specific to one target group. For example, "listing pros and cons" may be an effective ingredient for increasing motivation to use an app (an R target) but not for learning the habit of using it (an S target), whereas high-dose spaced practice with error control is effective for learning the habit but is unlikely to increase motivation to use the app in everyday life. Similarly, ingredients like heat and electricity that are used for organ function targets are likely to apply only to that group of targets. Most ingredients, however, can be used with more than one type of target, including clinician actions such as providing instructions, modeling, feedback, and cueing—and also objects such as digital devices and apps. The one rule in the RTSS is that every S target has the ingredient of *providing opportunities for practice*, as practice is essential for developing skills and forming habits.

Successful performance of any treatment task depends on three factors: (1) the client must be capable of doing the task, that is, must have the prerequisite skills and

TABLE 4.1. Target Groups in the Rehabilitation Treatment Specification System

Name of target group	Definition	Typical ingredients	Mechanisms of action	Examples of cognitive rehabilitation targets
Organ functions	Change or replace organ functions	• Electrical stimulation applied to the brain • Energy applied to soft tissues • Exercise schedules for strengthening or endurance training • Devices for limb or organ replacement	Depends on the organ (e.g., changes in electrical signaling, tissue stretching, increased cardiac efficiency, artificial organ features)	• Increased accuracy of recall on a list-learning task via transcranial direct current stimulation
Representations	Enhance knowledge, or modify attitudes or emotional responses	• Didactic instruction • Providing information in multiple modalities • Linking to previous knowledge • Prompts to evaluate task importance or self-efficacy	Cognitive or affective information processing	• Increased knowledge of facts about brain injury • Increased awareness of strengths and challenges • Increased self-rated motivation to complete a task
Skills and habits	Improve ability to perform a mental or physical activity	• Opportunities for repeated practice • Instructions • Modeling • Cues • Feedback	Learning by doing	• Increased accuracy in following steps in a task • Increased frequency of turning off the TV to reduce distractions at work • Increased frequency of entering to-do items in a digital reminder

knowledge; (2) there must be an opportunity to do the task (e.g., if the task is to practice with a partner, the partner must be available); and (3) the client must be motivated
(Michie et al., 2011). The last of these merits some special consideration, as motivation
can be a significant barrier in cognitive rehabilitation.

The subset of R ingredients that are specifically to increase client motivation are
called *volition* ingredients, as they are selected to increase the client's voluntary effort
in therapy. Fields such as health psychology and clinical psychology have identified and
tested many ingredients to increase volition. An excellent resource is the Behaviour
Change Taxonomy (BCT; Michie et al., 2011), published by the Centre for Behaviour
Change at the University College London. As part of the BCT project, Michie and colleagues created an open-access database of studies using behavior change ingredients,
with ingredients listed for each study. Common volition ingredients are listed in Table
4.2. Additional ingredients are included in Chapter 3 in the section "Motivational Interviewing."

Most clinicians use volition ingredients as a matter of good therapy practice: we
give clients encouraging and supportive feedback, choose targets that are meaningful to
them, and act in ways we believe will build rapport. In these cases, volition ingredients
are added to the O, R, or S target we are treating. Volition ingredients are particularly
important when we assign home practice and are not present to directly motivate the
client. To maximize the likelihood that the client will find the opportunity and be motivated to do the home practice, we might add volition ingredients like those in Table 4.2.
Other ingredients might include a tracking log or digital reminder system, or another
external aid as described in Chapter 8.

Sometimes adding ingredients is not enough, and lack of motivation or engagement
is the main barrier to the client's progress in therapy. In that case, the clinician might
specify a separate R target to increase motivation or engagement. For example, a client might be unaware of their cognitive limitations, feel self-conscious about using an
aid or strategy, or believe that they are incapable of change. In planning treatment, the
clinician might then set a target of increased accuracy of self-judgments of performance

TABLE 4.2. Examples of Volition Ingredients

- Identify the discrepancy between their current behavior and goal standard.
- Choose their own goals (aims and targets).
- Choose their own practice schedule (for home practice).
- List pros and cons.
- Imagine future outcomes.
- Identify themself as role model.
- Consider an identity associated with changed behavior.
- Reframe problems (e.g., as "typical" or "challenges").
- Mentally rehearse successful performance.
- Use positive self-talk.
- Focus on past successes.
- Agree to a behavioral contract.
- Identify barriers to task completion and strategies to overcome those barriers.

Note. Adapted from Michie, van Stralen, and West (2011); available under CC BY 2.0 license.

on a specific task, increased self-rated willingness to use an aid or strategy, or increased confidence in being able to achieve the target. The clinician would then choose ingredients that they hypothesize will help achieve that volition target and, critically, would measure achievement of that motivation or engagement target.

Additional examples of targets and ingredients in each category are shown in Table 4.1. Targets can be at any level of the ICF: personal factors (e.g., improving mood), environmental factors (e.g., increasing family members' knowledge about injury effects), body structures and functions (e.g., improving attention), activities (e.g., increasing skill in using strategies for note taking in class), or participation (e.g., increasing knowledge about support groups). The key is that clinicians theorize that what they do or provide will *directly* improve client functioning for that target. For example, if joining a support group is the target and the clinician addresses that target by providing information, that means that the clinician believes the *only* barrier to joining a support group is lack of information. If joining the support group also requires goal-management training to improve follow-through, improved conversation skills, and increased motivation and self-efficacy, then each of these may be a target for rehabilitation.

Key Advantages of the RTSS

One key advantage of the RTSS is that it ensures a match between ingredients and targets. Treatment is most efficient and effective when treatment ingredients match the target category. For example, if the target is for the client to always turn off the television when having a conversation (an S target), the clinician should *provide opportunities for practice* (an S ingredient) versus *explain how turning off the television can improve focused attention* (an ingredient for an R target).

In typical cognitive rehabilitation activities, there is sometimes a mismatch between ingredients and targets. For example, in a previous cognitive rehabilitation trial (Cooper et al., 2017), clients were provided with a list of strategies to "optimize attention." There were 15 types of strategies, most of which included two or more substrategies. For example, the strategy "modify times" included the following substrategies: choose your individual best time, such as morning or afternoon, to focus on a task requiring attention to detail; allow yourself time when changing tasks; when changing tasks, verbalize what you are currently doing; and if you know you will be interrupted, work on a very familiar mundane task. Providing a list of strategies is an appropriate ingredient if the target is *knowledge* about strategies (an R target), but if the target is for the client to habitually use an attention-optimizing strategy in everyday life (an S target), then the clinician must provide opportunities to practice (the essential ingredient for an S target). As noted above, there is strong evidence that practice is essential for learning new habits and skills. Clinicians need to guard against the temptation to provide education only and not do actual training and practice of the desired targets. Specifying R and S targets helps avoid this pitfall.

A second key advantage of using the RTSS is that it helps us identify commonalities and themes across interventions and targets. In many cases, different therapists are applying similar treatments, but the treatments go by different names. One clinician's "memory training" may be another clinician's "compensatory strategy training" and yet another clinician's "activities of daily living training." All of those interventions can have the same target (e.g., increased recall of steps in a routine) and the same ingredients (e.g., high-dose practice with error control, modeling, feedback), but because the terminology and descriptions differ, it can be a challenge for clinicians to communicate with each other. Differences in terminology also are a barrier to translating research findings into practice, as a clinician searching for treatment methods for one named treatment might not realize there are other studies that could apply. This makes intervention less efficient and more challenging to describe to critical stakeholders, like clients and payers.

Intervention for clients with mild traumatic brain injury (mTBI) provides an example of treatment that goes by many names. A theme across cognitive signs and symptoms in clients with a history of mTBI is *reduced information-processing capacity*. Common client complaints include difficulty listening in noisy environments, thinking when they have pain or fatigue, focusing on one source of information in the presence of multiple stimuli, and sustaining mental effort over time. All of these can be interpreted as "reduced capacity to manage information," but treatments for these problems can go by many different names (e.g., time management strategies, strategies to reduce distractions, strategies to reduce mental fatigue, mindfulness strategies). By specifying targets and ingredients using the RTSS, we can identify commonalities across these nominally different approaches, which allows us to communicate and share research results across clinicians, professions, and clinical populations.

RTSS Specification Examples

The following are two examples to illustrate how the RTSS can be used in intervention planning. The RTSS also is used throughout the application chapters in this text, so there are many additional examples for different types of intervention.

Example 1. Mental Fatigue after mTBI

Seiko is a mechanic who sustained a mild TBI in a shop accident. Her chief complaint is that she can't get work tasks done because the tasks often take more mental energy than she expects. She says she's "wiped out" after a few hours of work but wants to "keep pushing through it," but if she does so, she's exhausted the next day. The treatment aim is for Seiko to learn to pace her work activities to match her mental energy level. Targets and ingredients for this treatment are listed in Table 4.3. The first target is an R target, as the clinician wants to educate Seiko about options and collaborate with her to choose one that is most likely to be effective. Seiko and the clinician decide that a useful strategy could be for Seiko to self-evaluate her mental energy before she starts a task and take a break if she sees that her energy level is low. Seiko and the clinician come up with a visual analogue scale that looks like a gas tank, with "Low Fuel—Need a Pit Stop" (a rest break) at one end and "Full Tank—Ready to Go" at the other. The next target is for Seiko to develop skill in using the scale (an S target) and after that to practice using it with work-simulation tasks to begin to form the habit of using the scale and taking breaks (an S target).

Seiko is reluctant to use the visual analogue scale at work, as she says that if others make fun of it, she might not have the courage to use it. Thus, the clinician chooses a volition (R) target to increase Seiko's self-efficacy for overcoming social pressure to not use the scale, including asking Seiko to set what she believes is a reasonable expectation for practice the next day at work. Seiko uses the scale successfully for enough work tasks to manage her energy overall, so the next target is to increase the likelihood that she will continue to use the scale after discharge from therapy.

TABLE 4.3. Targets and Ingredients for Treatment in Example 1

Target	Target group	Ingredients	Outcome
Increased knowledge of strategies to self-evaluate mental energy	R	• Information • Weighing pros and cons • Ideas for different strategies • Trial and error using different strategies • Feedback • Modeling	Selection of strategy
Increased accuracy in using gas-tank ruler	S	• Opportunities for practice • Instructions • Feedback • Modeling • Gas-tank ruler drawing • Work-simulation task	Accurate use of gas-tank ruler on structured therapy task with cues
Increased automaticity of using the gas-tank ruler and taking breaks	S	• Opportunities for practice • Error-control methods • Gas-tank ruler drawing • Work-simulation tasks that require different energy levels	Independent use of gas-tank ruler on work-simulation tasks with a variety of mental energy demands
Increased self-efficacy for using gas-tank ruler at work	R (volition)	• Reframing strategy as "normal" • Imagining future outcome of having enough mental energy • Pros and cons • Copies of the ruler • Client-identified goals for practicing at work (e.g., two tasks per day)	Score of 4 or 5 on a 5-point self-efficacy rating scale
Increased likelihood of maintaining strategy use over time	R (volition)	• Focus on past success • Client-selected expectations for using strategy • Client-selected reminders to use strategy • Behavioral contract	Self-reported strategy use at 1 month postdischarge

Example 2. Client with Limited Insight

Kimbel is a psychiatrist who sustained a severe TBI from falling off a roof when attempting home repairs. His chief complaint is that his practice partners are blocking him from resuming work because they say his memory is poor. He claims he is being "forced to do cognitive rehab" by his partners before he can go back to work, though he doesn't see the point of it. He knows all about cognitive functions and the brain and can explain in detail why he has recovered. Kimbel's aim is to get back to work as soon as possible. The clinician chooses increased awareness of memory strengths and challenges as the first target of intervention. The therapy target and ingredients are specified in Table 4.4. Because Kimbel is an expert in cognitive function, the clinician invites Kimbel to

TABLE 4.4. Target and Ingredients for Treatment in Example 2

Target	Target group	Ingredients	Outcome
Increased awareness of memory strengths and challenges	R	• Asking the client to describe memory subtypes • Phrasing as "getting a sense of what you are capable of" rather than "showing impairments" • Collaboration to identify practice scenarios • Use of scenarios from a familiar, professional source • Videorecording role-playing • Datasheet for client to record recall errors • Prompts to self-evaluate • Prompt for client to create own memory profile	Accurate verbal description of his own memory strengths and challenges

describe memory subtypes in a working document and map them to memory functions needed in a client interview. The clinician then works with Kimbel to choose practice scenarios from the fifth edition of the *Diagnostic and Statistical Manual*, which is a fundamental text for Kimbel's profession. The clinician asks Kimbel to make specific predictions for performance, based on his previous work. The clinician and Kimbel record themselves role-playing the scenarios, with Kimbel taking notes as he would in his practice; then the clinician provides a datasheet and asks Kimbel to watch the videos and self-evaluate the accuracy of his questions, comments, and notes. Based on the data from this exercise, Kimbel is prompted to create a profile of his own memory strengths and challenges, which will become the foundation for identifying strategies and supports for accurate performance.

SYSTEMATIC INSTRUCTION

This book primarily focuses on instruction because that is the core therapeutic activity required for cognitive rehabilitation. Whether a practitioner is teaching the use of an assistive device, a metacognitive strategy, or a social communication behavior, effective instruction that considers the cognitive, psychosocial, and contextual domains is requisite to successful rehabilitation outcomes. A possible outlier is process-oriented interventions that attempt to directly intervene on cognitive processes, such as attention training. The examples of computer-based cognitive retraining in Chapter 11 illustrate this approach. While process-oriented therapies have a different theoretical orientation than instruction-based treatment, the existing literature on these types of interventions emphasizes the importance of focusing on functional goals and integrating strategy training with "re-training" cognitive functions (e.g., Sohlberg et al., 2014). Thus, instructions are still critical. We next describe the processes and techniques encompassing systematic instruction, an approach to teaching that underlies all aspects of cognitive rehabilitation.

The theory underlying systematic instruction is that persons with learning challenges benefit most from structured training that includes specific techniques designed to enhance the likelihood that information will be learned, stored in memory, and later applied. Key ingredients in systematic instruction include the use of *explicit models, massed* and *distributed practice, minimization of errors* during initial acquisition (to prevent the learning of errors), *strategies to promote learner engagement,* and *carefully guided practice* to enhance mastery, maintenance, and generalization across contexts (Powell et al., 2012). As such, systematic instruction requires mastery of clinical techniques that accommodate deficits in attention, memory, and executive function and promote motivation with an end goal of improved meaningful activity.

Systematic instruction contrasts with other instructional models that rely on the learner to experiment and draw conclusions from their performance. The latter models include *discovery learning* (i.e., exploratory learning) (Hammer, 1997) and *trial-and-error* learning (sometimes referred to as "learning through errors" or "learning from consequences"). In a trial-and-error model, the clinician sets up the environment to allow the client to explore and develop their own understanding of target concepts or strategies. The instructor's role is to observe errors and provide feedback. Readers may be familiar with this approach as the educational foundation of the Montessori method (Montessori, 1912). The assumption underlying this approach is that learners are capable of critically analyzing events and forming their own conclusions about their experiences; most importantly, it assumes that the learners are *able to learn from their mistakes.* Trial-and-error learning is the most common instructional method in rehabilitation; however, often it is not the most effective method for clients with significant cognitive impairments.

Systematic instruction may be particularly useful for clients who have significant declarative learning and memory problems, and for training skill and habit targets (Powell et al., 2012). By contrast, clients with relatively good declarative learning and memory might benefit from trial-and-error learning and need fewer explicit models and less practice to initially acquire information or develop skills. It is important to remember, however, that the opportunity for practice is an essential ingredient for skill and habit targets, and the treatment plan must include ingredients for transfer of learning to contexts outside of the therapy room.

The field of special education has generated a substantial body of instructional research showing the efficacy of systematic instruction. The two research-based approaches within special education that have most influenced training practices in neurorehabilitation are *direct instruction* and *strategy instruction* [see detailed reviews in Ehlhardt et al. (2008) and Sohlberg, Ehlhardt, & Kennedy (2005)].

Direct Instruction

The instructional model that has been subjected to the most experimental scrutiny is direct instruction (DI), pioneered by Engelmann and Carnine (1991). DI is a comprehensive, explicit instructional method shown to be effective in teaching a wide range of material across different populations with learning challenges, particularly individuals with learning disabilities (Engelmann & Carnine, 1991; Stein, Carnine, & Dixon, 1998). DI requires systematic design and delivery of instruction in order to facilitate efficient acquisition and generalization of a variety of targets, including knowledge of facts and concepts and use of cognitive strategies and external cognitive aids. The following key techniques are associated with the DI design–delivery process (Engelmann & Carnine, 1991; Marchand-Martella, Slocum, & Martella, 2004; Stein et al., 1998):

- Analyzing and sequencing instructional content (i.e., task analysis)
- Training in a broad range of examples
- Using simple, consistent instructional wording
- Establishing a high mastery criterion
- Providing models and carefully faded prompts
- Providing high amounts of correct massed practice followed by distributed practice
- Providing cumulative review

DI has been applied to the rehabilitation of individuals with acquired brain injury because of its effectiveness in teaching new facts and skills to people with profound anterograde memory impairments (Glang, Singer, Cooley, & Tish, 1992).

Cognitive Strategy Instruction

Strategy-based instruction for cognition is another instructional approach that has been experimentally evaluated within special education (Englert, Raphael, Anderson, Anthony, & Stevens, 1991; MacArthur, Graham, Schwartz, & Schafer, 1995). This approach, which can be integrated with the previously described DI approach, teaches learners to monitor their own thinking. Different terms are sometimes used to describe strategy-based instruction, including *procedural facilitators*, *scaffolded instruction*, *cognitive strategies*, and *metacognitive strategy instruction* (Baker, Gersten, & Scanlon, 2002; Dunlosky, Hertzog, Kennedy, & Thiede, 2005; Englert et al., 1991; Harris & Pressley, 1991; Stein et al., 1998). Core strategy instructional techniques (Baker et al., 2002; Kim, Vaughn, Wanzek, & Wei, 2004; Swanson, 2001) include:

- Establishing the context for learning (i.e., helping learners see the "big picture") by using tools such as graphic organizers or simple outlines of important themes or concepts
- Using questions and/or prompts to encourage learner self-assessment
- Teaching the learner to use self-regulation scripts to summarize and elaborate on content (e.g., "Have I checked my work?")

Although the principles of strategy training are included in most types of rehabilitation, the most direct application occurs in *metacognitive strategy training* (Kennedy et al., 2008), which is discussed in Chapter 7.

Several meta-analyses have attempted to parse out the most effective instructional practices and components within the special education literature (Adams & Engelmann, 1996; Kavale & Forness, 2000; Mastropieri, Scruggs, Bakken, & Whedon, 1996; Swanson, 1999, 2001; Swanson, Carson, & Saches-Lee, 1996; Swanson & Hoskyn, 1998; Walker, Douglas, Douglas, & D'Agostino, 2020). Particularly pertinent is the series of meta-analyses by Swanson and colleagues. Following an extensive search yielding over 900 data-based articles, the authors selected 180 studies that met specific inclusion criteria (e.g., inclusion of a comparison/control group, sufficient data to calculate effect sizes) (Swanson, 2001). These studies were categorized into one of four groups based on the instructional techniques employed. The results indicated that a model using both DI and strategy instruction techniques *in concert* produced the largest effect size. Strategy instruction alone, DI alone, and nondirect or nonstrategy instruction showed respectively smaller effect sizes. A meta-analysis by Graham and Harris (2003) also supported the effectiveness of self-regulation strategy development for a variety of students with and without disabilities. These meta-analyses are part of a rich experimental literature within the field of special education that supports the use of explicit, systematic instructional techniques to effectively teach individuals with learning disabilities (Sohlberg et al., 2005).

The field of neuropsychology has built on the special education research and evaluated instructional design and teaching procedures for people with acquired neurogenic memory disorders. Similar to the procedures just described, evidence-based instructional methods supported in the neuropsychological literature include scaffolding instruction, error-minimization methods, distribution of practice trials, and incorporation of metacognitive strategies (Haslam, 2018; Kennedy et al., 2008).

Taken together, studies in educational psychology and neuropsychology have demonstrated the effectiveness of a combined approach that incorporates the principles of DI and cognitive strategy instruction. This approach has been specifically evaluated in students with learning disabilities and in adults with a variety of cognitive impairments.

Error-Control Methods

As their name suggests, *error-control methods* are instructional methods that limit the client's opportunity to make errors, typically by scaffolding correct responses by providing models or other cues prior to task attempts. These methods were developed to capitalize on nondeclarative (implicit or procedural) learning processes reviewed in Chapter 2, which typically are intact in clients referred for cognitive rehabilitation. Perhaps the most commonly used error-control method in cognitive rehabilitation is *spaced retrieval* (SR) training. SR training is a method for both learning and retention of a target and involves initial presentation of the full target and then repeated retrieval of the target over progressively longer time intervals. It has strong support from the literature in TBI (Bourgeois, Lenius, Turkstra, & Camp, 2007; Ehlhardt et al., 2008; Hillary et al., 2003; Togher et al., 2014) and dementia (Hopper et al., 2005; Kessels, 2017), as well as growing evidence from other clinical populations with acquired brain damage (e.g., people with impaired declarative learning due to substance use disorders; Pitel et al., 2010). SR is described in Chapter 6 as an instructional method for clients with poor declarative learning and memory and relatively intact nondeclarative learning and memory, and for skill and habit targets for any client.

Summary of Instructional Methods

Figure 4.2 illustrates the relationships among client characteristics, degree of automaticity required, and effective ingredients. For clients with severely impaired declarative learning and memory, the main instructional method for training all skill, habit, and representation targets may need to be errorless learning (EL).

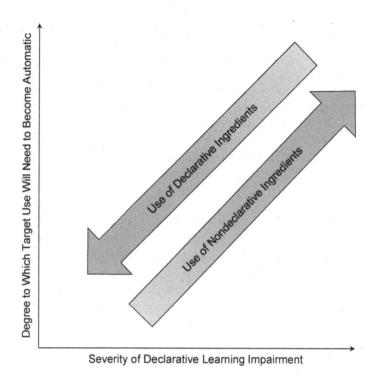

FIGURE 4.2. Summary of relations among instructional ingredients, client memory profile, and target characteristics. Ingredients for declarative learning include elaboration and visualization; ingredients for nondeclarative learning include error control and high-dose spaced retrieval practice.

CHANGING THE BRAIN: PRINCIPLES OF NEUROPLASTICITY APPLIED TO REHABILITATION

The notion that the adult brain can change was first proposed by William James (1890), and decades of research since that time have shown how brain structures and functions change in response to structured input and repetition (Kleim & Jones, 2008). The umbrella term for these brain changes is *neuroplasticity*, which encompasses the set of processes by which the healthy brain encodes experience and learns new behaviors and the damaged brain relearns lost behaviors or learns compensatory behaviors. Neurons have an extraordinary facility to modify their structure, connections, and function in response to differing internal and external forces across the lifespan (Kolb & Muhammad, 2014). A major focus of neuroscience research has been to explain the *underlying mechanisms* responsible for these changes so that they can be applied to improve rehabilitation outcomes.

Based on a review of neuroscience research until that time, Kleim and Jones (2008) generated a list of neuroplasticity principles that they believed to be especially relevant to rehabilitation after brain damage. Whereas this research focused primarily on motor skills, a follow-up paper translated these findings into rehabilitation for aphasia (Raymer et al., 2008) and generated a roadmap for rehabilitation research in the future. Table 4.5 lists the principles outlined by Kleim and Jones and suggests implications for cognitive rehabilitation and instructional practice.

TABLE 4.5. Principles of Experience-Dependent Neural Plasticity

Principle	Description	Implication for instruction
Influences on design of instruction: Planning matters		
Specificity	The nature of the training experience dictates the nature of the plasticity.	During initial acquisition training, strive to make stimuli and contexts as similar to target task as possible.
Interference	Plasticity in response to one experience can interfere with the acquisition of other behaviors.	During initial acquisition training, make sure that training does not address multiple salient targets simultaneously.
Salience matters	The training experience must be sufficiently salient to induce plasticity.	Target tasks and behaviors that are relevant and meaningful to the learner.
Time matters	Different forms of plasticity occur at different times during training: High-frequency intervention in the acute stage may be damaging to the brain but has been associated with significant benefits in the chronic stage.	Take careful data to evaluate response to intervention and do not assume that the opportunity for meaningful change ends after spontaneous recovery has peaked.
Age matters	The effects of intervention are different at different ages: Very young brains (<1 year) may have plasticity that is not adaptive; older brains (>65 years) are less plastic than younger brains (1–65 years).	Whereas younger brains may have a greater ability to substitute function, they have fewer established pathways to support learned behaviors. All ages can benefit from rehabilitation, but plasticity will operate differently at different ages.
Influences on implementation of instruction: Practice matters		
Use it or lose it	Failure to use specific brain functions can lead to functional decline in those functions.	Gains require maintenance over time or they may reverse. Consider long-term maintenance schedules.
Use it and improve it	Training that drives a specific brain function can lead to an enhancement of that function.	Focus on specific, functional targets.
Repetition matters	Induction of plasticity requires sufficient repetition.	Provide high amounts of practice.
Intensity matters	Induction of plasticity requires sufficient training intensity.	Provide intensive practice (e.g., massed practice) during initial target acquisition.
Transference	Plasticity in response to one training experience can enhance the acquisition of similar behaviors.	Actively promote generalization to similar treatment targets.

Note. Adapted with permission from Kleim and Jones (2008). Copyright 2008 by the American Speech–Language–Hearing Association; permission conveyed through Copyright Clearance Center, Inc.

The principles in Table 4.5 also suggest that a supportive rehabilitation environment will provide the opportunity for high-intensity, high-frequency repetition of meaningful and functional skills, in a context that is as similar as possible to the one in which those skills will be used and extending into the chronic stage post-onset with the opportunity for maintenance of skills. This environment will consider the age of the learner (a growing concern given the aging population and lack of experimental literature on neurorehabilitation in older adults) and will capitalize on skills and knowledge that have developed over each individual's lifetime. It will provide opportunities for learning but not overwhelm the learner, and it will limit interference effects from competing stimuli and goals.

Based on the principles in Table 4.5, Kleim and Jones (2008) suggested the following conditions to optimize recovery of function:

- Functional plasticity and recovery are use dependent.
- Plasticity requires pairing sensory input with feedback (top-down modulation and training with learning).
- Demonstration of plasticity depends on the availability of sufficient residual neural resources.
- Participants' motivation and attention are critical modulators of plasticity.

These tenets suggest that the brain changes in response to both internal input (e.g., medications that change neuronal responses, attention) and external input (e.g., training and instruction) as well as contextual factors such as people and places relevant to task completion.

With the exception of Chapter 11, this book reviews the evidence-based practice techniques supporting effective *external input* and identification of contextual factors to improve rehabilitation outcomes, with the understanding that effective instruction both promotes and exploits experience-dependent neuroplasticity. Many of the principles outlined in Table 4.5 match the instructional tenets articulated in this book. For example, effective instructional planning requires careful consideration of generalizable features (i.e., specificity and interference), personal factors (i.e., age and time post-onset), and environmental contextual factors (e.g., salience) that can enhance learning and motivation. Similarly, effective instruction can enhance neural plasticity by providing intensive practice (i.e., repetition and intensity) of targets that are used in everyday life (i.e., "use it or lose it"). In summary, there is a clear overlap between effective instructional practices and factors that enhance neuroplasticity.

SUMMARY

In this chapter, we discussed three foundations of effective cognitive rehabilitation: the importance of clearly specifying treatment targets and ingredients, use of systematic instructional methods, and the need to align therapy methods with the science of changing the brain. These are recurring themes throughout the remainder of the text.

CHAPTER 5

The PIE Framework

A Roadmap for Intervention

In this chapter, we describe a general therapy practice framework: Plan, Implement, and Evaluate (PIE). The PIE Framework describes key categories of clinical activities when treating clients with cognitive challenges and serves as the basis for designing and implementing therapy. The three phases of the PIE framework are shown in Figure 5.1.

Planning, implementation, and evaluation are neither linear steps nor static. For the sake of simplicity, we describe the three phases separately; however, the treatment variables to be implemented and evaluated must be planned *prior to* implementing and evaluating treatment, to optimize the effectiveness and efficiency of the therapy process.

Planning starts with assessment. Assessment tasks should be selected with the end purpose in mind (Murray & Clark, 2014). In rehabilitation contexts, the end purpose of assessment is usually to help identify meaningful therapy goals that will positively impact the client's everyday life and sense of well-being. As discussed in Chapter 1, the World Health Organization's International Classification of Functioning, Disability and Health (2001) provides a structure for person-centered assessment that focuses on success in meaningful everyday activities. The clinician will use the same structure to identify therapy aims and targets that will result in meaningful change for the client. Assessment with a purpose and selection of meaningful therapy aims and targets are critical elements in the planning phase, defining the "who, what, where, when, why" of the therapy process.

Implementation refers to methods that maximize the efficiency, durability, and applicability of learning. Until recently, implementation methods have often not been clearly defined in the rehabilitation literature, and likewise are not often specified in clinical practice. In the course of just one therapy activity, a clinician might use several different treatment actions simultaneously (e.g., explaining the rationale, linking to

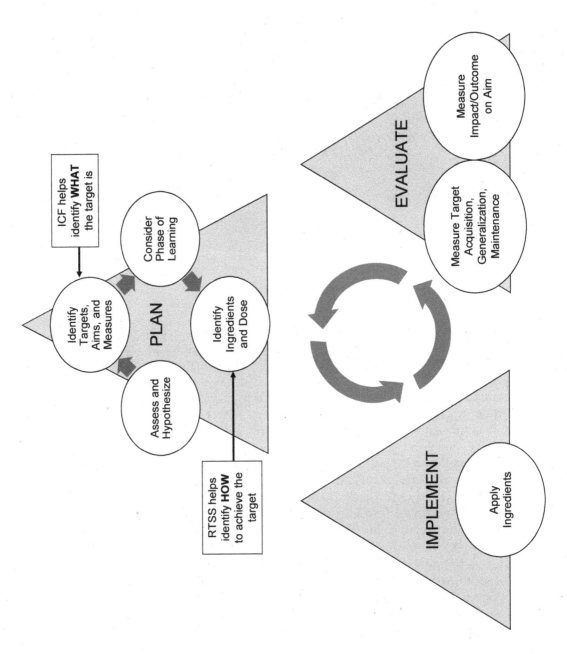

FIGURE 5.1. PIE framework.

prior knowledge, cueing, praising, correcting) without necessarily being able to articulate why they chose those actions or how they relate to the therapy target. The Rehabilitation Treatment Specification System (RTSS), described in detail in Chapter 4, provides a structure to help clinicians identify actions and objects (*ingredients* in the RTSS terminology) that they predict will help the client achieve treatment targets, defining the "how" of the therapy process.

Finally, *evaluation* of client performance is critical for both measuring outcome and also making decisions about when to continue, modify, or stop therapy. Clinical data are essential to evidence-based decision making. Dollaghan (2007) described three pillars of evidence-based practice: (1) client preferences, (2) evidence from the literature, and (3) evidence from the client's individual performance. While clinicians may be comfortable with the first two pillars, reliable and feasible analysis of client outcome has been more challenging. Fortunately, clinical tools have been emerging in recent years to support therapists in applying single-subject design methodology to the clinical setting (see PIE: Evaluation later), enabling evidence-based decisions about the therapy process.

Chapters 6 through 9 describe specific interventions, and elements of the PIE process that are particular to each are described in those chapters. Here, we provide a thorough overview of all key elements in planning, implementing, and evaluating our interventions, regardless of treatment target or method.

PIE: PLAN

Planning Step 1: Assess and Learn Client's Priorities

The clinical interview is perhaps one of the most important components of an assessment, as this is how the clinician begins to understand the client's world through the client's eyes. Results from the clinical interview will drive the rest of the assessment process. During the interview, the clinician will begin to paint a picture of *who* the client is: What are their interests and occupations? What are their sociocultural lived experiences, beliefs, values, and identities? What do they perceive as their current strengths and weaknesses or successes and challenges? What matters most to them right now and in the future? Ethnographic interviewing principles (Westby, Burda, & Mehta, 2003) may assist the clinician in developing rapport while simultaneously gaining a wealth of information about their client. Self-rating questionnaires can supplement this information and may help prompt clients to consider aspects of functioning that they were not able to draw to mind with open-ended questions.

The clinical interview should not be limited to the client but ought to also include everyday people who know the client well (Kay, Cavallo, Ezrachi, & Vavagiakis, 1995). It is important to identify family, friends, and community sources of support who might play a role in treatment and assess the client's level of connectedness to these individuals. Likewise, recognizing contexts and relationships that may produce barriers to recovery is important for planning. In some cases, treatment recipients may be individuals who support that client rather than the client themself. A common example is the training of conversational partners for people with aphasia, in which significant others or volunteers are trained in techniques to increase the engagement and participation of persons with aphasia (Kagan, Black, Felson Duchan, Simmons-Mackie, & Square, 2001; McVicker, Parr, Pound, & Duchan, 2009). Partner training is discussed further in Chapter 9, and Chapter 10 describes the importance of focusing on caregivers in the inpatient environment. In all settings, everyday people should be a part of the assessment and therapy process.

The clinical interview should allow the clinician to develop preliminary *treatment aims*. As described in Chapter 4, treatment aims, often called *long-term goals*, are broader aspects of daily functioning that involve more than one target and may involve more than one discipline's contribution. Aims often fall into the participation level of the ICF, but they could fall at any level. Here is an example of information obtained from a clinical interview that leads to a potential treatment aim:

Mr. Williams—Possible Treatment Aim

Mr. Williams is a sixth-grade classroom teacher. He sustained a moderate brain injury a year ago but has returned to teaching on a graduated basis this month. When meeting with his rehabilitation team to discuss progress, he reported that he was struggling to write points on the board during class discussions. He said this was embarrassing and contributed to him losing control of the classroom. He wanted his rehabilitation team to help him deal with the problem.

Mr. Williams's aim might be to "feel less embarrassed and more in control of his class," or "be better at writing points on the board during discussions." Achieving these aims could require multiple treatment targets (e.g., learning a note-taking strategy, training a classroom aide to take notes, disclosing his challenges to administration). Some aspects of the aim also could be beyond what therapy could help him achieve (e.g., if there is no classroom aide available).

Information obtained through the clinical interview also will help clinicians select appropriate rehabilitation assessment tools and procedures, which may include standardized, norm-referenced, or criterion-referenced tests; systematic observation methods; and dynamic assessment methods (Turkstra, Coelho, & Ylvisaker, 2005). These tools will provide additional clarity and context information about the client's strengths, weaknesses, and aims.

Consideration of client characteristics is critical to decisions about treatment candidacy, selection of appropriate targets, and design of the instructional plan. Listed below are the five domains that should be considered for each client:

1. *Sociocultural lived experiences, beliefs, values, and identities* represent the foundation of any therapeutic alliance (see Chapter 3). A deep respect for who the client is as a person will pave the way for collaborative and successful intervention.

2. The client's *cognitive strengths and challenges* must be clearly understood, particularly in attention, memory, executive functions, social cognition, and self-awareness. The client's profile in regard to auditory and reading comprehension, oral and written expression, and social communication are also important for the design of therapy.

3. *Motor functions* should be considered in intervention planning, including not only physical strength and endurance, but also qualitative aspects of movement such as fine motor control and balance, limb function, speech, and swallowing.

4. *Sensory functions* must be considered in planning, especially vision and hearing. Intake screening assessments routinely underestimate the prevalence and influence

of impairments in hearing and visuomotor functions among individuals with ABI, and these must be evaluated routinely and carefully.

5. *Psychosocial functioning* encompasses a large domain. The clinical interview should provide information about the client's emotional state, including feelings of anger, grief, or depression and the presence of factors such as emotional lability. Pre-existing conditions such as anxiety or depression will also be important to consider. It is essential to evaluate more than the presence or absence of psychological or mental health challenges. It is equally important to determine a client's attitudes and motivation toward therapy and recovery by learning about their interests and what gives them meaning and hope. Level of motivation, awareness of challenges, self-efficacy, and beliefs and expectations about treatment are key factors that should play a role in the design and implementation of therapy. As discussed in Chapter 3, many of these are critical to optimizing resilience.

One of the hallmark skills of a rehabilitation clinician is the ability to consider all of the interview and assessment data together and formulate a coherent and holistic summary of the client's characteristics. Once this summary has been prepared, the clinician can move onto the next phase of planning.

Planning Step 2: Hypothesize

In identifying targets for treatment, clinicians generate hypotheses about what is causing problems and develop treatment plans based on those hypotheses. These hypotheses often are not stated or communicated to other team members, however, or are not tested systematically. To support clinicians in systematically and explicitly testing hypotheses, Ylvisaker and Feeney (Ylvisaker & Gioia, 1998) introduced the concept of *patient-specific hypothesis testing* (PSHT). The aim of PSHT was to encourage clinicians to state their assumptions or hypotheses, compare their own hypotheses with what other team members might propose, select one, and use single-subject design methodology to test it. We return to methods of hypothesis testing when we discuss *evaluation* later in this chapter. Here, we consider Mr. Williams and generate hypotheses about factors contributing to his challenges:

Mr. Williams—Possible Hypotheses

Mr. Williams is struggling to write points on the board during class discussions. This could be related to:

- Impaired attention and/or working memory
- Anxiety
- Poor verbal formulation
- Reduced cognitive resources due to effort to maintain postural control
- Reduced cognitive resources due to effort to maintain fine motor control

When team members work in silos, this shared hypothesis-generation opportunity can be missed, leading to each individual discipline risking being overly influenced by their own clinical biases. As Maslow famously said, "I suppose it is tempting, if the only tool you have is a hammer, to treat everything as if it were a nail" (Maslow, 1966,

p. 15). For example, speech-language pathologists might tend to assume cognitive-communication impairments are the underlying factors because these are what they are accustomed to assessing and treating, whereas a rehabilitation psychologist might look first to mental health concerns, and an occupational therapist might focus on energy conservation strategies and intervention to improve fine motor control. An effective team will work together to share results, generate hypotheses using evidence and clinical judgment, and use hypothesis testing to select the best path forward. Assessment and hypothesis generation may occur in tandem. For example, the clinician might generate the hypothesis that Mr. Williams's difficulty writing points on the board is due to impairments in working memory while observing Mr. Williams's performance on a standardized working memory test. Hypothesis testing also may be carried out over a trial period of intervention, with new hypotheses generated as the client performs treatment tasks. Interprofessional collaboration and communication is key when generating and testing hypotheses (Waldrone-Perrine et al., 2022)

Planning Step 3: Define Targets

As discussed in Chapter 4, the RTSS distinguishes between treatment *aims* and treatment *targets.* Treatment aims tend to be participation-level activities that rely on the successful achievement of more than one target. For example, we determined above that a treatment aim for Mr. Williams might be to improve his ability to write notes on the board during class discussions. In contrast, the target is a specific aspect of function that the clinician hopes to directly change in one or more therapy sessions. The clinician's choice of targets to achieve aims will depend on their model or theory of cognitive functioning (see Chapter 2) and hypotheses about what is contributing to client performance. In addition to specifying the target itself, the clinician should specify the *aspect* of the target that is to be improved, such as accuracy, speed, quality, frequency, duration, or level of prompting or independence. The aspect of the behavior is what will be measured in therapy.

Aims and targets will usually be established collaboratively during the clinical interview process and assessment, and in consultation with other team members. As the clinician learns about the client's priorities and challenges, they can collaboratively set targets that reflect the functional domain that is being affected by changes in cognitive function.

To illustrate application of the RTSS to selection of treatment targets, consider two women aged 45 who have moderate anterograde amnesia after clipping of an aneurysm involving the middle cerebral artery. Celina is married and takes primary responsibility for managing the home and children and has a supportive wife. Linda is a manager in a software company and lives with her husband, who is retired. Collaborative goal setting might lead to identification of treatment aims for both women that include instructional targets to exploit procedural learning, but in different areas. Celina may have aims involving home management tasks, whereas Linda may have vocational aims as she goes back to work in a different capacity. Treatment targets for cognitive rehabilitation efforts thus would likely be strikingly different. Celina might be learning to use a cognitive strategy that emphasizes task completion and that can be applied to different household activities, while Linda may be learning to use a computer task-management system that can be integrated with her supervisor's system and help her be successful in completing her modified job duties. The strategy and tools trained in the cognitive rehabilitation sessions represent the treatment targets designed to help move the clients toward their treatment aims. Selecting targets that support the client in achieving their aims will help build meaningful engagement in the therapy process.

Important Considerations in Defining Targets

The initial specification of therapy target(s) requires consideration of two important factors. The first is to discern whether there are prerequisite behaviors or information that need to be taught prior to addressing the target. For example, when training a person to follow a phone procedure to call for emergency help, it may first be necessary to teach them what constitutes an emergency. Second, the clinician must work with the client to identify all the components or steps necessary for successful use of that target. In our example, the clinician and client need to generate a task analysis for the emergency phone procedure before beginning the actual training. Teaching targets involving learning a strategy or use of an external aid will typically involve a list of sequential steps for implementing that strategy or aid. Knowledge targets will include discrete facts or information. This task analysis is an important step in effective teaching and should not be overlooked. Reviewing the assessment results and the prerequisite and component skills of proposed targets will allow the clinician to define targets that are *within the client's reach for achieving* (Sohlberg & Turkstra, 2011).

It is also critical that targets *consider the context* (setting, people, timing) as well as any *facilitators and barriers in the environment*. Defining the ultimate target environment(s) at the beginning of intervention allows the clinician to identify the different training examples and contextual variability that will need to be programmed into therapy to ensure generalization. For example, consider a student with a memory impairment who needs to write down school assignments in a homework planner at the end of each class. The clinician could create training stimuli by having the student or parent record the school bell and use it as a cue for the student to practice writing in their homework planner. In terms of stimulus variability, treatment may begin with one type of assignment, such as a math assignment modeled after the format implemented in the student's math class. As the student is successful, other types of homework assignments may be added to the instructional plan (e.g., assignments from the student's language arts class). The field of direct instruction (Engelmann & Carnine, 1991; see Chapter 4) refers to this as *general case programming*. Treatment begins with the most general case example and then extends it in order to capture a sufficient number of scenarios to allow the client to generalize.

There may be more than one target context. Some rehabilitation targets have sequential target contexts in a progression. For example, the initial target context may be the hospital or therapy room or with the clinician, whereas home or with a family member is the ultimate target context. Similarly, there may be simultaneous target contexts. For example, the target for training a memory prosthesis may be to use it both at home with a spouse and also when at the doctor's office. Timing might be another contextual factor to consider (e.g., remembering to start dinner after turning off the news, implementing an escape routine when feeling angry). An effective treatment plan considers each of these contextual factors from the outset.

Environmental facilitators and barriers include people who interact with the client in the environment, competing demands on the client's time and attention, and facilitators or triggers of the desired client behavior. For example, there may be a natural prompt in the environment for a person whose target is to initiate using a specific memory aid, such as the school bell in the previous example (an environmental facilitator). An example of a barrier might be the limited time between classes, which does not allow sufficient time to write down assignments, necessitating the development of a template or checklist to decrease writing time.

Writing effective intervention targets is not easy, and too often the temptation is to jot something down quickly (e.g., "improve working memory") that ignores many of the criteria described above. However, spending a few extra minutes at the outset to clearly formulate treatment targets will contribute to improved client engagement and clarity of outcome (Dörfler & Kulnik, 2020; Kucheria, Sohlberg, Machalicek, Seeley, & DeGarmo, 2020).

SMART Targets and Goal Attainment Scaling

Reviewing the considerations above will help ensure that each target is *specific,* and *unambiguous.* The clinician, client, family, and team members must have a shared understanding of what they are striving for. Consider the following:

- **The client will maintain eye contact at least 50% of the time.** This target does not specify the context. Is the client expected to work on eye contact in one-on-one interactions with hospital staff, in group conversations with family members when on home visits, or all the time? This target is also ambiguously worded. Does "50% of the time" mean half of each conversation or half of all conversations? Ensuring that targets are specific and unambiguous helps everyone row together in the same direction. Another contextual element that may not be clear in this target is level of independence—is the client expected to maintain eye contact independently or with a certain level of prompting? Nobriga and St. Clair (2018) indicated that independence should be assumed if the target wording does not specify a level of support, but the clinician may wish to specify this to ensure clarity for all those involved.

Targets also must be *measurable and/or observable* so that it is clear when each target has been achieved. Consider the following:

- **The client will improve their confidence in starting conversations with peers at the brain injury clubhouse.** This target stipulates the context, but the outcome is not observable because confidence is a feeling rather than a behavior and "improve" is not operationally defined. The clinician could instead collaborate with the client to describe what confidence would look like in behavioral terms and then alter the target to reference those observable elements. Alternatively, the clinician and client could jointly create a 1–5 scale that would allow the client to reliably rate their perception of confidence, which, while not necessarily observable, is measurable. "Improve" could then be defined as the frequency of occurrence of the desired confidence behaviors or moving a specified number of intervals along the rating scale.

Finally, targets must specify the element of *time.* "Time" often refers to a deadline by which the target should be achieved (e.g., within 1 month, in time for a family wedding). While it can be difficult to precisely estimate the time required to achieve many elements of cognitive rehabilitation, it nevertheless remains important to do so in order to encourage both client engagement and funder support. "Time" also has a second meaning that refers to how often success needs to be demonstrated. Consider the following:

- **Within 2 months, the client will independently refer to their calendar before scheduling an appointment.** While a deadline for achieving the target is specified, the number of times the behavior should be demonstrated by the deadline is not indicated. As worded, the client could demonstrate the behavior one time within 2 months and be considered to have achieved the target. While that might be appropriate for some targets (e.g., preparing a speech), it would not be appropriate for a skill/habit target such as referring to a calendar. Examples of success criteria for the number of times a skill/habit target should be demonstrated include:

  - In at least X% of opportunities over the course of a week (or day, month)
  - Across at least X consecutive occurrences
  - At least X times weekly for Y weeks

The above list of target-specification principles is lengthy. Fortunately, the SMART acronym (Bovend'Eerdt, Botell, & Wade, 2009) is a well-known method to support effective target specification. While there are slightly different permutations, the acronym typically stands for:

- *Specific* (unambiguous, context and level of support specified)
- *Measurable* (and/or observable)
- *Attainable* (prerequisite skills in place, component skills identified, within client's reach)
- *Relevant* (meaningful, leading toward achievement of aims)
- *Time-based* (timeframe for achievement, number of times)

Returning to Mr. Williams, we can consider an example of a target that meets all of the SMART criteria:

Mr. Williams—Possible Target

Aim: Write notes on board accurately and efficiently.

Hypothesis: Working memory is reducing his ability to convert a student's comment into a shortened version for the board.

Target: After listening to a 10-second news story followed by a comment, Mr. Williams will independently use the "Play it again, Sam" strategy to efficiently paraphrase the comment onto a whiteboard in five consecutive attempts.

This target's context has been specified and is unambiguous, attainable, and time-based. It is relevant because news stories are typically 10 seconds long and the content being discussed in the classroom is similar to that of brief news stories. The target is also easily measurable (measurement options will be discussed in the "PIE: Evaluate" section later in this chapter). Importantly, this target also reflects the evidence supporting cognitive strategy training (Kennedy et al., 2008).

Another helpful target-specification approach that reflects all of the above principles is goal attainment scaling (GAS; Kiresuk & Sherman, 1968). GAS takes SMART targets and adds the notion of levels of success rather than having one achievement level. Krasny-Pacini, Evans, Sohlberg, and Chevignard (2016) and Grant and Ponsford (2014) both provide excellent overviews of the rationale behind GAS, its strengths and limitations, and the critical requirements in formulating reliable and valid goals using GAS methodology; and Kucheria and colleagues (2020) demonstrated the feasibility of outpatient speech-language pathologists learning and engaging in collaborative interviewing that resulted in valid Goal Attainment Scales for their neurogenic clients. The standard layout for GAS scales includes five levels:

−2	−1	0	+1	+2
Much less than expected	Less than expected	Expected outcome	Better than expected	Much better than expected

Using person-centered wording, the level descriptors could be:

−2	−1	0	+1	+2
If I decline	Where I am now	Where I hope to be following therapy	If I made really good progress	If I knocked it out of the park

The −1 level reflects the client's current performance that they hope to improve. The 0 to +2 levels reflect gradations of improvement, while the −2 level describes a worsening of performance. This is the standard scaling used in the research literature. In clinical practice, therapists sometimes use an alternative version:

−1	0	+1	+2
Below current performance	Current performance	Expected outcome	Better than expected outcome

This alternative version has the potential motivational advantage of all improvement levels showing a plus sign + (vs. aiming for 0 in the standard scale) and current performance being described neutrally as 0 rather than negatively as −1. Clinicians may find that they (or their clients) have a preference for one over the other, but if using GAS to obtain T-scores (Bouwens, van Heugten, & Verhey, 2009), the five-level version must be used.

Writing GAS goals requires careful attention to detail. In addition to ensuring SMART elements are reflected, clinicians must also ensure that:

- *The progression of skill is unidimensional,* such that only one variable is changing over time.
- *Each level is equidistant,* such that the "distance" between −2 and −1 is approximately the same as the distance between −1 and 0, 0 and +1, and +1 and +2.
- *There are no gaps between levels and all levels are mutually exclusive,* such that every possible outcome can be clearly mapped to the scale.

Unfortunately, there are many examples of Goal Attainment Scales that do *not* meet these criteria. Consider the following goal that seeks to help Diego, who is an inpatient with impulsivity challenges, stop getting out of bed independently:

−2 Much less than expected	−1 Less than expected	0 Expected outcome	+1 Better than expected	+2 Much better than expected
Diego doesn't refer to the reminder poster at all and never rings the call bell for help.	Diego looks at the reminder poster but still rings the call bell 33–50% of the time.	Diego looks at the reminder poster and rings the call bell for help 50% of the time.	Diego rings the call bell for help 90% of the time, only having to look at the reminder poster some of the time.	Diego rings the call bell for help 100% of the time, without having to look at the reminder poster at all.

The formulation of this Goal Attainment Scale violates all three criteria:

- Two variables are changing—making use of the reminder poster and frequency of using the call bell. These habits and skills may or may not correlate. If Diego ignores the reminder poster and rings the bell 50% of the time, there is no place on the scale to reflect this performance. Similarly, if he rings the bell 100% of the time but always relies on the reminder poster to do so, is that still considered success according to this scale?
- The distance between levels is unequal. In looking at the frequency of using the call bell, the five levels progress from 0% to 33% to 50% to 90% to 100%.
- There are gaps between levels. If Diego uses the call bell 70% of the time, there is no place on the scale to reflect this level. Some overlap also exists between levels −1 and 0 because if Diego uses the call bell 50% of the time, that level of performance falls into both levels.

A version of this scale that meets all criteria could be:

Aim: Improving personal safety

Context: When Diego is in bed in the hospital room and wants to get out of bed

Timeframe: Level 0 to be demonstrated across 3 consecutive days by 1 week from today

(Note that ingredients and a measurement plan also will be specified and are discussed later on in this chapter.)

−2 Much less than expected	−1 Less than expected	0 Expected outcome	+1 Better than expected	+2 Much better than expected
Diego rings the call bell for help less than 20% of the time.	Diego rings the call bell for help 20–39% of the time.	Diego rings the call bell for help 40–60% of the time.	Diego rings the call bell for help 61–80% of the time.	Diego rings the call bell for help more than 80% of the time.

Another example of a well-formulated Goal Attainment Scale, this time for a client resuming some social community reintegration, could be this:

Aim: Improving quality of social interactions

Context: When Jenene attends a weekday recreational group for individuals with ABI

Timeframe: Level 0 to be demonstrated across 3 consecutive weeks within the next 2 months

(The treatment ingredients and measurement plan will be additionally stipulated and are described later in this chapter.)

−2 Much less than expected	−1 Less than expected	0 Expected outcome	+1 Better than expected	+2 Much better than expected
Jenene has an anger outburst 4 times or more per week.	Jenene has an anger outburst 3 times per week.	Jenene has an anger outburst 2 times per week.	Jenene has an anger outburst 1 time per week.	Jenene has no anger outbursts in the week.

GAS is particularly helpful for measuring progress on *functional* targets that take place outside of the therapy room. For example, a speech-language pathologist may be targeting improved breath support and overarticulation to address dysarthria in a structured therapy context. These types of structured targets may be easily and simply specified as SMART. However, when the client is applying these strategies in more functional contexts, GAS may be more effective in capturing the desired levels of outcome, for example intelligibility ratings by a spouse.

As discussed earlier, engaging the client in defining aims and targets is a critical component in effective treatment specification. For GAS targets that are used in functional contexts, this discussion is helpful to both understand how the client perceives their current circumstances and educate the client on what different circumstances would look like in concrete, objective terms. The clinician must prompt the client to fully describe the contexts and behaviors they desire to change and then use the client's words as much as possible to describe the GAS levels. However, there will be times when using the client's words may result in level descriptions that violate the requirement to be unidimensional. Consider the following levels that were formulated using the client's words as they described their ability to answer questions after doing a presentation in class:

−2 Much less than expected	−1 Less than expected	0 Expected outcome	+1 Better than expected	+2 Much better than expected
"I answer, 'I don't know' when asked a question to avoid a rambling, nonsensical answer."	"I initially go blank when it comes time to answer questions, and then it takes me at least two tries to say what I want. I feel like I am rambling."	"It takes me no more than two attempts to say what I want. It feels like I'm rambling a bit, but at least I didn't go blank."	"I get my responses out on the first try. The responses are sometimes a bit long but are usually closer to what I want to say."	"My first response is good! My answers are shorter and to the point."

This client has included multiple factors to describe their current performance and what better and worse performance would look like. This does not meet the unidimensional criterion because we don't know that all elements will vary in concert with one another, and we may therefore be unable to clearly determine where their performance falls on the scale. One option is to choose one of the primary variables and formulate the levels using only that variable. Alternatively, if the clinician sees value in using the client's words, they should attempt to mitigate the multidimensionality problem by incorporating only the factors that seem most likely to correlate with one another and then using discussion at each measurement opportunity to determine the proper rating on the scale. Another option might be to generate a Likert-type scale using the client's descriptors.

In summary, defining the treatment target requires that the clinician and client collaborate to identify the targets and aims, operationally define the targeted behavior, and specify contexts and supports for the treatment plan. The research literature is clear on the value of such an approach; however, it is not yet routine in clinical practice (Prescott, Fleming, & Doig, 2015). To support clinicians in generating effective aims and targets, Forms 5.1 and 5.2 at the end of the chapter contain checklists for SMART and GAS formulation. Fillable versions are available in the digital files accompanying this book.

Planning Steps 4 and 5: Plan Implementation and Evaluation Phases

As discussed at the beginning of this chapter, the planning phase includes planning the implementation procedures and the evaluation measures. For the sake of simplicity, we will discuss these two phases in the "PIE: Implement" and "PIE: Evaluate" sections below, but it is critical for the clinician to recognize the importance of determining the procedures and measures up front in order to approach the intervention plan methodically. In today's rehabilitation context, where clinicians frequently are not afforded sufficient time to work with their clients and have busy caseloads pulling them in multiple directions, the importance of systematic planning to maximize chances for efficient target and aim achievement cannot be overemphasized.

PIE: IMPLEMENT

Implementation, or *how* the rehabilitation target will be taught, flows from the outcome of the planning steps described earlier. The clinician has identified the client's characteristics and worked with them to define the target context and specify the desired outcome. Implementation planning is based on these factors in conjunction with environmental factors such as the availability of services.

The two categories of treatment targets in the RTSS that are most common in cognitive rehabilitation are: (1) skills and habits and (2) representations (e.g., knowledge and attitudes). To learn or reestablish skills and habits, one method with strong evidence of validity for individuals with memory and learning impairments is *systematic instruction*, described in Chapter 4. Systematic instruction methods apply to many targets described this book, as we focus on effective teaching of tools and strategies that help clients achieve functional targets. Teaching these tools and strategies will involve using systematic instruction to establish skills and habits, as well as techniques such as didactic instruction for knowledge targets (see Chapter 6) and motivational interviewing and cognitive reframing to increase motivation and engagement (see Chapter 3). For systematic instruction, the nature of the client's cognitive impairments will determine the level of specificity needed in the instruction plan. Clients with profound declarative learning and memory impairments will require different levels of task analyses, practice regimens, and generalization than those with mild learning challenges who might not need this level of specificity.

In the next section, we provide an overview of the treatment framework used throughout this text, with primary consideration for clients with moderate to severe challenges in learning and memory. These principles apply to all individuals with brain injury, and Chapters 3 and 12 describe additional considerations for those with mild brain injury whose cognitive impairments may be secondary to other physiological or psychological factors such as fatigue or anxiety.

The key RTSS element in designing implementation is the choice of treatment *ingredients*. As described in Chapter 4, ingredients are clinician actions or clinician-selected objects that the clinician hypothesizes will help achieve the targeted change in function. Ingredients include the materials chosen (e.g., photos vs. objects, communication supports like a pencil and paper), as well as clinician actions such as providing instructions, verbal and nonverbal support and feedback (e.g., hand-over-hand cueing, modeling, corrective feedback), opportunities for practice (e.g., repeating a task 20 times to increase skill), and praise and encouragement. Thus, while the targets are "what" we are trying to achieve, the ingredients are "how" we are going about achieving them. If the clinician does not clearly specify what they are doing in a session, it becomes impossible to understand which elements may be positively, neutrally, or negatively impacting change, which, in turn, reduces the efficiency of target attainment.

Returning to Mr. Williams, we can now add ingredients to our plan:

Mr. Williams—Possible Ingredients

Target: After listening to a 10-second news story followed by a comment, Mr. Williams will use the "Play it again, Sam" strategy to efficiently paraphrase the comment on a whiteboard.

Ingredients: Clinician actions include instructing Mr. Williams to restate the comment verbatim or close to verbatim and then, while starting to write, paraphrase the comment into key word chunks; explaining repetition and chunking as memory supports; modeling the strategy with multiple examples; providing opportunities for massed practice of using the strategy; and providing corrective feedback, praise, and encouragement. Materials include multiple 10-second video news clips, each with an associated comment; written or pictographic reminders of the strategy; and whiteboard and dry erase marker.

In reviewing our earlier plan for Diego, to increase his frequency of using the call bell for help in exiting the bed, ingredients could include:

- A visual reminder posted prominently in his line of sight when exiting the bed
- Opportunities for massed practice with therapy and nursing staff of reaching for the call bell before exiting the bed
- Education about the importance of not falling
- Feedback when the call bell is not used

- Rapid response and praise when the call bell is used
- Daily feedback about progress toward the target

In addition to specifying the ingredients, clinicians must consider therapy *dose*. Just as different individuals may need 50 milligrams versus 100 milligrams of a drug to achieve the desired effect, different clients may need a higher or lower dose of therapy ingredients. Dose needs to be considered on multiple levels:

- Number/amount of ingredients (e.g., number of repetitions per target in each therapy session, amount of cueing, frequency of instructions)
- Duration of each therapy session (e.g., 45 minutes) as well as each target's activity within the therapy session (e.g., 15 minutes for target 1, 20 minutes for target 2)
- Frequency of therapy sessions (e.g., once per week)
- Length of intervention plan (e.g., 3 months)

The remainder of this implementation section describes the three phases of training (acquisition, mastery, maintenance). It is important for the clinician to recognize their client's current training phase so they can accurately specify ingredients and dose. For example, a client in the acquisition phase likely needs a much higher dose in regard to minutes of therapy than a client in the maintenance phase and also is likely to need a higher dose of ingredients such as modeling and cues. Importantly, clients with significant memory impairments will require specific instructional ingredients such as error-control methods (see Chapter 6) to learn skills or concepts. The selection of ingredients may vary over time as a client develops greater independence. It is for this reason that our PIE diagram in Figure 5.1 has a reminder for the clinician to confirm the phase of therapy before proceeding to specify ingredients and dose.

A key concept in the RTSS is ensuring internal consistency across targets, ingredients, and outcome measures, and this mental checkpoint is one step toward ensuring that consistency. Across all three phases of training, the clinician must be intentional about using practice tasks and corresponding protocols and outcome measures that reflect the client's needs and aims as well as optimizing therapeutic rapport and client engagement strategies that will increase client's sense of self-efficacy and motivation.

Implementation Phase 1: Acquisition

The term *acquisition phase* refers to the initial learning (or relearning) of the rehabilitation target. As discussed in Chapter 4 and applied below, when first teaching a target concept, skill, or behavior, it is important to consider the training stimuli, practice regimen, and client's level of cognitive engagement.

Training Stimuli

At this stage, the clinician's planning has identified the target, prerequisites, training materials, cues and prompts, and context in which training will occur, and the clinician is ready to begin training. Clients with more intact declarative learning or recall ability or for whom the target skills are familiar may require less or no acquisition training, as they may be able to learn and retain a behavior or information after several demonstrations. However, clients with cognitive impairments that affect learning and retention will benefit from systematic acquisition training. Another consideration will be whether there is a need to unlearn or extinguish a previous behavior. A client who used a complex electronic planner to organize meetings and travel preinjury might need to unlearn some procedures in order to use a simple digital aid for tracking medications. Unlearning will also require systematic instruction.

To begin acquisition training, the clinician selects a range of training or practice stimuli that will elicit the behavior. Initially, instruction will focus on the most common or simple exemplar. For example, when instructing a client to use a phone calendar to record appointments, the clinician would have the client practice with the most frequent appointments (e.g., therapy sessions) and then add other examples (e.g., friend visits). Similarly, the clinician can vary dates and times of the appointment to systematically introduce a range of appointment characteristics.

Clinicians often assign *home practice* as an ingredient to increase opportunities to practice the target behavior. There are four important considerations for home practice:

1. Home practice can be used to increase opportunities to practice a skill or habit, in which case it is the same target but practiced at home.

2. Home practice can be a way to transition from a skill learned in therapy (e.g., learning to enter appointments in a planner) to a habit of using that skill automatically (e.g., entering new appointments in the planner every day). In this case, the clinician should specify a separate target for the habit and add ingredients accordingly. For example, ingredients such as modeling, self-reflection, and review of feedback can be effective for skill acquisition but are less effective for developing habits, which benefit from high-dose practice of correct responses.

3. Home practice is sometimes assigned with the expectation that the client will generalize what they learned in therapy to novel contexts and tasks. As noted throughout this text, a main finding across cognitive rehabilitation studies is that most clients do not spontaneously generalize what they learn in therapy to their everyday lives without support. If the target is generalization, then the therapy session should include ingredients specifically selected to promote generalization, such as variability in training stimuli during the session.

4. A common occurrence in rehabilitation is that clients do not do their homework. While this is often attributed to the client (i.e., the client's lack of adherence or compliance with treatment recommendations), it is the responsibility of the clinician to employ ingredients that specifically target motivation. For this reason, the RTSS guidelines recommend adding a separate target for motivation to complete the homework, with appropriate ingredients. Ingredients to increase client motivation and the likelihood that the client will voluntarily complete tasks out of the view of the clinician (i.e., *volition* ingredients) are described in Chapters 3 and 4.

When teaching a concept or other information (e.g., safety awareness), the clinician should also provide a range of examples, beginning with positive examples (e.g., lock the brakes on your wheelchair before standing) and moving to negative examples (e.g., do not walk while wearing slippery socks).

Practice Regimen

During the acquisition phase, when a person with declarative memory impairments is first acquiring a target concept, skill, or behavior, the following three training conditions will maximize learning potential:

1. **Error-control methods.** The clinician is attempting to *establish* the target. While it may not be possible to prevent all errors from occurring, errors are minimized during acquisition by the use of error-controlled instruction techniques. These techniques include ensuring an appropriate level of task difficulty, clinician modeling with prompts or cues prior to task attempt that are gradually faded, and use of immediate corrective feedback with knowledge of performance when an error is made. When errors are made, the clinician will model the correct response and have the client demonstrate it until the client demonstrates the response accurately. The clinician will then back up to the last step or component that the client performed correctly and have them start there and add the correctly practiced step so that it is chained to the previously learned step. These procedures are described in reference to training facts and simple routines (Chapter 6) and the use of external aids (Chapter 8).

2. **Massed practice.** When first establishing the target, the clinician engages the client in massed practice trials. The goal of these trials is to ensure that the client is able to successfully produce the target in response to the stimulus, without assistance from the clinician, which might take several repetitions of the target in a row. This intensive schedule has been shown to enhance initial target learning (Huckans et al., 2010). If the target has multiple steps or components, the clinician chains them together but may need to isolate difficult steps or concepts and provide specific intensive practice on each. This acquisition training is systematic and relatively fast-paced to provide sufficient learning opportunities and keep the client engaged.

3. **Intensive practice.** In addition to massed practice, it is critical to provide sufficient repetition of practice when first establishing the target. For some clients and instructional targets, the acquisition phase may be very short—for example, a portion of one session, as the client might learn the target with one demonstration. Other training scenarios may take considerable time. For instance, teaching a person with a severe declarative memory impairment a complex behavioral sequence (e.g., doing laundry) might require several weeks of acquisition training in steps. As noted above, home programs can play a critical role in providing practice opportunities, especially for establishing habits and skills. It is important to keep in mind, however, that clients who are learning via nondeclarative processes will learn what they perform most often, so errors in the home environment must be controlled and the support person in the client's home environment should receive training to implement error-control techniques. The importance of error control outside of the therapy session cannot be overestimated: Many training programs fail because learning conditions at home "undo" what has been trained in therapy. Although there currently are no evidence-based guidelines for caregiver training in cognitive rehabilitation (Boschen, Gargaro, Gan, Gerber, & Brandys, 2007; Fisher, Lennon, Bellon, & Lawn, 2015), there is growing evidence that caregivers can learn to manage cognitive impairments in children and adults (Fisher, Bellon, Lawn, Lennon, & Sohlberg, 2019; Judge, Yarry, & Orsulic-Jeras, 2009; Sander,

Clark, Atchison, & Rueda, 2009; Wade, Carey, & Wolfe, 2006), and that this can significantly decrease stress and burden at home (Sander et al., 2009; Wade et al., 2006). It is noteworthy that successful caregiver training programs offer *ongoing* support by health care professionals. Without this support, caregivers may experience an increased burden because they feel that they are "on their own" managing both maintenance of treatment gains and also new problem behaviors (Hoepner & Turkstra, 2013).

Client Motivation, Engagement, and Self-Efficacy

The third consideration during initial target acquisition is the level of client motivation and engagement. Motivation and engagement will have been enhanced by selecting targets and ingredients that are meaningful to the client and reflect their lived experiences, beliefs, values, and identities. Resilience-enhancing techniques that can optimize motivation and engagement and be embedded in instruction are reviewed in Chapter 3. Successful rehabilitation depends on a client's belief that they can do what is being asked of them, and that when they do so, it will result in meaningful changes in their lives. Promoting these beliefs is part of building client self-efficacy through therapeutic rapport, use of counseling techniques such as motivational interviewing, and selection of appropriate targets and instructional examples. These motivational factors are reviewed in detail in Chapters 3 and 4.

Effortful processing techniques (e.g., semantic elaboration, visualization, self-generation of responses) as well as metacognitive strategies (e.g., prediction and reflection) have been shown to enhance engagement and therefore learning. There can be a tension between minimizing errors and encouraging effortful processing; ultimately, it is necessary to use clinical judgment to strike a balance for an individual client, context, and targets. Most importantly, clinicians should avoid passive learning. For example, if teaching a client a cooking routine, a clinician might have the client periodically taste the recipe and evaluate whether it needs more flavor rather than only reviewing and practicing the recipe steps.

Implementation Phase 2: Mastery ("Fluency") and Generalization

The goal of the mastery and generalization phase is to consolidate new learning so that the client can use it reliably. For example, a person may be able to use a strategy in a quiet room but not when distracted or tired or may still need occasional prompting. The clinician should probe the client's performance at the start of each session. When the client demonstrates the ability to complete the target skill or concept during a session but does not necessarily recall the skill or concept later in that session or in the next session or does not implement the target consistently in the desired contexts, it will be helpful to implement instructional techniques in the mastery phase of training.

It should be noted that failure to establish mastery of new skills is a common occurrence in rehabilitation, where lengths of stay are becoming progressively shorter and opportunities for practice in everyday contexts are limited. This phase, however, is critical for generalization and maintenance and requires careful attention in rehabilitation. Establishing target mastery and generalization requires manipulation of the same three factors discussed in "Implementation Phase 1: Acquisition," that is, consideration of training stimuli, practice regimen, and client engagement and motivation.

Practice Stimuli

Incorporating stimulus and contextual variability is critical at this point. During the planning process, the clinician and client identify the environments and contexts in which the target will be implemented, which, in turn, allows for the identification of antecedents in each context that can trigger the desired skill or concept. During the acquisition phase, a general response has been established. During the mastery phase, target responses for all of the conditions are practiced, requiring the clinician to provide more varied training stimuli and ensure that practice occurs in the client's natural environments. While this may seem impractical, the characteristics of procedural learning required for individuals with moderate to severe declarative learning difficulties stipulate that the learning context be similar to the context in which the skills will be used. Therapy that does not consider this basic learning rule is unlikely to generalize and thus is not a cost-effective use of rehabilitation. Similarly, incorporation of everyday people in the client's life will be critical.

Practice Regimen

The clinician makes active modifications to these three elements:

1. **Error-control methods.** The clinician continues to use error-control instructional methods. Given that the client has already acquired the target, modeling is limited to instances in which the client makes errors, to prevent *drift*—the tendency to move away from the target response over time. The clinician should continue to provide guided practice through occasional prompting with general or opportunity cues, while gradually fading cues based on client performance. Feedback also can be adjusted to move from immediate corrective feedback to delayed general feedback, using knowledge of results (e.g., "Did you complete all the steps?"). When errors are made, the clinician can have the client practice the correct response and then back up and chain it to the new step.

2. **Distributed practice.** Fundamental to the mastery phase is the introduction and gradual lengthening of distributed practice trials so that the client is able to implement the target independently over increasingly longer periods of time. It may be that, as training conditions are altered (e.g., by changes in the prompt or environment), it will be necessary to drop back to acquisition training and provide some massed practice. Keeping careful session data will reveal this need. Spaced retrieval (SR) training, discussed further in Chapter 6, is an example of a specific treatment procedure that provides structure to distributed practice trials.

3. **Intensive practice.** The clinician maintains high levels of practice during the mastery phase to establish fluency with the instructional target. The goal is for the target to become automatic and natural in a variety of contexts. Continued practice is essential. The clinician should continue to monitor and document home practice to ensure that correct practice is completed with sufficient intensity.

Client Motivation, Engagement, and Self-Efficacy

The techniques used to optimize motivation, engagement, and self-efficacy during the acquisition phase are also useful during the mastery phase. They are reviewed in Chapters 3 and 4. During the mastery phase, the clinician incorporates additional metacognitive components to facilitate active engagement during practice sessions. A sample metacognitive technique is to ask the client to predict and then reflect on accuracy of their performance by taking session data and comparing their own performance across trials and sessions. The client also may predict which aspects will be easy or challenging, then reflect on how those factors operated during performance. The clinician and client may choose to modify the target or the environment based on this self-assessment. It should be noted that there is a necessary tension between enhancing client involvement and limiting errors. As the client gains more control in the process, there will be more opportunities for error; hence, the clinician must gauge whether error responses will be intrusive or instructive as the client is learning the therapy targets. Correct responses are most critical during initial acquisition. It is also important to keep in mind that previous declarative knowledge and reasoning skills may be preserved in individuals with profound anterograde memory impairments. That is, the person's ability to tell you what they *would* do in a given situation often does not correlate with actual performance. Thus, for this population we recommend minimizing discussion of target behavior, instead focusing on rehearsal of correct responses.

Implementation Phase 3: Maintenance

The maintenance phase occurs once the client has demonstrated the training target reliably and fluently in their desired contexts. Distributed practice trials and probe data during the mastery phase will have revealed this outcome. Recidivism and abandonment of targeted strategies or behaviors are common rehabilitation problems, and there are ingredients that clinicians can use to increase the likelihood that a rehabilitation target will be retained beyond the cessation of therapy. In most cases, this phase of therapy is not conducted by the clinician in a therapy setting. Significant others in a client's naturalistic settings will often be enlisted to support maintenance. Clinicians may space out their sessions and conduct check-ins to ask about maintenance and offer "tune-ups" as indicated. Below we list factors that the clinician can build into the instruction process to promote durability of learning. This can take considerable planning, as often the clinician enters the maintenance phase for one target while beginning the acquisition phase for another.

Instructional Context

During this phase, the clinician may train natural supports, which are the people and contexts that promote ongoing use of the instructional target. These supports will have been previously identified and trained during therapy; for example, an educational assistant may be trained to encourage ongoing use of an assignment completion strategy, or a colleague may be trained to support the use of a memory system in a supported work environment. There might also be factors that are part of the client's natural environment that have been exploited to provide ongoing facilitation, such as the school bell noted earlier as a signal to use a memory aid. Careful investigation of opportunities and people in a person's natural environment can be the key to that person's long-term use of a target skill. Providing these everyday supports with written reminders and prompts can help to ensure maintenance of support.

Practice Regimen

The need for cumulative review of instructional targets is often overlooked. Even without a cognitive impairment, people do not behave as robots and automatically continue implementing all intended and learned behaviors. The implementation of diets, exercise programs, and mental health strategies all have peaks and valleys, and most people need ongoing support and adjustments to maintain desired habits (Michie et al., 2011). People with cognitive impairments require periodic review and support (Powell et al., 2012). So-called booster sessions have been shown to facilitate maintenance of gains after therapies such as SR for memory impairments in adults with dementia (Cherry, Hawley, Jackson, & Boudreaux, 2009) and often are cited as a necessary ingredient in effective clinical treatment trials (e.g., Bourgeois et al., 2007; van Hout, Wekking, Berg, & Deelman, 2008). People and their contexts and aims will change, and adjustments in a schedule, routine, or behavior are likely to be necessary. Clinicians must consider how follow-up and adjustments might take place and who will be involved in this process. Planning for cumulative review should be part of the therapy process and built into the training of natural supports.

Client Motivation, Engagement, and Self-Efficacy

The same engagement and motivation strategies used in the acquisition and mastery phases of training also apply to the maintenance phase. Supports may be tailored to anticipating difficulties that may cause cessation of strategy use. Building in accountability to a support person for strategy use beyond therapy may be helpful. Scheduling booster sessions or enrolling the client in community classes or activities that support targets are other options to promote motivation to maintain skills.

Overview of Session Structure

Clinicians need efficient systems that can be replicated across clients for effective instruction to be practical in everyday settings. Having a systematic way of planning the session and documenting the data can help streamline decisions and information. The typical instructional session consists of four parts:

1. **Check-in.** The clinician reviews any homework or relevant information since the previous session and adjusts the session plan accordingly.

2. **Retention probe.** Most sessions begin with a probe that measures the client's retention of previously taught concepts, skills, or behaviors. The probe will typically list the steps or components for the target and measure parameters such as accuracy of completion of each step with overall percent correct. This information is used to pinpoint where to begin in the training sequence in that session and as a measure of

therapy progress. For example, if a retention probe indicates that the client has forgotten some components or previously trained steps in a sequence to use a strategy or device, the clinician will back up and begin training at the step prior to the error. The clinician can use the therapy session data form and progress monitoring form to record client performance on the probe, which can then become a measure of therapy progress for the target (see the "PIE: Evaluate" section that follows).

3. **Practice.** Based on performance during the retention probe, the clinician engages the client in practicing therapy targets, which comprises the bulk of the therapy session. As outlined above, the amount and type of practice will vary with the client's learning characteristics, learning phase, and nature of the task. Practice results may be used as a measure of client progress (e.g., an average of performance across trials or performance on the final trial in the session), in addition to or in place of the retention probe results (see the next section).

4. **Review.** Sessions typically end with a review and final probe and perhaps homework or planning.

At the conclusion of this chapter, several forms are included to support the clinician in applying a systematic approach to intervention planning. These forms are also included in the digital files accompanying this book:

- Form 5.3 is a progression planning worksheet to support systematic planning to advance a client's skills through increased independence, increased breadth of participation across contexts, and/or increased complexity of contexts.
- Form 5.4 is a sample therapy session data form for the acquisition, mastery, and generalization phases of learning. Clinicians may use this form to document session results in detail, and the content should transfer easily to the clinical note for the session. Versions customized for each category of intervention described in Chapters 6–8 are available in those chapters.
- Form 5.5 is a sample session-to-session progress monitoring form for the acquisition, mastery, and generalization phases to assist the clinician in analyzing progress over time (see the section that directly follows). There are also customized versions in each category of intervention described in Chapters 6–8.
- Form 5.6 is a sample progress monitoring form for the maintenance phase, which can be used for all types of interventions.

Having a protocol for implementing effective instructional methods during therapy sessions increases the ease with which a clinician can implement therapy and may thereby improve effectiveness and productivity.

PIE: EVALUATE

As discussed earlier, evaluation is not something that is introduced at the end of intervention. Preparing for evaluation is an integral step in the planning phase. Clinicians must decide at the outset how progress and achievement of targets will be measured. "Outcome" data are the ultimate determiner of the impact of treatment. "Progress" or "session" data reflect the steps along the way to achieving the outcome and are critical to testing hypotheses and therefore implementing effective intervention. Evaluation occurs at the level of both targets and aims.

As noted earlier in this chapter, the *target* should specify the skill or behavior along with the aspect of the skill/behavior that is expected to change (e.g., speed, accuracy, frequency, quality, duration, amount of prompting or independence). Recall that if prompting is not specified, independent performance is assumed. The target should also specify the context (e.g., on a sample stimulus in therapy, in a semi-structured activity in the clinic, in the classroom, with a peer). The target should be specific as well as observable and measurable. It should be meaningful to the client and within the client's reach for achieving.

In contrast, the *aim* is a broader aspect of daily functioning that involves more than one skill and may involve more than one discipline's contribution. Aims are often reflected in person-centered outcome measures (PCOMs) that engage clients in the process of identifying priorities and measuring rehabilitation success in the field. The use of PCOMs has been linked to decreased health care costs, higher goal attainment, and improved self-efficacy (Prescott et al., 2015). Despite agreement about the need for PCOMs, however, they remain underused in brain injury rehabilitation (Kucheria et al., 2020). In fact, some clinicians continue to rely on standardized assessment tools to provide evidence of outcome. As far back as 1984, McCauley and Swisher described the limitations of standardized tests as measures of progress or outcome:

> The use of norm-referenced tests to assess progress can result in the underestimation or overestimation of change. . . . [N]orm-referenced tests, which by definition are designed to look at differences between individuals, will almost always be composed of items that can be expected to result in a broad range of performances and, therefore, will rarely be sensitive enough to behavioral change to document progress in therapy. . . . [S]ome amount of change in test scores can occur as a result of the test's imperfect reliability. . . . [T]he client may simply "learn" the test because of repeated administrations. (McCauley & Swisher, 1984, p. 346)

Scores on standardized cognitive tests cannot fully capture functional outcomes of the heterogeneous ABI population (Chaytor & Schmitter-Edgecombe, 2003). Therefore, while standardized tests do contribute important information for the clinician's formulation of a treatment plan, scores on these tests are rarely appropriate indicators of progress or outcome.

Earlier we reviewed the process for developing collaborative SMART targets and the use of GAS (Krasny-Pacini et al., 2016), which can provide relevant and objective measures of the impact of cognitive rehabilitation on both treatment targets and functional aims. In GAS and SMART targets, the outcome is built right into the target wording, so it is clear to all involved when the desired outcome has been achieved. Some examples of SMART targets with built-in outcomes include the following:

- Shanice will independently check her calendar at least 3 times per day, for 14 consecutive days.
- In the final week of therapy, Taylor will use circumlocution to manage conversational word-finding difficulties 80% of the time they occur in session.

Following up on an earlier example of GAS for Diego, we can now add in a measurement plan to support documenting the outcome level achieved:

Aim: Improving personal safety

Context: When Diego is in bed in the hospital room and wants to get out of bed

Timeframe: Level 0 to be demonstrated across 3 consecutive days by 1 week from today

Ingredients: A visual reminder posted prominently in his line of sight when exiting the bed, massed practice with therapy and nursing staff of reaching for the call bell before exiting the bed, education about the importance of not falling, feedback when the call bell is not used, rapid response and praise when the call bell is used, daily feedback about progress toward target

Measurement plan: Nursing staff to document all occurrences that come to their attention of Diego's use and nonuse of the call bell in a daily tracker within his patient chart

−2 Much less than expected	−1 Less than expected	0 Expected outcome	+1 Better than expected	+2 Much better than expected
Diego rings the call bell for help less than 20% of the time.	Diego rings the call bell for help 20–39% of the time.	Diego rings the call bell for help 40–60% of the time.	Diego rings the call bell for help 61–80% of the time.	Diego rings the call bell for help more than 80% of the time.

This is now a complete target with the process and outcome clearly specified. There are other formulations of targets that permit an array of possible outcome measures, and the clinician should work collaboratively with the client to determine the best measures to meet their needs. Recalling Mr. Williams, we generated the following as a target for him:

After listening to a 10-second news story followed by a comment, Mr. Williams will independently use the "Play it again, Sam" strategy to efficiently paraphrase the comment on a whiteboard in five consecutive attempts.

Possible progress measures for a target such as this include:

- Percent of time the strategy is used accurately and independently
- Percent of time the comment was correctly repeated the first time and repeated in chunks while writing
- Length of time between original comment and paraphrase
- Length of paraphrased sentence relative to original
- Quality rating, 1–10, of paraphrased sentence

It was additionally hypothesized that gains made on this target would support Mr. Williams in achieving his aim of writing notes on the classroom whiteboard efficiently and accurately. Just as there are many options for measuring the effectiveness of the strategy during structured tasks in the therapy sessions, there are many options for measuring the ultimate impact of the target in the classroom:

- A rating scale of 1–10, completed at the end of each class where this task occurred, identifying satisfaction with performance
- Self-reported percentage of time the strategy was applied during this type of classroom task
- 1–5 rating of conciseness plus 1–5 rating of accuracy of paraphrased comments
- Rating or timed measure of efficiency from time comment is made to when paraphrased sentence is completed
- GAS rating that reflects the various stages of improved written paraphrasing

Targets are typically evaluated via session-to-session data tracking (in both practice trials and retention probes), but the carryover into additional practice contexts is evaluated by generalization probes and, later, by maintenance probes. In contrast, aims are typically evaluated via impact data. These accumulated data points are critical for making clinical decisions about moving from the acquisition to generalization and maintenance phases of training.

Target Acquisition Data

The bulk of time during treatment sessions is spent providing practice opportunities for the client. The clinician should keep data on parameters relevant to the specific target, such as the number of correct practice trials and the associated level of support provided, length of time, and quality of performance. As discussed earlier, retention of the prior session's learning should be probed at the outset of the session to document the client's recall of the strategy, aid, or new learning and to ensure that the target is addressed at the appropriate starting point in the current session. In addition, the clinician should document the results of practice trials completed in the session. Analysis of these data together (session-to-session retention and within-session performance; see sample forms at the end of the chapter and in the digital files accompanying this book) can provide insights into treatment modification. For example, data may reveal that prompts were faded too quickly to allow for errorless practice or that there were not enough practice opportunities to allow for target acquisition. These session data are particularly critical during the initial acquisition phase.

Earlier in this chapter we listed the three pillars of evidence-based practice according to Dollaghan (2007): client preferences, evidence from the literature, and evidence from the client's individual performance. The last pillar is often confused with so-called clinician experience, and that is a pitfall to avoid. A clinician's prior experience is important and informative but may not always predict what will work with the next client. Similarly, the research literature may not always predict what will work with an individual client. Therefore, gathering objective, unbiased data from each individual client is crucial to making informed decisions. This is often called "practice-based evidence" (Horn & Gassaway, 2010).

The following principles underlie effective data collection for practice-based evidence:

1. Data must be *valid*. This principle is observed via the collaborative goal-setting process described earlier.

2. Data must be *reliable*. This principle is managed via the creation of SMART- and GAS-scaled targets and the careful stipulation and application of ingredients.

3. Data must be *objective and free from bias*. Clinicians should not selectively choose which data to include. This means recognizing and mitigating both biased thinking patterns and pressure from outside sources. Gambrill (2012) describes common decision-making errors that are frequently related to bias. For example, if you ask clinicians why they think therapy worked, they are likely to credit the quality of their therapy, whereas they tend to attribute lack of progress to poor client motivation (Cicerone et al., 2005). In contrast, clients tend to ascribe progress to their hard work and supportive family and lack of progress to ineffective therapy (Cicerone et al., 2005). Using valid, reliable, and objective data is important in order to make good decisions about therapy programs.

4. Data must be collected *predictably and frequently*. The clinician should make it a routine expectation to gather data at every session. Collecting data on an intermittent basis risks introducing bias into the data, and it also leaves insufficient data points with which to reliably evaluate gains. For an analysis of progress to be robust, multiple data points across similar intervals (e.g., every day, once per week) are required. Ideally, the clinician would obtain three baseline data points *prior to* initiating intervention to feel confident that there is a stable starting point (Lane & Gast, 2014). Unfortunately, this is often not realistic in the time-constrained world of clinical practice. Therefore, in a treatment-only data-gathering context, clinicians should have a minimum of 10 data points in order to maximize reliability of treatment gain analyses (Higginbotham & Moulton, 2017).

Returning to Mr. Williams, we know from our planning stage that principles 1–3 above were met. For principle 4, let's consider the following data scenario, in which we took within-session practice measures twice weekly over the course of 5 weeks on Mr. Williams's implementation of his "Play it again, Sam" strategy (note that we could have alternatively or additionally documented retention probe results for this analysis):

	Session Number									
	1	2	3	4	5	6	7	8	9	10
% accurate, independent use	30	40	30	50	40	60	60	80	70	80
1–10 quality rating	2	3	3	2	5	5	4	3	4	5

This dataset meets principle 4 because we have a predictable, equal spacing of measurements, with 10 occurrences of each.

Now that all data collection principles are met, what do these data tell us? Is Mr. Williams progressing well toward his target, or should we be reevaluating one or more elements of our original plan? Too often when it is not clear that the target is attained, clinicians resort to either assuming more time is needed or randomly altering ingredients or targets. Both approaches risk wasting important client and clinician time, as well as funds for intervention.

Fortunately, we can draw from single-subject design methodology (SSDM) to help answer our clinical question: Has Mr. Williams's behavior changed beyond what we would expect from normal variability? In SSDM, data are divided into Phase A and Phase B. As discussed, in the research literature and in optimal clinical contexts, Phase A includes baseline data and Phase B includes treatment data. Without baseline data, we cannot say with certainty that it was our intervention approach that caused the change in behavior (Lane & Gast, 2014). However, a treatment-only design can still provide insight into whether a change is occurring and whether that change is clinically significant (Higginbotham & Moulton, 2017). In a treatment-only design, we split the treatment data set in half, labeling the first half as Phase A and the second half as Phase B. Always choosing the halfway point to divide the data ensures a predictable and unbiased method of comparing performance over time.

Figure 5.2 shows Mr. Williams's results for percent accurate and independent use of his "Play it again, Sam" strategy when plotted in two phases (the first five sessions in Phase A and the last five in Phase B). We can then use visual inspection from SSDM to evaluate changes in level, trend, and stability. Lane and Gast (2014) provide detailed procedures for obtaining these measures, but an overview follows.

Level

Level refers to measures of the central tendency of performance data, such as mean and median. Median is the better choice for a single-client scenario because it is less affected by outliers. If working with the list of session data, we order the data points in Phase A from the lowest to highest and find the middle point (if there is an uneven number of data points) or calculate the average of the two middle points (if there is an even number). Using the graph, we plot a line such that half of the data points in Phase A fall above the line and half fall below it. This process is repeated for Phase B. Figure

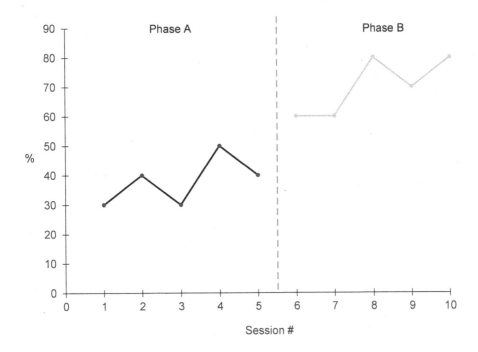

FIGURE 5.2. Mr. Williams's results for percent accurate and independent use of his "Play it again, Sam" strategy when plotted in two phases.

5.3 shows the median lines added to Mr. Williams's data graph, highlighting that his median performance was 40% in the first half of treatment and 70% in the second half.

Trend

Trend refers to the direction of change (flat, increasing, decreasing). The mathematical calculations for trend are more complicated (see Lane & Gast, 2014), but to plot the trend lines, we can simply draw a line following the direction of the trend, where about half the data points are above the trend line and half below it. When the trend lines are added to the graph, as shown in Figure 5.4, we can see that the trend is increasing in both phases, but the pace of change, or the slope of the trend line, is steeper in Phase B.

Stability

Stability refers to how variable performance is around the median or trend lines. Range is the measure used to assess stability; it is evaluated by inspecting the difference between the lowest and highest numbers in each phase (full range) or by narrower bands, for example, the range where 50% or 75% of data points fall. For Mr. Williams, there is little change in median stability between Phase A and Phase B, with the full range of data points equaling 20% in both cases (30–50% in Phase A and 60–80% in Phase B). A similar calculation can be completed for variability around the trend line.

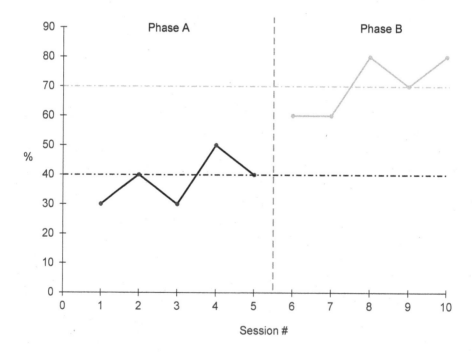

FIGURE 5.3. Mr. Williams's results for percent accurate and independent use of his "Play it again, Sam" strategy when plotted in two phases, with median lines added.

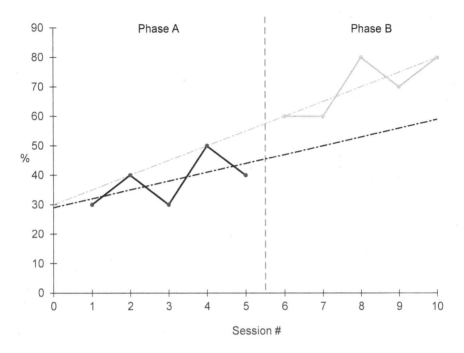

FIGURE 5.4. Mr. Williams's results for percent accurate and independent use of his "Play it again, Sam" strategy when plotted in two phases, with trend lines added.

We can now consider all visual inspection results together:

- Median performance (level) increased from 40% in the first half of treatment to 70% in the second half.
- Pace of change (trend) increased in the second half of treatment.
- Variability appeared low in the first half and was maintained in the second half.

Although limited by the lack of baseline data, these results do provide good support for Mr. Williams making clinically significant changes.

Time-intensive data setup and analysis will not be feasible for many clinicians, so it is important to have repeatable systems and templates in place. The above procedures are simple enough to complete by hand or with a word-processing spreadsheet program. However, clinicians may opt to purchase commercially available software programs that will automate all of these procedures, such as Therapy-Science (*www.therapy-science.com*). In addition to the above visual inspection procedures, Therapy-Science can provide the following information quickly and simply:

Trend (Direction of Change)

- What is the average session-over-session change?
- Approximately how long will it likely take to achieve the target?
- Is an improvement in stability clinically significant?

Level (Median Performance)

- Is a change in performance from the first half of treatment to the second half clinically significant?

Evidence of Systemic Change

- Is there evidence that overall change (level and trend considered together) is clinically significant?

Although clinicians would need to spend time reviewing the instruction sheets in Therapy-Science to refresh their memory about significance levels and other statistical concepts, the explanations provided are geared toward practicing clinicians and easy to follow. From that point, it is simply a case of entering the session data and looking at the results.

Examples of results obtained when we enter the data from Mr. Williams's performance are shown in Tables 5.1 and 5.2. In our PIE flowchart in Figure 5.1, we have a decision point to evaluate the evidence of change. The data will help us decide if we should continue with the current approach and phase of implementation, continue with the current approach but advance the phase of implementation, or go back to review all the elements of planning to decide which component(s) may need to be adjusted in order to achieve the target.

The results in Table 5.1 tell us that Mr. Williams is making clinically significant progress on his accurate and independent use of the "Play it again, Sam" strategy, as evidenced by the combined impact of changes in level and trend (Tau-U Fully Corrected pEst ~ 0.008). The trend line also suggests that Mr. Williams will likely achieve 90% accuracy within a few sessions. In contrast, Table 5.2 shows that the improvements in quality of

TABLE 5.1. Results of Data Analysis Generated by Therapy-Science for the Percent of Accurate and Independent Use of Strategy Measure

% Accurate and independent use of strategy	Phase A (first half)	Phase B (second half)
Trend		
Average session-to-session change	5.0%	
How many more sessions are likely required to obtain 90%?	2–3	
Trend (slope)	3.75%	5.00%
Level (median)		
Level	40%	70%
Is change in level clinically significant?	Yes, Mann–Whitney pEst ~ 0.004	
Overall systemic change		
Is overall change in level + trend clinically significant?	Yes, Tau-U Fully Corrected pEst ~ 0.008	

TABLE 5.2. Results of Data Analysis Generated by Therapy-Science for the 1–10 Quality Rating Measure

1–10 Quality rating	Phase A (first half)	Phase B (second half)
Trend		
Average session-to-session change	0.33	
How many more sessions are likely required to obtain 8/10?	8–9	
Trend (slope)	0.58	0.00
Level (median)		
Level	3	5
Is change in level clinically significant?	Yes, Mann–Whitney pEst ~ 0.029	
Overall systemic change		
Is overall change in level + trend clinically significant?	No, Tau-U Fully Corrected pEst ~ 0.102	

the paraphrased sentence have been slow and seem to be stalling. Mr. Williams did make significant gains going from an average rating of 3/10 in the first half of treatment to an average rating of 5/10 in the second half, but the trend began to flatten at the 5/10 rating level. This tells us that Mr. Williams can remember and apply the strategy, but we may need to provide him with more instruction and practice in how to paraphrase.

In summary, acquisition data are of critical importance in the evaluation phase, allowing clinicians to make needed changes in targets and/or ingredients in order to maximize the effectiveness and efficiency of intervention. While the procedures above may appear daunting at first, they are very manageable, and there is immense value in transforming them into a clinical habit to best support client needs.

Target Generalization Data

The clinician should also determine whether the specific skill or information taught in session is used in the identified naturalistic environments. This can be accomplished through periodic use of naturalistic probes, which are samples of the target behavior in the relevant context (e.g., testing a face–name association in that person's workplace). Probe data do not have to be collected in every session, but as described earlier, they should be collected systematically to avoid error bias (e.g., only probing on "good" days or in certain contexts). These data are important for testing generalization and can reveal the need for additional training in a specific context and also influence selection of treatment stimuli. Forms 5.4 and 5.5 at the end of the chapter may be used for tracking generalization data in addition to acquisition and mastery data. The single-subject evaluation methods described above should be implemented when evaluating performance on generalization probes.

Target Maintenance Data

Once generalization has been demonstrated for a target, it is important to collect probe data to determine if the learning is durable over time. These probes could be obtained during a session that focuses on acquisition or mastery of other targets or collected via phone or videoconference check-in appointments. Instead of analyzing for gains, we would use the single-subject design methodology described above to determine maintenance versus regression of performance on a target. Form 5.6 at the end of the chapter provides a progress monitoring form to help the clinician visualize maintenance of gains over time.

Impact Data (Aims Outcome Measurement)

A critical clinical question is whether the target improves the client's daily functioning, once it is executed in natural settings. Improvement in daily functioning is the ultimate goal of rehabilitation and motivates the initial choice of training targets, and we select targets because we believe they will contribute to achievement of the client's aims. Improvement in daily functioning is measured with *impact data*, often referred to as *outcome data*. Impact data are generally collected at two points in time: pretreatment (baseline) and at the conclusion of treatment. For example, if the goal of training is the use of a calendar app to increase attendance at medical appointments, then the impact data would determine whether the client has fewer missed appointments after learning to use the app. There is little point to independent use of a calendar app if it does not result in increased attendance at scheduled events. Furthermore, third-party payers routinely deny coverage for impairment-level cognitive targets (e.g., "Improve short-term recall to 90% accuracy") and instead expect targets that are directly linked to improvements in everyday outcomes, such as independence and employment (e.g., "Use a memory aid to complete work tasks with 90% accuracy," provided that meets the minimum standard for the workplace). Form 5.6 at the end of the chapter contains a section to document impact data during the maintenance phase, although impact data may also be collected during the mastery and generalization phases.

Example of Complete Data Use

Table 5.3 provides several clinical examples illustrating the different domains of outcome measurement across the categories of instructional targets discussed in upcoming chapters, and let's discuss one target here in greater detail.

Imagine we are training the rehabilitation target "using a smartphone calendar app to record appointments" for a client with moderate to severe declarative learning impairments following an anoxic event. Session data reveal the client's ability to use the calendar app as taught during the acquisition phase of therapy, measured by either the number of calendar entries or steps in the calendar event-entry procedure completed independently in the session. The clinician would take a probe at the beginning of the session to evaluate whether the client had retained the previously taught steps in order to know where to begin the training. Another level of measurement is whether the skills to use the app are implemented outside of therapy in real-world contexts (i.e., generalization probes). This could be assessed both by looking at entries made outside of therapy

TABLE 5.3. Sample Evaluation of Outcome before, during, and following Intervention for Targets in Different Training Categories

Sample targets	Sample target acquisition data	Sample target mastery/ generalization data	Sample target maintenance data	Sample aim outcomes
Facts and routines: *increased accuracy of naming grandchildren*	Percent of correct recall of grandchildren's names from photos (SR data)	Percent of correct uncued naming of grandchildren on a video call	Percent of correct recall of grandchildren's names 1 month after discharge from therapy	Patient reports decreased worry about forgetting names of grandchildren.
Cognitive strategies: *use of goal completion strategy at home (Stop, Plan, Do, Check, Repeat)*	Number of strategy steps client independently demonstrates during therapy with opportunity cues	Number of times client uses strategy at home, as recorded on strategy log	Number of times client uses strategy at home, as recorded on strategy log 2 weeks after treatment is completed	Increased number of home tasks completed on caregiver log.
External aids: *use of voice recording app for adding events to daily schedule*	Percent of correctly following steps to use app to add events to daily schedule	Number of new schedule entries made at home between therapy sessions	Number of new entries each day for 1-week period following treatment withdrawal	Client reports improved employer ratings for being on schedule.
Social communication partner training: *increased time waiting for person with TBI to speak in a conversation*	Number of times partner waits for person with TBI to speak, in a semi-structured conversation at clinic	Partner's logs documenting examples of pausing during dinner table conversations	Partner's responses on questionnaire mailed 3 weeks after cessation of therapy indicating ongoing use of pausing strategy	Partner reports decreased arguments with person with TBI about not being able to say what they want to say.
Social communication training for person with TBI: *use of strategy to promote increased processing time by saying, "I need a minute" in conversation with partner*	Number of times person with TBI says, "I need a minute," in a semi-structured conversation at clinic	Partner's logs documenting examples of person with TBI saying, "I need a minute" during dinner table conversations	Partner's responses on questionnaire mailed 3 weeks after cessation of therapy indicating ongoing use of "I need a minute" strategy	Person with TBI reports increased feeling of being heard in conversations.

and by client or care provider report of real-world use. The clinician would continue to take probe data at the beginning of sessions during the mastery phase to evaluate maintenance following distributed practice training. Ultimately, assuming calendar app use is mastered and implemented in daily life, the clinician could measure the functional impact of the training to determine whether there is an increase in the frequency of getting to appointments. The functional measure may have been set up as a GAS scale showing the number of calendar entries that the client attended. Collecting pre- and post-data on outcome of aims through the logging of appointment successes and failures demonstrates potential impact. Collection and analysis of data at these different levels during the therapy process allow the clinician to adjust intervention and targets accordingly.

SUMMARY

This chapter has reviewed the PIE framework that can be used to create a customized therapy plan for teaching a wide variety of targets to a wide variety of clients. The framework incorporates methods of instruction that have been empirically shown to be effective in teaching children and adults with cognitive impairments. Figure 5.1 provides a graphic summary of the PIE components, and Form 5.7 (at the end of the chapter and in the digital files accompanying this book) provides a PIE treatment planning checklist that incorporates the PIE elements as well as concepts presented in earlier chapters. Forms 5.1 and 5.2 include checklists with key reminders for effective goal writing. Form 5.3 offers a template to systematically plan to advance a client's skills through increased independence, increased breadth of participation across contexts, and/or increased complexity of contexts. Forms 5.4 through 5.6 provide sample within-session and across-session datasheets. In the chapters that follow, the PIE framework is applied to specific interventions, and materials are provided for clinical use when instructing on each type of target.

In the next four chapters, we apply the PIE framework to specific types of targets, using the instructional methods described in Chapter 4 and considering the client cognitive and psychological characteristics described in Chapters 2 and 3. The last three chapters focus on special considerations for inpatient rehabilitation (Chapter 10), computer-based cognitive training (Chapter 11), and patients with functional cognitive symptoms (Chapter 12).

SMART Target Checklist

☐ **S**pecific   Target is worded specifically and unambiguously; context and level of support are specified.

☐ **M**easurable   Behavior is observable and/or measurable.

☐ **A**ttainable   The client has the prerequisite skills; any needed component skills have been factored in; the target is within the client's reach.

☐ **R**elevant   The target is meaningful for the client and will lead toward achievement of their aims.

☐ **T**ime-Based   Deadline and/or number of times to be completed are specified.

Goal Attainment Scaling Checklist

☐ All possible outcomes have been considered.

☐ Only one variable is changing across levels.

   ☐ If two variables are changing, they are clearly correlated and likely to change in concert.

☐ The amount of change between levels is clinically important.

☐ The expected outcome is realistically attainable (not too difficult, but also not too easy).

☐ All levels are mutually exclusive.

☐ There are no gaps between levels.

☐ There are approximately equal intervals between levels.

☐ Each level is defined in terms that are:

   ☐ Concrete

   ☐ Non-ambiguous

   ☐ Observable and/or measurable

☐ There is a set timeframe for goal achievement.

Based on McDougall and King (2007) and Grant and Ponsford (2014).

Progression Planning Worksheet

A client's skills can be progressed by advancing one or more of the following aspects of the target:

- **Increasing independence** (e.g., physical/hand over hand, modeling, specific verbal prompt,* subtle verbal cue,* visual cue,* independent)
- **Increasing variety of contexts** (e.g., one location only, two similar locations with same communication partner, two similar locations with two communication partners)
- **Increasing complexity of setting contexts** (e.g., therapy room, clinic reception area, small shop, big-box store, mall), **partner contexts** (e.g., clinician, familiar individual, unfamiliar individual, familiar group), **and/or linguistic contexts** (e.g., response to questions, structured conversation, unstructured conversation)

In the acquisition phase of training, only the first two aspects should be considered, and when increasing variety of contexts, only small increases in variety are appropriate to ensure the client effectively and efficiently acquires the new skill with minimal errors. In contrast, in the generalization and maintenance phases, the full range of advancement options may be appropriate for the client.

Current Target:	Training Phase:	Associated Aim:

Hierarchy to increase <u>independence</u>:

Hierarchy to increase <u>variety of contexts</u>:

Hierarchy to increase <u>complexity of contexts</u>:

*There are different definitions of "cue" versus "prompt," and often they are used interchangeably. Here, we use "cue" as a hint; something that doesn't directly assist the client in performing the target behavior but gives them a general reminder. Cues can be in the environment (e.g., a visual schedule, hearing the bell ring at the end of class) or can be a subtle hint from the communication partner (e.g., pointing, asking "what happens next"). In contrast, a "prompt" is direct support to complete the behavior, such as physical assistance (e.g., opening the calendar app on the phone) or specific verbal direction (e.g., "summarize the paragraph before moving to the next one," "go get your phone to check your schedule").

Therapy Session Data Form—Target Acquisition, Mastery, Generalization

Client Name:	Date:	Location:	Others Present:

Target:	Associated Aim:	Training Phase:

Ingredients—Items:	Ingredients—Actions:	Ingredients—Motivators:	Measurement Plan:

Check-in Info and Results of Homework:

Practice Data:

Comments/Observations:

Session Summary/Analysis of Progress:

Feedback and Homework Provided (task, context, ingredients, tracking):

Plan for Next Session:

Progress Monitoring Form—Target Acquisition, Mastery, Generalization

Client Name: **Target:**   **Training Phase:**

Select the summary measure being tracked (must use the same from each session):

☐ Retention probe result from start of each session

☐ Average of each session's practice trial results

☐ Other:

	Summary Measure			
	Date 1:	Date 2:	Date 3:	Date 4:
Task Description/Steps:				
Ingredients:				
Prompts and Supports:				
Motivational:				
Other Measures:				

Progress Monitoring Form—Target Maintenance and Therapy Impact

Client Name:

Target: **Aim:**

Data obtained via: ☐ Direct observation   ☐ Client report   ☐ Significant other report

Review Date:			
Task:			
Context:			
Ingredients • **Prompts and Supports:** • **Motivational:**			
Results:			
Comments:			
Recommend:	OR ☐ Active monitoring no longer required	OR ☐ Active monitoring no longer required	OR ☐ Active monitoring no longer required

Impact Data:

Treatment Planning Checklist

PLAN

Assess and Hypothesize

☐ Interview to learn who the client is, determine possible treatment aims that reflect sociocultural lived experiences, beliefs, values, and identities, and select assessment tools and procedures.

☐ Administer assessment tools and procedures to obtain clarity on client strengths, weaknesses, and goals.

☐ Prepare a holistic summary of assessment results and client characteristics.

☐ Review all possible underlying factors that could be responsible for the client's presenting characteristics.

☐ In collaboration with team members, state assumptions and select a working hypothesis.

☐ Test hypothesis with assessment measures or a trial of therapy.

Define Targets, Aims, and Measures

☐ Confirm functional and meaningful treatment aims.

☐ Select behaviors to address in therapy (targets), including which aspect of behavior is to be modified (accuracy, speed, quality, frequency, duration, level of cueing) and in which context(s).

☐ Ensure targets contribute to achieving aim(s).

☐ Ensure targets reflect assessment results and underlying cognitive model/theory.

☐ Ensure target group (S vs. R) addresses client needs.

☐ Ensure client has prerequisite skills and insight/awareness needed to achieve targets.

☐ Complete task analysis to specify all steps required to achieve target.

☐ Prepare a plan to advance independence in and/or complexity of target behaviors and contexts.

☐ Identify stakeholders to support the intervention process.

☐ Identify facilitators and barriers.

☐ Formulate targets using SMART or GAS formatting.

☐ Select target measures (acquisition, generalization, maintenance).

☐ Select impact measures.

Identify Phase of Learning, Ingredients, and Dose

☐ Identify implementation phase for target (acquisition, generalization, or maintenance).

☐ Describe ingredients (clinician actions and materials) required to advance the client toward achieving targets.

☐ Ensure ingredients are appropriate for the target group (e.g., distributed practice for S targets, self-reflection for R targets) and are consistent with theorized mechanism of action.

(continued)

☐ Ensure ingredients are appropriate for the client's skills, sociocultural beliefs and values, and psychological status.

☐ Ensure ingredients and variety of stimuli match phase of implementation.

☐ Include ingredients for motivation or awareness, if needed (required for homework).

☐ Determine stakeholder role in supporting intervention ingredients.

☐ Determine length of intervention program, frequency of therapy sessions, duration of each therapy session, number of repetitions per target in each session.

IMPLEMENT

Apply Ingredients

☐ Prepare session data and progress monitoring forms.

☐ Determine practice starting point via retention probe results.

☐ Implement practice stimuli and methods in required contexts.

☐ Provide sufficient opportunity for practice within sessions.

☐ Provide sufficient opportunity for practice across sessions.

☐ Incorporate team members and other stakeholders in training opportunities, as appropriate.

☐ Optimize client motivation, engagement, and self-efficacy.

☐ Ensure homework takes into account opportunity for practice, partner and environmental supports, and client motivation.

EVALUATE

Measure Target Acquisition, Mastery, Generalization, and Maintenance

☐ Document target acquisition data.

☐ Analyze progress on acquisition measures to test working hypothesis or ongoing progress.

☐ If progress is not being made, reevaluate the plan (hypothesis, target, ingredients) and reimplement.

☐ If progress is being made, continue with acquisition phase or advance to mastery and generalization phase.

☐ Probe for target generalization.

☐ Analyze target generalization probe results, adjusting plan or learning phase as needed.

☐ Probe for target maintenance.

☐ Analyze target maintenance probe results, adjusting plan or learning phase as needed.

Measure Impact/Outcome on Aim

☐ During mastery/generalization or maintenance phase, obtain objective data of changes in daily functioning.

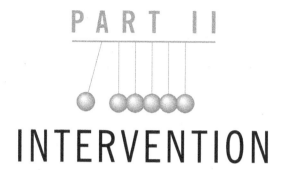

PART II

INTERVENTION

CHAPTER 6

Training Discrete Facts and Routines

Occasional memory lapses happen to most of us: it's not uncommon to forget the name of a new acquaintance, or a phone number or password. In fact, it's so common that there are legions of books and tricks available to help remember important bits of information. These memory lapses may be an inconvenience for most people, but for those with acquired memory disorders they are a source of major frustration and have significant effects on independence, employment, and education.

In this chapter, we focus on instructional methods the clinician can use to help structure information so clients with declarative learning and memory problems can learn and remember discrete facts or concepts and simple routines. A fact may be defined as something that has objective reality, that is done, and can be proven (*Merriam-Webster's Collegiate Dictionary*, 1986). A concept is an idea or notion that exists in the mind, a unit of knowledge linked to a symbol that can be shared, such as a word (*Merriam-Webster's Collegiate Dictionary*, 1986). These "bites" of information are typically short and serve specific purposes, but may be both simple (e.g., recalling a home address, the name of a physician a description of the injury) and complex (e.g., explaining what is meant by "rehabilitation" or "social network"). Facts and concepts are types of knowledge targets, which are included in the group of representation (R) targets, as introduced in Chapter 4. R targets also include beliefs and attitudes, and these are discussed in Chapter 3.

Sometimes a simple routine functions as a fact, in that it is learned as a single piece of information that is used with a cue. For example, the simple routines of checking a daily calendar each time you enter the kitchen or pressing a call bell when you need help are akin to learning a fact—the behavior is learned via repeated practice and prompted by a simple cue. These simple routines are S targets (habits), but because they benefit from some of the same instructional methods used to train facts and concepts, we are including them in this chapter and information about facts and concepts applies to these routines as well.

A client may need to learn a discrete fact, concept, or routine to accomplish a specific task (e.g., learning vocabulary for an upcoming driver's test, remembering medication names to report to physicians, remembering to turn left to get to the dining room). Sometimes a client requires an R target for facts they need to know prior to carrying out training on the associated strategy (Chapter 7) or external aid target (Chapter 8). For example, a client may need to learn which bills are paid on which days of the month in order to carry out a bill payment strategy, or a client may need to remember what the icon for a smartphone app looks like in order to use the external aid when needed. In these situations, the primary targets of strategy and external aid use are skills and habits, but the R fact targets are building blocks required to achieve the new skills and habits. The same is true for social skills and social communication (Chapter 9): the nature of social skills and social communication is such that knowledge and attitude targets are deeply intertwined with skill and habit targets, and clients might need to learn specific concepts or simple routines as targets to achieve their social participation aims. The techniques discussed in this current chapter are therefore important for training R targets across all categories of cognitive rehabilitation, whether in a primary role (learning facts, concepts, and simple routines) or in roles supporting the implementation of skills and habits (carrying out strategies, using external aids, implementing social behaviors). However, R targets relating to strategies, external aids, and social communication will be discussed in their respective chapters.

The methods emphasized in this chapter are mostly designed to capitalize on nondeclarative learning and memory, requiring relatively little conscious effort on the part of the client other than engaging in the intervention. This stands in contrast to Chapters 7, 8, and 9, in which we discuss training methods that typically require sufficient perception and awareness to identify when to implement the trained skill, as well as sufficient declarative memory to learn and generalize the steps involved. We do, however, include discussion of techniques to train R targets that rely on declarative memory, as these will be pertinent for individuals with milder cognitive impairments.

In addition, the methods described in this chapter are designed to train recall of the *information bites* mentioned above—short pieces of information and quick, simple routines. This is similar to a *stimulus–response* method to elicit an overlearned response to a specific verbal or situational cue. By contrast, Chapter 7 describes memory *strategies*, which may be applied to learning longer factual material (e.g., study strategies to learn from a biology textbook chapter for a test) and are designed to generalize across contexts (e.g., any textbook content). It is important for the clinician to distinguish between methods for training specific facts or concepts for a specific purpose (this chapter) and training strategies to learn longer or more complex material across a range of contexts (Chapter 7).

The overall aim of training facts and concepts, as well as the other components of the treatment plan, is to minimize demands on impaired memory processes, mostly declarative learning and retrieval from long-term memory, so that the client may more fully participate in their desired activities; that is, we are working to make access to information and simple routines more automatic and thereby increase the probability that the client will be successful.

This chapter begins with a brief overview of declarative and nondeclarative learning characteristics and the associated ingredients required for training facts, concepts, and simple routines. We then apply the PIE (Plan, Implement, and Evaluate) framework to provide clinicians with the needed clinical implementation processes.

THE NATURE OF LEARNING FACTS AND CONCEPTS

There is some debate about how facts and concepts are learned, particularly the extent to which different types of memory are involved (see Martins, Guillery-Girard, Jambaque, Dulac, & Eustache, 2006). As described in Chapter 2, declarative learning is the conscious process of acquiring new memories, whereas nondeclarative learning is the process of acquiring memories through automatic association or repeated practice, without conscious awareness of the learning process. Declarative instructional methods like elaboration, visualization, chunking, and self-explanation are not helpful for nondeclarative learning and, in fact, can interfere with learning, especially if the client spends time on these declarative methods at the cost of practicing the correct response. For example, instructing a client with a severe declarative memory impairment in techniques to visualize their address will be less effective than using spaced retrieval or other error-control methods that provide structured practice remembering the actual address. Declarative learning methods require the type of long-term learning and memory that are impaired in such a client; hence, instructional methods that rely on nondeclarative memory can be more effective. This is not to say that declarative learning methods are not effective for clients with cognitive impairments—to the contrary, there is evidence that declarative learning methods can be as effective as nondeclarative methods for clients with milder memory impairments (Haslam, 2018)—but rather that use of these methods requires careful consideration of the learner's strengths and challenges.

In everyday life, declarative and nondeclarative learning and memory interact: Clients typically will use some combination of both on any given task, depending on their memory strengths and challenges, the instructional method used by the clinician, and the to-be-learned facts and concepts. The type of memory involved in fact and concept learning also depends on what is meant by "remembered." Declarative memory appears to be necessary for conscious recollection of facts and concepts, that is, the ability to recall information in response to a question that triggers a conscious memory search, such as "What is your work address?" Nondeclarative learning leads to a sense of familiarity (Anderson & Craik, 2006), which could be evidenced by the client's ability to walk to the correct work address without being able to state it correctly.

Declarative Learning

Declarative teaching and learning are commonly used in education: a teacher explains facts and concepts in class, assigns material for students to consciously memorize outside of class, and evaluates acquisition using tests that require conscious recall. This type of declarative learning can involve a combination of episodic and semantic memory: we might remember learning a fact or concept as an event (e.g., remembering when the teacher explained it), but over time and with repetition, the "date stamp" of that event might fade and the information might become a semantic memory.

A common ingredient for declarative learning is providing opportunities to learn by trial and error, that is, allowing the client to try and potentially fail and then learn from their mistakes. Trial-and-error learning [also called error-based learning (Ownsworth et al., 2013) or discovery learning (Vereijken & Whiting, 1990)] engages both memory processes and executive functions, as we monitor our performance and shift thoughts and behaviors to be more successful on subsequent trials. Trial-and-error learning does not always require multiple training trials: learning can occur with only a single trial if that one trial was sufficiently salient. For example, if you left a client's file in your car once and the file was stolen, that single instance might be sufficient to change your knowledge of safe file storage methods forever. In most cases, however, providing opportunities to learn by trial and error and providing error-correction feedback alone (e.g., telling the client what they did wrong) are insufficient for clients to achieve a target, especially when the target is to recall or recognize a fact or concept independently. Clients need opportunities to practice the correct response. In fact, for some clients with severely impaired declarative learning, trial-and-error approaches can result in the client learning the error response.

Other ingredients that facilitate declarative learning include elaboration (e.g., linking the idea to the client's existing, related knowledge), visualization (e.g., having the client use an image to depict the characteristics of a fact or concept), and self-explanation (e.g., having the client explain the meaning of the fact or concept to themself or others). The Case Applications at the end of this chapter provide examples of training facts and concepts via these declarative methods. *Teach-back* is an example of self-explanation where the clinician asks the client to explain or demonstrate what they have just been shown or taught (Talevski, Wong Shee, Rasmussen, Kemp, & Beauchamp, 2020). The teach-back method is reviewed in Chapter 7, in the "Use of Strategies Following Mild Traumatic Brain Injury/Concussion" section. Like other ingredients that support declarative learning, teach-back can be effective for teaching facts to clients who have relatively good declarative learning and memory and primarily need education about strategies to manage cognitive challenges.

Distributed practice is a particularly important ingredient when teaching or training facts and concepts to learners with and without declarative memory impairments. There is strong evidence for a spacing effect in typical learners (Cepeda, Pashler, Vul, Wixted, & Rohrer, 2006; Donovan & Radosevich, 1999; Kim & Xu, 2019); that is, the act of successfully retrieving a fact or concept over progressively longer time intervals increases the likelihood of successfully retrieving it in the future (see Cepeda et al., 2006, for discussion of the theoretical mechanisms underlying this effect). The spacing effect is highest for low-complexity, low-cognitive demand targets (Donovan & Radosevich, 1999), such as recalling simple facts and concepts (e.g., one's address, names of coworkers), and lowest for complex facts and concepts like *justice* or *personalized care*. The length of retrieval interval is correlated with the length of the spacing interval (i.e., people recalled better after longer intervals if similar intervals were incorporated into training), and the effect is stronger if the test is recognition (as in multiple-choice questions) versus free recall (Kim, Wong-Kee-You, Wiseheart, & Rosenbaum, 2019).

Table 6.1 shows examples of common ingredients for declarative instruction. These ingredients have been shown to be effective for typical students learning facts and concepts (Dunlosky, Rawson, Marsh, Nathan, & Willingham, 2013).

TABLE 6.1. Ingredients for Declarative Learning

- Provide information in multiple modalities.
- Provide semantic or other related cues.
- Provide feedback (e.g., evaluative, corrective, encouraging).
- Use information organization methods (e.g., chunking, outlining, scaffolding).
- Link or encourage client to link to-be-learned information to prior knowledge.
- Encourage client to generate semantically associated facts or concepts.
- Use Socratic questioning.
- Provide mnemonics.
- Encourage client to visualize correct response.
- Encourage client to problem-solve.
- Prompt client to self-test and encourage distributed self-testing.
- Use teach-back (i.e., ask client to teach the content to the clinician).
- Provide opportunities for trial-and-error learning (e.g., provide least-to-most cues).

When contemplating using ingredients that rely on declarative memory to train facts and concepts, the clinician should consider the following:

- **Information that is more meaningful to the learner is learned and retained better.** This includes information that the person believes is important and also information that can be connected meaningfully to the learner's previous knowledge (Dewar, Patterson, Wilson, & Graham, 2009). For example, a tennis player would be expected to learn new tennis terms more easily than geology terms because they have an existing knowledge context for the new information.

- **Abstract concepts are more difficult to learn than concrete concepts.** For example, the concept of *executive dysfunction* is more difficult to learn than the concept of *failing school if you don't get your work done* because the notion of executive function is abstract, whereas failing in school has concrete repercussions. Even abstract concepts may be made concrete, however, as in the use of metaphors described by Ylvisaker and Feeney (2000). These authors collaborated with adults with traumatic brain injury (TBI) to develop personally relevant metaphors, often in the form of people they admired, that captured complex behavior and personality profiles desired by each client. For example, one client, Jason, had severe behavior problems, which he learned to control by internalizing a self-image of "Jason the Marine" and "Jason as Clint Eastwood." This was a way to make very abstract concepts such as control, independence, and competence concrete and accessible to the learner.

- **Concepts that the learner can visualize are learned and remembered better than concepts that are more difficult to visualize** (e.g., *traffic accident* is an easier concept to learn than *defensive driving*). This is related to the previous principle: concepts that are easier to visualize are generally more concrete, although not always (e.g., the client might have a memory of a person performing a brave act, which can help them visualize courage).

• **Facts and concepts that come from highly populated categories are more difficult to recall than those from less-populated categories.** The number of closely related items in a given category is referred to as *neighborhood density*: the more highly similar items there are within that category, the more difficult it may be for a person with a memory problem to retrieve the specific item they need. For example, "small dogs" is a highly populated category—197 dog breeds were officially recognized by the American Kennel Club in 2021 (*www.akc.org*), and about half of these are small dogs. By contrast, "famous Scottish philosophers" is a relatively small category: there are about 20 who are internationally recognized, but most people have heard of only two: David Hume and Adam Smith. If a person who is not an expert in the area is trying to recall the name of a single category member, the name of a small dog breed will be harder to remember than the name of a Scottish philosopher because there are more potential competitors among small dog names than among Scottish philosopher names.

In addition to semantic neighbors, other types of neighbors influence the probability of correct recall of a given fact or concept. This includes sound-alike (i.e., phonologically similar) neighbors (e.g., "dog," "clog," "cog"), look-alike neighbors (e.g., similar-appearing dogs), or written words with similar forms (e.g., "harrier" vs. "terrier"). Neighborhood density effects are probably why *unicorn* is easier to learn and recall as a distinct concept than *Romano cheese*, although they are similar in frequency of occurrence in written English. There is only one type of unicorn, but Romano is one of many similar-looking types of cheese that are used with the same foods. Romano also has competition from a commonly used phonologically and graphemically similar neighbor: "Parmigiano cheese." Thus, a person trying to learn the concept of Romano cheese might recall Parmigiano cheese in error.

We all have experienced neighborhood density effects with numbers and passwords, which have proliferated in our everyday lives and are becoming more and more difficult to sort out from each other. Neighborhood density effects should be kept in mind when choosing targets for training: targets from high-density neighborhoods might be more difficult to learn and recall accurately, depending on the individual client's knowledge and expertise and the type of training approach to be used.

• **Face–name associations are particularly difficult to learn.** Face–name associations are completely arbitrary and require the person to learn not only the association between a name and a face but also the association between a first and last name (Thoene & Glisky, 1995). Face–name learning methods that work for individuals without memory problems, such as connecting the name to a characteristic of that person (e.g., "Bob bobs his head when he says 'yes.'"), are generally not practical for people with memory disorders, mostly because they forget to use them or remember the strategy but not the name. The requirement to first generate an image then link it with a name, and then retrieve both when needed, is taxing for an already impaired cognitive system and can be impractical when meeting people in everyday life. While few studies have examined face–name learning in acquired brain injury (ABI; e.g., Bourgeois et al., 2007; Manasse, Hux, & Snell, 2005), evidence from studies in dementia suggests that error control and spaced retrieval are more effective ingredients than association and visualization, particularly for adults with moderate to severe declarative learning and memory impairments (Hawley, Cherry, Boudreaux, & Jackson, 2008; Hopper, Drefs,

Bayles, Tomoeda, & Dinu, 2010). The next section explores these nondeclarative training ingredients.

Nondeclarative Learning

Facts, concepts, and simple routines also can be learned via nondeclarative (implicit) methods. Nondeclarative methods are probabilistic; that is, the person learns whatever they do the most, whether it is correct or incorrect. Thus, for nondeclarative learning, the critical ingredients are providing opportunities for practice of correct responses and using methods for error control or error minimization (Baddeley & Wilson, 1994).

Two methods that rely mostly on nondeclarative memory and error control are spaced retrieval (SR) training and the method of vanishing cues (MVC; Haslam, 2018). SR training is a method for both learning and retention of a target and involves initial presentation of the full target and then repeated retrieval of the target over progressively longer time intervals. It has strong support from the literature in TBI (Bourgeois et al., 2007; Ehlhardt et al., 2008; Hillary et al., 2003; Velikonja et al., 2014) and dementia (Hopper et al., 2005; Kessels, 2017), as well as growing evidence from other clinical populations with acquired brain damage [e.g., adults with impaired declarative learning from alcohol use (Pitel et al., 2010)]. Using SR requires skill in identifying stimulus–response pairs that are important in the client's everyday life, are natural for the client to produce, and occur in natural settings with enough frequency and consistency that there is sufficient opportunity for practice.

In SR training, the clinician points to or states the stimulus (e.g., "What is your address?") and provides the target response (e.g., "135 Reese St., Denby"), and then asks the client to repeat the target response immediately. If the client answers correctly, the clinician waits for 30 seconds and then provides the stimulus again. If the client cannot produce a correct response after 30 seconds, then the delay can be shortened or MVC (see below) can be used for initial acquisition of the stimulus–response pairing, again with the goal of minimizing errors. With each correct response, the clinician doubles the time interval. When the time interval reaches 2 minutes, the clinician introduces a distractor activity during the time interval to prevent the client from attempting to use declarative methods to remember it. If doubling the time interval is too long, the clinician can increase the interval by a smaller amount. Similarly, the clinician may start with a *continuous visual cue* to support the client in retrieving the correct response. A continuous visual cue is an image or word that is visible to the client throughout the training, such as leaving a card with the target response on the table until the client has learned the target (Benigas, Brush, & Elliot, 2016).

At all times, the client is discouraged from using a conscious mental search to think of the answer: if they do not answer immediately, the clinician stops them from using the conscious strategy, gives the correct answer and asks them to repeat it, then goes back to the last time interval at which they were successful. This process continues until either some practical upper limit is reached (e.g., the end of a 30-minute therapy session) or the client makes an error. If the latter occurs, the clinician immediately models the correct stimulus–response pair and then asks the client to repeat it, returning to the last delay interval at which they were successful. The response is considered "learned" when some criterion time has passed and the client can produce the correct response to the stimulus. This time might be a day or a few hours. At the end of the session, the client must have produced more correct responses than errors. If the client has made more errors than correct responses, the clinician should consider changing the target immediately, before the client learns an incorrect response.

Figure 6.1 shows an example of tracking performance across seven trials in the first session a client is learning their new address. Each trial consists of repetitions of the stimulus–response over increasing intervals until the client makes an error. Looking horizontally across Trial 1, we can see that a continuous visual cue was used and the client was successful at recalling the address after 30 seconds, but not after 1 minute. In Trial 2, a continuous visual cue was again used and the client was successful at the 30-second and 1-minute intervals, but not after the 2-minute interval, during which a distractor activity was introduced (the client had volunteered to prepare candy gift bags for an upcoming party). In Trial 3, the continuous visual cue was faded and the client successfully recalled their address after 1 minute but not after 2 minutes. Each time the client made an error, the clinician modeled the correct response, had the client repeat it, then began the next trial at the last successful interval (e.g., on Trial 4, the client erred at the 4-minute interval so the clinician began Trial 5 at the last successful interval, which was 2 minutes). With two consecutive errors at the 4-minute mark, the clinician decided to reduce the increase in interval for the sixth trial. In the final two trials before the session ended, the client struggled to manage the increase from 3 minutes to 6 minutes, so the clinician made a note to consider reducing the size of that interval increase in the next session.

For a detailed description of SR and instruction on how to use it, we refer readers to the SR training manual by Benigas, Brush, and Elliot (2016; also see Cepeda et al., 2006, for evidence that typical learners additionally benefit when intervals are spaced over time). The text is highly recommended for helping screen candidates, plan therapy, and track progress over time.

MVC is a method for the initial acquisition of a target and involves gradually fading cues after a complete initial presentation of the target. While MVC has a long history of use for teaching facts and concepts to adults with brain injury (see the review in Haslam

Date: April 3
Target: Accurately recall new home address
Stimulus/Cue: "What is your address?"   **Response** (verbal) physical, both): 135 Reese St., Denby

Trial	CVC?	Time Interval							Comments/Observations	Administration Notes
		30s	1m	2m	4m	8m	16m	32m		
1	Y	✓	✗							CVC = Continuous Visual Cue
2	Y	✓	✓	✗					Began with CVC (address written on index card) for error control purposes but was able to quickly fade CVC.	
3	N		✓	✗						Put ✓ in response line when interval achieved; continue on that line until error occurs (✗); then start next trial at last successful interval
4	N		✓	✓	✗				Distractor activity = preparing candy gift bags	
5	N			✓	✗					
New Time Int:		30s	1m	2m	3m	6m	12m		Next session—may need to further reduce interval increase between 3 and 6 min.	
6	N			✓	✓	✗				Add distractor activity at 2 min+
7	N				✓	✗				

FIGURE 6.1. Example of tracking SR performance across seven trials in a session for a client who is learning their new address.

and Kessels [2018]), there is mixed evidence supporting its use. The few studies directly comparing SR and MVC have shown a significant advantage of the former for teaching facts and concepts to clients with declarative learning and memory impairments (Haslam, 2018). We include it here because it is thought to be helpful for clients who need information presented in units smaller than the stimulus–response pairing typically used in SR and because SR training includes a continuous visual cue option that can be implemented similarly to MVC (Benigas et al., 2016).

On the first trial in MVC, the clinician presents the client with the stimulus (e.g., "What is your address?") along with a cue card showing the target response (e.g., "135 Reese St., Denby") and asks the client to answer the question by reading the response aloud from the card. In Trial 2, the clinician presents the stimulus with the cue again, but this time the cue offers less information (e.g., the city name or some letters from the city name have been removed). This process of reducing the level of cueing support continues until the client can complete the stimulus–response pair without a cue, in which case SR training can commence. Similar to what is done in SR training, if the client gives an incorrect response on any trial, the clinician returns to the previous successful stimulus length (e.g., adds a letter or word), and begins again. When used independently, rather than as a precursor to SR training, the learning proceeds until there are no visible cues, then distractors are introduced systematically until the response can be recalled in contexts similar to the client's daily life.

Table 6.2 summarizes ingredients that facilitate nondeclarative learning. When contemplating a nondeclarative approach such as SR to train facts and concepts, the clinician should consider the following:

Simpler is better. SR and other error-minimization methods are based on classical conditioning, where the clinician and client identify a stimulus that will trigger a specific response and the response must be produced correctly each time. Based on their study experience, researchers who used SR with adults with TBI (Bourgeois et al., 2007) recommended that the stimulus and response be as simple as possible. If the client's goal is to learn a long, complex piece of information, the probability of producing it correctly is lower than if the information is short and simple, and the likelihood of learning is lower as well. Recall that nondeclarative learning methods require high rates of correct responses and minimal errors, so it is critical to identify a response that the client can produce successfully and consistently. If the information to be learned is complex, it might be more efficient and effective to train a procedure that the client can use to access that information (e.g., putting an autobiographical statement in a notebook, and training the client to access the notebook when asked about their personal history). Complex

---

TABLE 6.2. Ingredients for Nondeclarative Learning

- Use specialized error-control training methods (e.g., spaced retrieval with most-to-least cues, chaining).
- Choose a therapy target that has the same features as the target in everyday life (e.g., same visual layout, same words).
- Incorporate variability in everyday life into training (e.g., if target must be produced with different cues in everyday life, incorporate those cues into training).

---

facts and concepts may be broken down into pieces and trained via chaining (discussed in Chapter 8), but the client must be able to produce each piece successfully.

Generalization of nondeclarative learning is limited. The results of many studies of nondeclarative learning in amnesia have shown that this type of learning is hyperspecific, that is, it is specific not only to the information learned but also to surface features such as the materials used and the physical context (Stark, Stark, & Gordon, 2005). The following example shows how declarative learning might operate in a person with intact declarative learning:

> It is relatively easy to learn the fact that Allyson Felix became the most decorated athlete in U.S. track and field history during the 2021 Olympics. Having learned this piece of information, you immediately understand that she won Olympic medals. This knowledge will be available to your conscious recollection, and, if your declarative memory is intact, it will automatically be linked to related facts, such as knowledge that the Olympics took place in Tokyo, during the pandemic amidst much controversy.

The processes engaged in declarative learning such as this are automatic and underlie the flexible use of new semantic information in a variety of contexts. By contrast, a person who learns only via nondeclarative mechanisms might learn, literally, the statement "Allyson Felix became the most decorated athlete in U.S. track and field history." This specific response will be triggered only by the cue with which it was trained, and the information will not automatically be linked to previous knowledge. For this reason, when training persons with declarative memory impairments, each link to previous knowledge should be taught directly, and the clinician should not assume generalization to other contexts (e.g., other persons asking the prompt question or other prompt questions).

From a rehabilitation perspective, limited generalization is perhaps the most critical feature of nondeclarative learning, as it has serious implications not only for where training is conducted, but also for counseling stakeholders about the limits of new learning. Most clients have some residual declarative learning, as true anterograde amnesia is relatively rare. Even for individuals with milder declarative memory impairments, however, generalization must be planned early in the training process, and the clinician should consider conducting training in the context of where the learning ultimately will be used and with the materials and people that will be involved in its everyday use.

Declarative and Nondeclarative Memory Interact in Everyday Life

In everyday learning situations, declarative and nondeclarative memory interact not only with each other but also with other cognitive processes, including executive functions, and this can be a challenge to disentangle when setting treatment goals. As an example, consider a staff meeting at your workplace. The day after the meeting, you recall some details of the event (e.g., how one team member monopolized a discussion about client privacy), which is an episodic memory. You also recall facts about how privacy laws apply to clients in general, which has become a semantic memory, and a new acronym for health care privacy laws, another semantic memory. To complicate matters, at the same time as these declarative memory processes are engaged, you might be unconsciously influenced by previous negative feelings about the team member (nondeclarative memory for emotional associations). The meeting also provided the opportunity to rehearse interpersonal negotiation skills (nondeclarative memory for skills and habits) as you debated the best methods to ensure privacy of electronic medical records. At the end of the day, your future behavior is shaped by all of these processes together, which will be integrated and deployed via your skills in executive functions. A large part of the process of cognitive rehabilitation is deconstructing tasks just this way: figuring out which cognitive functions the client needs to use in which contexts, so we can capitalize on preserved skills and make learning more efficient and effective for that person. Also, as noted earlier, the fact and concept target being trained could be part of a multistep routine that also includes a strategy for identifying when such information would be needed, or access to an external aid that would provide supportive cues.

Summary

The take-home message for clients with memory impairments is that, as discussed in Chapter 2, most "memory impairments" in cognitive rehabilitation clients are impairments in declarative learning and recall. Because facts, concepts, and simple routines can be learned via both declarative and nondeclarative methods, clients with impairments in the former and strengths in the latter can learn without ever remembering the learning event itself. This has been shown in many studies of individuals with declarative memory impairments (see the review by Dewar et al., 2009). For example, Vargha-Khadem and colleagues (1997) found that children with severe memory impairments from a young age had nevertheless learned new concepts over several years of schooling, although they had no conscious memory of the learning events. This dissociation between semantic and episodic memory has been hypothesized to reflect the different roles of hippocampal structures versus nearby brain regions in these two types of learning (Irish & Vatansever, 2020; Tulving & Markowitsch, 1998) and has led to several studies showing good semantic learning in clients with little memory for events. In practical terms, this might lead us to expand our assessment questions so that we do not only ask clients to recall event-related facts (e.g., asking, "What did you learn from the nutritionist today?"), but also look for evidence that the person is applying the new information, even if they can't consciously retrieve it (e.g., if they can't recall what the nutritionist said but nevertheless change their food choices).

PIE FOR TRAINING FACTS, CONCEPTS, AND SIMPLE ROUTINES

Chapter 5 describes the key elements involved in the treatment process. Here, we review the elements that are specific to teaching facts, concepts, and simple routines. Consistent with Chapter 5, we describe the elements of *planning* (assessment and target selection), *implementation* (treatment ingredients and approaches), and *evaluation* (measurement of targets and aims) in distinct categories. It is important to remember, however, that the selection of ingredients, approaches, and measures is determined in the planning stage and that the evaluation stage may result in revisiting elements of the planning stage. Chapter 5 highlights how the PIE process is circular and iterative, but for the purposes of simplicity, we describe the three phases as discrete clinical processes.

PIE: Planning for Training Facts, Concepts, and Simple Routines

Assess and Hypothesize

To choose the appropriate ingredients, the clinician will first consider the neuropsychological profile of the client, as well as personal factors such as motivation and premorbid knowledge base, and environmental factors such as available supports. Assessment of client characteristics should include formal memory testing, given the importance of this information to treatment planning. Observation in everyday performance also is critical: standardized tests often reveal optimal performance, which may differ substantially from performance at the time and in the context where the facts and concepts will be used. Interviews with the client and important others in that person's life will inform the selection of aims and targets, and also provide insight into that person's awareness and motivation for therapy.

The following questions will guide the assessment and interview:

1. **What is the specific need?** There is no point in teaching facts, concepts, and simple routines for their own sake. All learning must be in the service of achieving a life-participation aim. Thus, the clinician should begin by identifying the client's aims and then analyzing activities related to that aim to identify places where learning facts and concepts would be helpful. For example, if the aim is for the client to have a social conversation, they might wish to recall autobiographical information to share with others or might like to tell a joke or talk about world events. If the aim is safety in the community, the client might need to know their address and phone number and the name of an emergency contact person. If the aim is related to work, face–name associations or job titles might be relevant information. For school, it might be academic knowledge or vocabulary. As noted above, training of facts and concepts likely will be part of a plan that includes other training methods and targets as well. A social conversation might require partner training, as well as teaching the client facts to share, and independence in activities of daily living likely will require not only facts and concepts but also multistep procedures and strategies. Thus, identifying the specific need means determining which facts and concepts should be taught in addition to recognizing other training methods that will be needed.

2. **Where is the information going to be used?** The context where information is going to be used may serve as an important cue to the retrieval of facts and concepts. Therefore, it is important to identify the situation in which targets will need to be used. This includes the *physical* context, such as a classroom or office; the *person* context, such as with a family member or stranger; and the *activity* context, such as at mealtime or in response to a question from another person. The importance of context cues increases in proportion to the severity of the client's declarative memory impairment: individuals with more severe declarative memory impairments are going to rely more on nondeclarative learning, which is highly context-specific. In this case, generalization to novel contexts is going to occur only to the extent that the novel context resembles the context in which the fact or concept was taught. For example, a person with profound anterograde amnesia might learn to give a brief description of their injury in response to the question "What happened to you?" If the question changes, however, to "Tell me about your injury," the new phrasing might not serve as a cue to the trained response without generalization training. Likewise, a student learning a new vocabulary word in school

might not automatically use that word in a variety of different ways. Later in this section, we will discuss how to plan for generalization in therapy, as this is possible, even with individuals who have profound declarative memory impairments, but it is important to know in advance how flexibly the client will have to use the fact or concept.

3. **When is the information going to be used?** A critical question in training is whether the target fact or concept is going to change in the future. Facts and concepts, once learned, may be very difficult to extinguish, particularly for individuals with severe anterograde memory impairments. For example, in a previous study (Bourgeois et al., 2007), care staff at a participant's residence requested a training target of "recalling that bowling was scheduled for Wednesdays." The aim was to reduce the resident's repetitive questions about bowling on Tuesdays, which had been the bowling day the previous year. This resident had dense anterograde amnesia, so she learned primarily by nondeclarative methods. The researchers used SR training to teach the new bowling day, but after three or four sessions, it was proving difficult to extinguish the previous Tuesday response, and the resident was learning a response of "Tuesday . . . no . . . Wednesday," which was confusing to everyone. The care staff then shared that bowling would be changing to Thursdays the next month. Clearly, the best approach in this case was to teach the simple routine of checking a planner for the bowling date. That way, the routine would stay the same despite changes in facts. One general rule of thumb is that *if the facts or concepts are likely to change in the future, train a routine or procedure to access the information, rather than training the information itself.*

The clinician must integrate the assessment information, along with knowledge about declarative and nondeclarative learning, to select the best approach to meet the client's needs. As described earlier, because of the conflicting literature on optimal approaches for training facts and concepts, the clinician may need to conduct dynamic assessments or trial intervention periods to test their hypotheses about which ingredients, declarative or nondeclarative, are best for their client.

Define Targets, Aims, and Measures

An important part of the planning process is to identify the desired outcome. The clinician must be clear on why they are teaching this fact, concept, or simple routine and how success will be measured. At this juncture, the clinician will specify measurable targets and aims and plan for multilevel evaluation. Examples of measurement are described later in the "PIE: Evaluation of Training Facts, Concepts, and Simple Routines" section.

CONFIRM TREATMENT AIMS AND IMPACT MEASURES

As described in Chapter 4, treatment aims are typically broader aspects of daily functioning and often involve more than one target. This is especially true for facts and simple routines, as it is rare for clients to want to learn these simply for their own sake. More typically, the fact or routine needs to be learned as part of a larger plan to complete an activity. For example, a student may need to learn new vocabulary items in order to submit reading comprehension assignments, or an adult may need to learn a script of their accident history in order to provide information at medical appointments. In both of these examples, the part following "in order to" represents the aim of the intervention, and outcome measures to reflect the impact of intervention on the aim, such as a Goal Attainment Scale (GAS), should be included in the plan (see the "PIE: Evaluation of Training Facts, Concepts, and Simple Routines" section below).

CONFIRM TREATMENT TARGETS AND PROGRESS MEASURES

In many ways, facts and concepts are among the easiest treatment targets to define: the target is for the person to recall the information independently, use the information in a given context, or produce a response when cued. Progress measures then simply capture the frequency of accurate production of the target response in the training context as well as the length of the interval over which the target response is retained. In some ways, however, facts and concepts may prove difficult to train: It can be challenging to determine the fact or concept that will have the desired functional impact and, given the conflicting literature, it can be difficult to select the best approach (declarative vs. nondeclarative) for each treatment target. Additionally, the match between target and ingredients needs to factor in the characteristics described earlier (e.g., selecting concrete concepts when using a declarative approach, training in context when using a nondeclarative approach). Nevertheless, in all circumstances, it is critical that the facts and concepts selected for training should relate to the achievement of the aim. Clear links among aims, targets, and outcome measures, and selection of appropriate ingredients will increase the likelihood that the intervention will be successful and meet the client's expectations.

GOAL (TARGET AND AIM) WRITING

Chapter 5 outlined the components necessary for writing treatment targets and aims, including treatment approach, treatment target, objective performance measurement, criteria, level of independence, and conditions/context. See Forms 5.1 and 5.2 in Chapter 5 for target and aim writing checklists using Specific, Measurable, Attainable, Relevant, Time-based (SMART) and GAS requirements.

PIE: Implementation of Training Facts, Concepts, and Simple Routines

The planning process reviewed in the above section lays the groundwork for effective and efficient training that will be carried out in the implementation phase. The planning process will have generated the target fact, concept, or simple routine to be taught; the context in which it will be used; and the choice of approach (declarative or nondeclarative) to best match the client's cognitive profile; as well as measures to monitor performance and measure outcome. The next phase is to begin training, starting with the acquisition phase.

Initial Acquisition Phase of Training

Methods used in the initial acquisition phase of training will be dictated by answers to the considerations in the previous paragraph. In regard to dose (frequency and duration), the rehabilitation literature provides few specific guidelines for teaching facts and concepts, particularly for the initial acquisition phase. The dose needed varies greatly, depending on factors such as the complexity of the information to be trained, severity of the client's memory impairment, type of training approach used, and concomitant cognitive impairments (e.g., in language, attention, or executive functions). This gap in knowledge exists primarily because study methods are so underspecified (Lambez & Vakil, 2021). While nondeclarative methods like SR training have prescribed training schedules in the acquisition phase, there are few guidelines for doses when using declarative methods like trial-and-error learning or for use of ingredients like visualization or elaboration.

Fortunately, one useful finding is that massed practice is effective for initial acquisition of complex information (Donovan & Radosevich, 1999), whether using declarative or nondeclarative approaches. Consider what is involved in using declarative learning ingredients like visualization or association: it might take a client some time to make the association between a visual image or mnemonic and the target information to be recalled, and they also might need to spend time thinking about the concept and practicing using it in context. Consider a target like learning about brain functions (a common education target for people with acquired brain injury and their families). The clinician and client might collaborate to generate a visual image that helps the client remember different functions and link that to examples from everyday life, and then the client might practice explaining brain functions the way they would in a future context (e.g., to an employer or peers). Similarly, when implementing a nondeclarative approach such as SR training, a client with severe declarative memory impairments will need repeated opportunities to retrieve the correct information to create an automatic response.

For some clients, acquisition of the fact, concept, or simple routine takes place within the therapy session, where there are no distractions and the clinician is providing cues. For others, particularly clients with severe declarative memory impairments, training includes features of the context in which the fact, concept, or simple routine will be used. The "context" is where, when, and with whom the client will be using the target information or demonstrating the target behavior. For example, if the client is learning a face–name association for a caregiver, the session might take place in a therapy room using a photograph of that person, providing the visual image that looks like the actual person. However, if a client is learning a routine for leaving the house with important items (e.g., "1-2-3 phone, wallet, key," cued by three windowpanes in the front door), training should incorporate features of the context that will cue the target behavior in real life (e.g., the client's home environment: their phone, wallet, and key).

Figure 6.2 is a sample completed therapy session form for tracking client data during SR training that is based on recommendations in the text by Benigas and colleagues (Benigas et al., 2016) (see Form 6.1 at the end of the chapter for a blank version, as well as a fillable version in the digital files accompanying this book). The client, Yusuf, was a retired executive who had severe declarative learning impairments after a cardiac arrest. He wanted to learn the name of the personal support worker (Tina) who worked in his home. In this session at the outset of the acquisition phase of training, the clinician elected to begin with a 10-second interval paired with a continuous visual cue based on assessment results, suggesting that this approach was most likely to be successful in preventing errors. Over the course of the six trials completed in the first session, the continuous visual cue was faded, and Yusuf was successful in retaining Tina's name for 2 minutes. Importantly, 75% of Yusuf's responses were correct, so errors were minimized. Error-minimization ingredients included the clinician repeating the correct stimulus–response pair immediately, when Yusuf made an error, and then asking Yusuf to repeat the correct response.

Therapy Session Data Form—Target Acquisition, Mastery, Generalization (Facts, Concepts, Routines—Spaced Retrieval)

Client Name: Yusuf	**Date:** Aug. 10
Location: Retirement home	**Others Present:** N/A

Target: Accurately recall name of personal support worker (Tina) in response to visual image

Associated Aim: Improve positive social connections with staff and other residents	**Training Phase:** Acquisition
Stimulus/Cue: Video image (~2 secs) of Tina	**Response ((verbal,) physical, both):** Tina

Ingredients—Items: Video image of Tina Cue cards for MVC and CVC Timer Distractor activity (checkers)	**Ingredients—Actions:** Play video image Provide reducing cues for MVC, if needed Spaced practice with error control
Ingredients—Motivators: Enjoys Tina's company Checkers is favorite game	**Measurement Plan:** Longest interval achieved Ratio of correct to incorrect responses

Check-in Info and Results of Homework: Yusuf greeted the clinician with, "You! I thought the other girl was coming today." (Tina arrives at the end of session.) Care log on coffee table was completed by Tina, as requested, and she indicated that Yusuf had asked her her name 5 times the day before.

Practice Data

Trial	CVC?	Time Interval

Trial	CVC?	10s	20s	30s	1m	2m	4m	8m	16m	32m
1	Y	✓	✓	✓	✓	✗				
2	Y				✓	✓	✓	✗		
3	Y						✓	✗		
4	Y						✓	✗		
5	N			✓	✓	✗				
6	N				✓	✓	✗			
7										

(continued)

FIGURE 6.2. Example of completed Therapy Session Data Form—Target Acquisition, Mastery, Generalization (Facts, Concepts, Routines—Spaced Retrieval).

Therapy Session Data Form—
Target Acquisition, Mastery, Generalization (Facts, Concepts, Routines—Spaced Retrieval) *(page 2 of 2)*

Comments/Observations	Administration Notes
Did not need MVC, started right into SR, but began with CVC and 10 sec interval for error control purposes given this is first session of practice. When CVC removed, started that trial at 30 sec for error control purposes. Yusuf was engaged throughout—definitely likes playing checkers for as long as possible. Tina arrived at end of session and Yusuf spontaneously stated her name correctly!	CVC = Continuous Visual Cue Put ✓ in response line when interval achieved; continue on that line until error occurs (✗); then start next trial at last successful interval Add distractor activity at 2 min+

Session Summary/Analysis of Progress: Longest interval achieved with CVC = 4 min, without CVC = 2 min. Ratio of correct to incorrect responses = 13:6, so 2.17.

Feedback and Homework Provided (task, context, ingredients, tracking): Provided Tina with easily visible name tag in large print to wear for now. She will continue documenting frequency of name-asking when she works her shifts with Yusuf.

Plan for Next Session: Enter longest interval without CVC in Therapy Science to track significance of gains over time; daughter will join us tomorrow for next session; start with 30 secs and no CVC; consider 3 min interval to assist with transition from 2 to 4 min.

FIGURE 6.2. *(continued)*

Mastery and Generalization Phase

To master the retrieval of facts or concepts, it is critical that the client has the opportunity to practice, regardless of how the information was taught. The optimal frequency of retrieval practice varies across studies; however, as discussed earlier in this chapter, for both declarative or nondeclarative instructional methods, there is strong evidence of a *spacing effect* in typical adults (Kim et al., 2019). The spacing effect means that opportunities for successful retrieval over determined time intervals should be built into any intervention. The spacing time interval typically is chosen by the clinician, though methods like SR training (Benigas et al., 2016) have a prescribed training schedule (see Figure 6.2 above). Most therapy schedules do not allow for the amount of practice needed to consolidate a new fact or concept, so home practice also may be needed. Chapter 4 discussed the importance of including *volition* ingredients when assigning home practice. Examples of volition ingredients are provided in Table 4.2 and include ingredients such as the client choosing their own practice schedule, using a log to track practice, and identifying barriers to home practice and strategies to overcome those barriers.

The mastery phase occurs when retrieval of the fact or concept has been demonstrated in optimal conditions (e.g., in the therapy room or the most structured everyday context) but has not generalized to the conditions present in everyday life or is not yet used consistently and automatically. Again, for clients who have relatively intact declarative learning and memory, moving to the mastery/generalization phase may occur after one session or demonstration. Ironically, this also might be true for clients with profound declarative learning impairments who learn by nondeclarative mechanisms only: these individuals experience no "interference" from declarative learning and may master some facts and concepts in a single session using error-control learning methods (Bourgeois et al., 2007). For these individuals, however, generalization will be dependent on the similarity of the target context to the one in which they were trained. If they are expected to use their new learning in an even slightly different context, it will be critical to follow the procedures outlined below for systematically varying stimuli.

The target of the mastery phase is to increase fluency or automaticity of retrieving the target fact or concept or using the simple routine, including in the context in which it will be needed. In general, mastery and generalization of the target are accomplished by attending to three variables:

1. **Fading learning supports.** Depending on which learning supports were introduced and the severity of the client's memory and executive function impairments, the mastery phase will involve fading the supports and helping the client achieve automatic recall of the target information or performance of the target behavior. For example, if the client's target is to retrieve a health card from their wallet if they are asked for their health information, then the clinician could begin with the cue "Can I see your health card that is in your wallet in your pocket?", then fade that cue to "Can I see your health card that is in your wallet?", and then ask the question most likely to be asked at a health care appointment: "Can I see your health card?" In the example from Figure 6.2 above, the special name tag worn by Tina would be discontinued.

2. **Incorporating or increasing stimulus variability.** If the target needs to be used in a variety of contexts, this is addressed during the generalization phase. The important context variables to manipulate will depend on the target. For the health card example above, the "context" might be different people, so the client could practice with different people at the rehabilitation facility, then different people in his everyday life. For the example given earlier in Figure 6.2, the face–name association was being trained in the exact context where it needed to be used, so no generalization was required. The more severe the impairment in declarative learning, the more that client will rely on cues to trigger recall. Cues may be physical (e.g., a blank email, if the target is to use specific politeness markers in an email), spoken (e.g., a question about the person's accident, if the target is to produce a scripted description), or related to other types of context.

3. **Maximizing engagement.** Individuals with limited awareness of their deficits can still learn new information, particularly with errorless techniques such as SR training, but the response will be automatic and stimulus bound. The therapy process is likely to be more successful if the client is actively engaged in the selection of targets and aims and can see evidence that therapy is working.

Maintenance Phase

The maintenance phase begins after target information has been consolidated in long-term memory. Clients with memory problems need practice to maintain new facts and concepts over time, and the clinician must actively plan how to achieve this once therapy is no longer available. The clinician should look at the client's environment and everyday routines for opportunities to practice recall. For example, a client with diabetes who wants to recall the names of low-carbohydrate foods when talking with family members could do their own grocery shopping or meal selection, so they have the opportunity to label items on a regular basis. If that isn't possible, the opportunity to make food choices could be added to their everyday routine. It is much more effective to have natural cues trigger recall of the information in context than to ask a hypothetical question in a drill format. Very few people enjoy being tested! The use of diaries, logs, and "check-ins" can be helpful for tracking maintenance of learning, provided everyday support people are trained in how to use them: it is unrealistic to expect a person with a memory impairment to remember to note when they forget.

In terms of long-term retention of facts, concepts, and simple routines, it is important to acknowledge that contexts and information change. Mechanisms need to be in place for reevaluating learning targets and adding new targets as the need arises. The optimal model for long-term service delivery may be a "train the trainer" approach, in which the caregiver learns how to train new facts, concepts, and simple routines, with guidance from a clinician. In this way, new information can be added as the need arises, with the added benefit that the caregiver is in the target context so generalization is efficient.

PI**E**: Evaluating Learning of Facts, Concepts, and Simple Routines

As described earlier, the planning process results in measurable targets that contribute to the client's aim. Success in achieving each target should be evaluated at multiple levels.

The most common measures of progress at the acquisition phase of training are percent accuracy of producing the target fact or concept and type and amount of cueing needed; response latency (how long it takes the client to produce a response after a cue is given); and, for error-control methods, the longest interval at which the client produced the correct response. These are the *target acquisition data*. If the training takes place somewhere other than the target context, or there are multiple contexts in which the information will be used, then the clinician will need to collect *generalization data*, which are similar measures as used in the acquisition phase but taken during progressively less structured and supported contexts (e.g., with no cues, different partners, or the real person vs. a photograph). If the training took place in the context where the facts and concepts are to be used, then generalization is automatic.

Facts, concepts, and simple routines are only useful if they are remembered over time. Thus, the third type of data to be collected is *maintenance data*. Often, clients are discharged from therapy soon after they initially master a goal, and the clinician never knows if the information is used over time. Long-term retention cannot be assumed, however, so it is important to find some mechanism for checking that the client can still remember the target information when they need it. This information not only helps that individual client, but also informs the therapist's future clinical practice. Maintenance data typically are versions of the acquisition and generalization data, for example, does the person produce that fact or concept in the same way over time?

Perhaps the most important outcome measure is whether the training had a positive impact on the client's aims. If the client memorized a script to make appointments, are they successful in making their own appointments independently? If they learned a script to describe their own memory impairments, could they use it effectively to self-advocate for accommodations at work? These *impact data* may be obtained via interviews with stakeholders, or from memory logs or other types of journals recorded by the client, with data compared to baseline evaluation before training began.

PUTTING IT ALL TOGETHER: CASE APPLICATIONS

This section describes two client examples to show the use of the PIE framework in training facts, concepts, and simple routines. The first example is from the research literature (Oberg & Turkstra, 1998) and uses elaborative encoding for two adolescents with TBI. We chose this study because it revealed the strengths and limitations of semantic learning in individuals with declarative memory problems, and also illustrates the process of choosing functional goals. We then follow with a clinical example, the first Case Application in this text. In this Case Application, we support the reader in working through the stages of applying the information in a structured manner, making use of the various forms presented in this book. We also supply sample completed forms. Both the research and clinical examples illustrate the use of declarative methods, as examples using nondeclarative methods were presented earlier in this chapter.

A Case Example from the Literature (Oberg & Turkstra, 1998)

Description of Clients

BW and SN were two adolescents with severe TBI who participated in a study of elaborative encoding for learning new vocabulary. BW was an 18-year-old male who had been injured at age 5. A recent CT scan showed evidence of bilateral necrosis of prefrontal cortex, left more than right. He had below-average scores on all tests of cognitive function, including memory and language, particularly abstract language comprehension and use. SN was a male 18 years old who had been injured 1 month prior to his enrollment in the study. He had a right frontal hematoma and required a left temporal lobectomy at the time of the accident, and a follow-up CT scan showed encephalomalacia (softening of the brain) in the left temporal region. Like those of BW, SN's scores on tests of language and memory were below average. He also showed perseveration in words, gestures, and ideas. For example, his definitions for *brave, precise,* and *strenuous*—when he was asked to define one after the other—were "honest and power inside," "happenings within," and "strength used within." Perseveration would prove to be a challenge when choosing and training vocabulary items (recall the discussion of *neighborhood density* above). Important for the purposes of this chapter, both of these adolescents were outgoing, sociable individuals who were interested in learning new words that would help them in school. Also relevant in retrospect, both had excellent nondeclarative learning and memory, which turned out to be significant factors in the study results.

Choosing Treatment Targets

For each adolescent, the authors chose 100 words that were needed at work or in school. For BW, these were newspaper and school-text words that were relevant to his curriculum; for SN, they were words related to his goal of working in the field of ophthalmology. Each participant was asked to generate definitions for the 100 words, and of those defined incorrectly, 40 target words were chosen. These were divided into 20 treatment words and 20 control words that would be used to test treatment efficacy.

Implementation

In the acquisition phase, treatment included the following elaborative encoding strategies:

- Reviewing words and definitions
- Matching words to synonyms
- Matching words to definitions
- Filling in blanks within sentences with target words
- Generating definitions with help from the dictionary
- Generating synonyms with help from the dictionary
- Using each word in a self-generated sentence
- Giving self-generated definitions to a classmate for feedback

Based on previous studies of elaborative encoding in TBI, stimuli were spaced rather than massed (e.g., each word was reviewed once, then the list was repeated, rather than repeating the same word several times before moving on to the next). To maximize generalization, the investigators emphasized multiple word meanings and using the words in a variety of sentences. BW completed ten 30-minute sessions over a 5-week period, and SN completed eighteen 30-minute sessions over 6 weeks.

Evaluation

Both participants learned 11 of the trained items versus 1 to 2 of the control items, and both maintained these gains after 1 month without treatment. Even after 1 year, SN was able to produce the exact definitions he had learned in treatment. In addition, both acquired partial knowledge about additional words on the training list. Most often, this partial knowledge was the ability to use the word in a syntactically correct sentence but with the wrong meaning. For example, SN was taught the word "formation" in the context of geology. Over the course of therapy, he produced these definitions:

- "In Utah, there are a lot of Jurassic formations."
- "Triceratops is found in the Jurassic; that's a good formation."
- "Triceratops are found a bunch in the Jurassic formation."
- "The formation of the Santa Rita Mountains has some matrix upon it."
- "The formations in those mountains are really prolific."
- "Iron is the most important formation in my vehicle."

The concepts of *matrix* and *prolific* were other items on the training list and appeared above as perseverations. When asked to use the word "assume" in different sentences, SN provided these definitions:

- "I assume too much."
- "Out of life I assume way too much."
- "You assume too much is going to happen when in reality it won't."
- "I assume too much out of life."
- "Some vehicle places assume too much with engine products."
- "She assumed a lot of money from her job."

These examples show that SN extracted syntactic information about the items—appropriately, as this is a nondeclarative (procedural) aspect of language—and learned some associations with the items (e.g., one meaning of "assume" is to take on, and being paid for a job might be linked to taking on money). BW showed the same pattern. This was perhaps the most important message of the study: correct production of the trained concept did not equal full understanding of and ability to use that concept in all contexts. For clients with declarative memory impairments this severe, "what you see" might be "what you get."

CASE APPLICATION—JENNIFER

Below we provide a clinical case example. We describe the stages of intervention and direct the reader to practice applying the information in a structured manner, making use of the various forms presented in this book (fillable forms for each item are included in the digital files accompanying this book). Completed Case Application Sample Answers are included at the end of this chapter.

Description of Client

The client, Jennifer, was a 24-year-old Métis woman who was seen for therapy 6 months after a bicycling accident. Jennifer had started a furniture restoration business out of a large workshop on her parents' alpaca farm just over a year before the accident, but physical injuries prevented her from engaging in most furniture restoration tasks. Jennifer had been diagnosed with a mild to moderate brain injury at the time of the accident, but the emphasis had been on her physical injuries. As she engaged in more activities, Jennifer's family reported noticing frequent forgetfulness, to the point that multiple tasks were not being completed. Jennifer and her family requested intervention to support her cognitive functioning. Her insurer approved funding for an assessment and four intervention sessions.

Planning

During the clinical interview, Jennifer emphasized that her aim was to engage in some form of meaningful, productive activity until she could resume her regular vocation. Her parents indicated that a family friend owned a small local hardware store and they wondered if working at the store for a couple of hours a day might be an option. The clinician had reviewed the original assessment results from 6 months prior and decided to conduct updated attention, memory, and executive function testing to determine what could be contributing to Jennifer's "forgetfulness." The assessment revealed the following client profile:

Sociocultural values. Jennifer greatly valued her family and community. She enjoyed living in a small town where everyone knew and helped everyone else.

Cognitive findings. Jennifer's scores on standardized memory and attention tests were in the moderately impaired range. Scores on tests of executive function were within normal limits when working memory demands were low. Jennifer was observed to independently attempt methods to support her memory when providing recent historical information (e.g., when asked the name of the hardware store at which she wanted to work, she said, "It has a shiny floor, and it rhymes with floor— Shore! Shore Hardware").

Physical and sensory functions. Jennifer had sustained a complicated fracture in the right wrist that required open reduction with internal fixation. She also had a full tear of her right anterior cruciate ligament and medial collateral ligament, and additional surgery was likely. These physical injuries limited her mobility, endurance, and ability to complete motor tasks with her right (dominant) hand. She fatigued easily, often needing intermittent breaks if required to stand for more than 30 minutes.

Psychosocial functioning. Jennifer reported that she was extremely embarrassed at her forgetfulness. She said she was relieved when her parents raised the issue because she had been too nervous to admit to them that she was struggling. She was worried that she would "go stir crazy" if she didn't do something meaningful, but at the same time was avoiding activities because she was afraid of forgetting and letting someone down. She also reported feeling guilty for being 24 years old and living with her parents, without contributing financially to the household.

Environmental variables. With Jennifer's reduced mobility, she was only able to climb two or three stairs before pain and fatigue became problematic. Her parents' house, the workshop, and the hardware store were all accessible with one or two stairs.

With Jennifer's permission, the clinician reached out to Andrea, the owner of Shore Hardware, to discuss possible options for Jennifer to assist at the shop. Andrea had the idea of Jennifer becoming a greeter to direct customers to the correct aisle to find what they were looking for. Andrea knew that Jennifer had extensive knowledge of most products in the shop from when she worked there as a teenager, and from when she would buy supplies there before the accident. Andrea had rearranged the store a few months earlier, but she felt confident that Jennifer would learn the new system quickly. Andrea was willing to be Jennifer's "coach" to help her succeed in the store and, if things went well, she would consider offering paid employment until Jennifer could return to her furniture restoration business. Andrea requested that Jennifer work at the store for 2-hour shifts on Wednesday and Thursday evenings, as well as Saturday afternoons, as that was when Andrea would also be present.

Knowing the context of Jennifer's aim to achieve independence in a work trial where she would greet and direct customers to the correct aisle at the hardware store, the clinician reviewed the assessment results to determine if Jennifer could best capitalize on declarative or nondeclarative learning for this task. Learning the categories of four aisles could easily be done via SR training, but given the range of product types in each aisle, Jennifer would need to engage in a more elaborative encoding process to optimally respond to customer inquiries. Also, although Jennifer had moderate memory impairments, she did have strong existing product knowledge and she had already independently used visualization and a rhyme to recall the name of the hardware store. The clinician therefore decided to take a declarative approach.

Application Practice

Document the aim and target on Form 6.2: Therapy Session Data Form—Declarative. Brainstorm ideas of ingredients (items and actions) that would support Jennifer in encoding the aisle locations of common hardware store items. Target acquisition, generalization, and maintenance will be measured by accuracy in identifying the correct aisle. Add the ingredients and measurement plan to the form. Compare your form to the Case Application Sample Answer: Form 6.2 at the end of the chapter, but don't peek at the data sections yet!

In addition to measurement of performance in session, Jennifer wanted a measure to reflect her success in responding to actual customer inquiries in the store.

Application Practice

Based on the information above and using the checklist in Form 5.2 in Chapter 5, create a GAS to measure the ultimate impact of training these facts on the success of Jennifer's work trial. Compare your scale with the Case Application Sample Answer: Goal Attainment Scale at the end of the chapter.

Implementation

The acquisition phase of training began by engaging Jennifer in the process of encoding the facts to be learned. In the first session, Andrea brought photos of each of the four aisles in the store along with lists of common items in each aisle. Encoding was completed for two of the aisles using three declarative learning ingredients:

- *Elaboration:* Instructing Jennifer to subcategorize items in an aisle, name each subcategory, then name the overall category for the aisle
- *Visualization:* Instructing Jennifer to scan the photos of each aisle into photo editing software, add the category name with a visual image, and list the subcategory names
- *Self-explanation:* Asking Jennifer to explain and repeat back her organization and naming system to the clinician

The clinician had Andrea randomly select 35 items from the lists for each of the two aisles and ask Jennifer questions in the form of "Where can I find . . ." and

"Do you have. . . ." Jennifer was required to answer with the category name and aisle number (e.g., "Décor items are in Aisle 1," "Fasteners are in Aisle 2"). Jennifer correctly answered 25 out of 35 questions. When she provided the wrong aisle, the clinician had Jennifer look at the visual image on her laptop and then immediately asked the question again until Jennifer provided the correct response. No difference in performance was noted between the two forms of questions.

Application Practice

Document the practice results from the first session on Form 6.2: Therapy Session Data Form. Generate ideas for the homework you'd like Jennifer to complete and for what you would like to do in the next session. Compare your form to the Case Application Sample Answer: Form 6.2 at the end of the chapter.

During the third session, Jennifer achieved 90% accuracy for items belonging to all four aisles. Andrea reported that when the same items were practiced sitting in a quiet office at the back of the store, Jennifer achieved 80% accuracy, and for the remaining 20% of items, Andrea directed Jennifer to the laptop images in order to get her to immediately generate correct answers after any incorrect responses. The clinician provided guidance to Andrea on how to promote increased generalization through fading learning supports, practicing in the busier storefront area, increasing the variety of items practiced, and using a distributed practice schedule. The clinician asked Jennifer to keep a logbook detailing their practice results.

Evaluation

The initial evaluation included the acquisition and generalization data described above. Four weeks later, Jennifer attended the final session with the clinician to review her logbooks and Goal Attainment Scale results, and plan for maintenance. The logbooks revealed that Andrea had discontinued use of the laptop images 3 weeks before and each day had added new products to the list of items practiced. Andrea and Jennifer initially completed practice in the storefront area twice during each 2-hour shift but had reduced practice to once per shift in the prior week. Jennifer shared her results on her Goal Attainment Scale: by the previous week, she had only needed to call Andrea for help once every three to four customers. Andrea then decided to hire Jennifer as a part-time employee in the greeter role, which had proven to be very popular with local residents, and added weekly inventory tasks to the job.

Together, Jennifer and the clinician created a plan to help Jennifer stay on track with her gains. She would continue with her logbooks, involve another store employee in completing intermittent practice and providing back-up support so that she could work shifts when Andrea was off, and reach out to the clinician if she felt a booster session was needed to maintain or expand her role within the store.

Therapy Session Data Form—Target Acquisition, Mastery, Generalization (Facts, Concepts, Routines—Declarative)

Client Name: Jennifer	Date: Aug 20	Location: Clinic	Others Present: Andrea (owner of Shore Hardware)

Target: 90% accuracy in recalling name of aisle when given the name of a hardware item, independently in therapy	Associated Aim: Improve independence during work trial as a store greeter	Training Phase: Acquisition

Ingredients—Items:	Ingredients—Actions:	Ingredients—Motivators:	Measurement Plan:
Photographs of 4 aisles List of common items in each aisle Photo editing software	Elaboration to categorize aisle items Visualization to map categories onto photographs of aisles Client explanation of categories Massed practice selecting categories	Potential for paid employment High interest and knowledge in hardware and DIY projects	% correct responses

Check-in Info and Results of Homework: Andrea brought item lists and aisle photos as requested (to assist in creating categories that accurately reflect commonly requested items in each aisle). Jennifer brought laptop with photo software as requested.

Encoding Process: Started with Aisles 1 and 2 today. Had Jennifer sub-categorize items in each aisle and generate a name for each sub-category (support provided to ensure names were unambiguous). Ex: Aisle 1 had subcategories Paints, Stains, Brushes, Fillers, Decals and she chose "Décor" as the overall category for this aisle. Same process for Aisle 2, named as "Fasteners." Had Jennifer scan the photos of the aisles into her photo editing software and insert labeled images for her main category and sub-categories. Asked Jennifer to then explain back the organization and naming system.

Practice Data: Andrea role-played the customer and asked questions in the form of "where can I find . . ." and "do you have . . . ." and Jennifer responded with "Décor items are in Aisle 1" or "Fasteners are in Aisle 2." Completed 35 practice reps (different item each time but would always go into either the Décor or Fasteners aisle): 25/35 correct. When incorrect, directed Jennifer to look at her visual display on laptop and then immediately asked question again and had Jennifer answer correctly. No difference observed between 2 forms of questions asked.

Session Summary/Analysis of Progress: 71% accurate for selecting between 2 aisles.

Feedback and Homework Provided (task, context, ingredients, tracking): Jennifer will meet Andrea at the store tomorrow to complete additional practice, with Jennifer explaining her categorization system as a warm-up and then Andrea administering the same 35 items as today, following the identical procedures.

Plan for Next Session: Have Jennifer explain her categorization system for Aisles 1–2. Complete encoding process for Aisles 3–4. Complete at least 20 practice trials for items belonging to all 4 aisles. Enter results in Therapy Science to track speed of progress toward 90%. Plan to move toward distributed practice.

Goal Attainment Scale

Jennifer's Goal Attainment Scale—to be achieved in 4 weeks

Independence in Directing Customers to Correct Aisles over Past Week

−2 Much less than expected	−1 Less than expected (baseline)	0 Expected outcome	+1 Better than expected	+2 Much better than expected
Requires assistance from Andrea more than 75% of the time.	Requires assistance from Andrea 51–75% of the time.	Requires assistance from Andrea 26–50% of the time.	Requires assistance from Andrea 5–25% of the time.	Requires assistance from Andrea less than 5% of the time.

Therapy Session Data Form—Target Acquisition, Mastery, Generalization (Facts, Concepts, Routines—Spaced Retrieval)

Client Name:	Date:
Location:	Others Present:
Target:	
Associated Aim:	Training Phase:
Stimulus/Cue:	Response (verbal, physical, both):
Ingredients—Items:	Ingredients—Actions:
Ingredients—Motivators:	Measurement Plan:
Check-in Info and Results of Homework:	

Practice Data										
		Time Interval								
Trial	CVC?									
1										
2										
3										
4										
5										
6										
7										

(continued)

Comments/Observations	Administration Notes
	CVC = Continuous Visual Cue Put ✓ in response line when interval achieved; continue on that line until error occurs (✗); then start next trial at last successful interval Add distractor activity at 2 min+

Session Summary/Analysis of Progress:

Feedback and Homework Provided (task, context, ingredients, tracking):

Plan for Next Session:

Therapy Session Data Form—Target Acquisition, Mastery, Generalization (Facts, Concepts, Routines—Declarative)

Client Name:	Date:	Location:	Others Present:

Target:		Associated Aim:	Training Phase:

Ingredients—Items:	Ingredients—Actions:	Ingredients—Motivators:	Measurement Plan:

Check-in Info and Results of Homework:

Encoding Process:

Practice Data:

Session Summary/Analysis of Progress:

Feedback and Homework Provided (task, context, ingredients, tracking):

Plan for Next Session:

Cognitive Strategy Instruction

In this chapter, we discuss how to help individuals regulate their behavior or their thinking by supporting them in the selection and use of cognitive strategies. Strategy training is one of the most commonly used approaches in cognitive rehabilitation across the severity continuum. Strategies may be simple, for example, coaching a person with an attention impairment to develop a self-reminder phrase such as "focus." Strategies may also be complex and contain multiple steps and phases. For example, there are numerous strategy packages that guide a person with executive function impairment through a process of defining a goal, selecting an approach, monitoring outcome, and revising as necessary (e.g., Miotto, Evans, Souza de Lucia, & Scaff, 2009). Additionally, some strategies may be used in conjunction with an external aid as a prompt or reminder for strategy use. Effective use of strategies requires clinicians to be skilled in how to collaboratively select and match strategies to a client's needs and abilities and implement instructional methods that support learning and adoption of strategy use in the naturalistic environment. Cognitive strategy instruction may be delivered as the sole approach in a cognitive rehabilitation regimen, but often it is part of a therapy program that includes other approaches such as the use of external aids.

Strategy use on the part of clients requires that they understand when and how to use a strategy and are able to monitor strategy impact. Clients essentially must engage in an internally generated cognitive process. Strategy use, at least until it becomes automatic, thus depends on some degree of intact *metacognition*. Metacognition is our ability to think about our own thinking. Kennedy & Coelho (2005) described the complex metacognitive skills that are by-products of *self-regulation*, which is fundamental to the effective use of strategies for task completion: (1) setting goals, (2) comparing performance with goals or outcomes (i.e., self-monitoring), (3) making decisions to change one's behavior in order to reach the desired outcome (i.e., self- control), and (4) executing the change in behavior (e.g., implementing an alternative solution). As described in Chapter 2, individuals with moderate to severe acquired brain injury (ABI) often have deficits in metacognition that can impact their self-regulation. Reduced awareness of deficits and being able to change one's own thinking to respond to changing demands are common challenges that may be helped by strategy training but will require careful selection of strategies and systematic training in order to manage these deficits (Kennedy, Linhart, & Brady, 2006; Sohlberg & Turkstra, 2011).

This chapter focuses on the independent use of cognitive strategies by clients who have sufficient metacognitive ability to recognize when and how to optimally employ the strategy. Depending on the complexity of strategies, there is a prerequisite degree of metacognitive ability that must be intact or cultivated for strategy training to be an effective treatment approach. As described in Chapters 2 and 3, reduced self-awareness is a common consequence of brain injury and can result from multiple sources, including damage to the brain networks and structures that allow us to understand disabilities (anosognosia), as well as psychological states where clients are not able to endorse changes in function because it is too emotionally painful (denial). Strategy use requires an internally generated, cognitive-behavioral response, so clients need sufficient awareness of their disability to initiate strategy use outside of therapy. Typically, the clinician will assess the client's level of self-awareness during a clinical interview, using a tool such as the Self-Awareness of Deficits Interview (SADI; Fleming, Strong, & Ashton, 1996). Clients will also need to be motivated and able to initiate strategy use at the required time and will need either some external prompting or internally generated initiative. Kaschel and colleagues (2002) provided caveats about using cognitive strategies as a therapy approach, including that strategies can be too complex for people with cognitive impairments and that they can be unnatural and difficult to apply to everyday life activities.

Matching a strategy to the individual client profile and using instructional techniques that accommodate cognitive challenges are key to a successful outcome in which clients employ the strategies to improve everyday functioning. The first section of this chapter describes different strategy options. This is followed by application of our Plan, Implement, and Evaluate (PIE) framework to help clients select, learn, and adopt strategies that will promote functioning in ways that are meaningful to clients' everyday lives.

STRATEGY OPTIONS

Providing effective strategy instruction requires the clinician to know the range of strategy options. Strategies can be grouped using a variety of schemas. For example, they may be categorized based on the type of cognitive impairment(s) they support (e.g., memory strategies) or by the type of task they are designed to facilitate (e.g., homework strategies). The field of neuropsychological rehabilitation provides strong evidence supporting the training of cognitive strategies to assist with goal completion for people with a variety of cognitive impairments (Kennedy et al., 2008; O'Neil-Pirozzi, Kennedy, & Sohlberg, 2016; Tate et al., 2014). Most studies have focused on evaluating strategy use for managing impairments in three cognitive domains: attention (e.g., sustaining and shifting attention), executive functions (e.g., problem solving, inhibition/impulse control, self-correction), and memory (e.g., recall and retention of information and procedures). At the core of cognitive strategy training is teaching an individual to self-regulate thoughts and actions—that is, "think about their own thinking"—and self-monitor performance during an activity (Kennedy & Coelho, 2005). The goal is for the client to use methods that will provide some control over their own learning, thinking, and/or behavior. Below we begin with a description of options for cognitive strategy training that target different cognitive processes and then review strategies designed to improve performance on specific functional tasks.

Sustained Attention Strategies

Vigilance or sustained attention is a very common area of cognitive impairment following ABI and responds well to strategy training (Sohlberg & Turkstra, 2011). There are countless strategies that can be generated with a client to assist with maintaining attention over time. Many basic attention strategies are straightforward and often tied to specific tasks. Table 7.1 lists example attention strategies taken from a manual from an attention training program and applied to specific client aims (Sohlberg & Mateer, 2011).

Executive Function Strategies

Most of the evidence supporting strategy instruction for improving executive functions comes from studies of metacognitive strategy instruction (MSI; Kennedy et al., 2008). MSI uses direct instruction to teach individuals to regulate their own behavior and deliberately monitor how they are performing a target task and change their behavior if performance is not optimal (Sohlberg et al., 2005). To self-regulate, individuals need to identify an appropriate goal and anticipate what they need to do to reach that goal, then

TABLE 7.1. Examples of Cognitive Strategies for Maintaining Attention

Strategy	Examples from clients
Visualization	Picture myself completing my homework.
External self-talk	Say "click save" out loud each time I enter one set of data.
Internal self-talk	Tell myself "focus" if my mind starts to wander while I'm reading.
Close eyes	If my mind wanders while I am working on my electronic bill pay, close my eyes for a brief time.
Breathe/relaxation	To clear my mind and refocus while at work, use my breathing techniques.
Body alert (sitting straight, facing material)	Before I start eating my meal, get my body in a ready position.
Double-check	Stop after each step of my washing routine and look at my progress.
Predict hard and easy steps	Before it's my turn in bridge, remind myself of the hard and easy parts of the turn.

identify possible solutions to challenges, self-monitor and evaluate progress, and modify their behavior or strategy use if they are not making adequate progress. MSI thus can be used to address difficulties with problem solving, planning, initiation, organization, and task persistence, all of which are commonly impaired in individuals with ABI and other acquired cognitive disorders. Table 7.2 lists examples of MSI techniques evaluated in the literature and shown to produce positive clinical results.

Metacognitive strategy training has a relatively long history within the field of cognitive rehabilitation. Von Cramon, Cramon, and Mai (1991) developed a problem-solving therapy (PST) group program, with the aim of enabling clients to be more effective in breaking down problems and adopting a slowed down, controlled, and stepwise approach, in contrast to the clients' more usual impulsive approach. Subsequent studies have used components or principles from PST (e.g., Miotto et al., 2009). A similar treatment approach that is heavily dependent on strategy training and has been supported by research is goal management training (GMT; Levine et al., 2000). This technique was derived from Duncan's concept of goal neglect (Duncan, Emslie, Williams, Johnson, & Freer, 1996) and involves training clients to develop a mental checking routine (using the metaphor of checking a mental blackboard), combined with a strategy of very clearly defining a goal to be achieved, learning the steps required to achieve the goal, and then regularly checking progress as part of the mental checking routine (Duncan et al., 1996).

More recently, GMT has been adapted to include mindfulness techniques. Participants learn how to use mindful attention and goal setting to recognize and stop "absent-mindedness" and "automatic pilot" approaches and adjust goals accordingly. Reviews evaluating GMT efficacy studies have concluded that GMT can have a long-term positive effect on executive functions when used in combination with other rehabilitation approaches, including external aid training and awareness training (Krasny-Pacini et al., 2014; Tornas et al., 2016). Other strategy training approaches have incorporated components of GMT. For example, the Goal-Oriented Attention Self-Regulation (GOALS) training protocol, shown to positively impact functional goal completion, was based on metacognitive problem-solving and goal-management interventions and features a prominent mindfulness component (Novakovic-Agopian et al., 2019). In contrast to training via practice on isolated tasks, GOALS involves application of attention regulation skills and strategies to support participant-defined goals in real-life, ecologically valid settings.

A wide variety of strategies have been used to address impairments in attention and executive functions. As shown in Table 7.2, a strategy may emphasize problem solving, goal management, self-regulation, or a combination of these. In the corresponding research studies, all participants used the strategy protocol being investigated, with variable results. In practice, clinicians can evaluate the specific cognitive profiles and functional demands of their individual clients and collaboratively select the strategy components that best match their clients' needs. For example, a client who has primary difficulty with impulsive behavior might benefit from strategy components that include training in problem recognition and refraining from an immediate response (Rath, Simon, Langenbahn, Sherr, & Diller, 2003), whereas a client who has primary difficulty with maintaining attention and focus during task completion may benefit from components in the GOALS strategy (Novakovic-Agopian et al., 2019).

There is substantial evidence that MSI can improve everyday functioning in young to middle-aged adults with ABI affecting memory and executive functions (Kennedy et

TABLE 7.2. Examples of Cognitive Strategies Addressing Executive Function

Metacognitive strategy	Description	Supporting research evidence
Problem-solving therapy (PST)	*Problem-solving process:* Participants are taught steps for sequences such as "problem identification and analysis"; "generation of hypotheses and decision making"; "evaluation of a solution."	von Cramon et al. (1991); von Cramon & Matthes-von Cramon (1994)
Time pressure management (TPM)	*Problem-solving process:* Intervention first helps with increasing self-awareness and acceptance of disability; then participants are taught step-by-step problem-solving approach rehearsed under increasing distractions.	Fasotti et al. (2000)
Problem solving with impulse control	*Problem-solving process:* Participants are taught to document impulsive reactions to problem situations and identify strategies to avoid reactions.	Rath et al. (2003)
Verbal mediation	*Self-instruction process for problem solving and goal completion:* Participants are taught to verbalize steps of multistep tasks and fade talking to whispering and then inner speech.	Cicerone & Giacino (1992); Cicerone & Wood (1987)
Goal attainment	*Goal-setting process:* Participants are taught steps to set goals and actively monitor progress toward goals.	Webb & Gluecauf (1994)
Goal management training (GMT)	*Goal-completion process:* Participants are taught six steps: stop, define main task, list steps, learn steps, execute task, check results.	Krasny-Pacini et al. (2014); Levine et al. (2000); Tornås et al. (2016)
Self-monitoring	*Self-monitoring process:* Participants are taught to make predictions and monitor performance via anticipating their own performance and/or recording task progress.	Cicerone & Giacino (1992); Suzman, Morris, Morris, & Milan (1997)
Self-monitoring (WSTC)	*Self-monitoring process:* Participants taught self-monitoring steps associated with acronym WSTC: What am I supposed to be doing? Select a strategy. Try the strategy. Check the strategy.	Lawson & Rice (1989)
Integrated attention regulation and goal management training programs (GOALS)	*Goal-Oriented Attention Self-Regulation (GOALS):* Attention regulation strategy using Stop-Relax-Refocus (SRR) is followed by training in application of identification, selection, and execution of self-selected complex functional tasks.	Novakovic-Agopian et al. (2019)
APS	*Attention and problem solving (APS):* This is a combination of PST (von Cramon et al., 1991) and GMT (Levine et al., 2000).	Miotto et al. (2009)
Strategic Memory Advanced Reasoning Training (SMART)	*Five sequential strategies:* Filter (attend to key information and ignore less relevant information). • Focus and chunk (combine important details). • Link (identify the gist or meaning). • Zoom (consider the broader context and also the details that support the gist). • Generalize (evaluate the gist from different perspectives).	Han et al. (2020); Vas et al. (2011)

al., 2008). While there is evidence that participants maintain gains from therapy over time, research suggests that variability exists in the extent to which participants generalize strategy use beyond the targets trained in therapy (Kennedy et al., 2008; Novakovic-Agopian et al., 2019). Furthermore, the treatment protocols for many of the research studies are delivered in group formats and have duration and session lengths that would not be feasible in clinical practice.

Memory Strategies

Memory strategies, commonly called *mnemonic* strategies, are techniques or methods employed by a person to enhance or improve their learning and/or recall of target information; specifically declarative information. Memory strategies tend to emphasize either semantic or verbal associations, both of which tap into semantic networks. They are often called *internal* strategies because they rely on conscious thought by the user and are contrasted with *external* strategies like notebooks and planners, which compensate for memory changes within the learner and attempt to lessen cognitive demands (see Chapter 8). In general, memory strategies require individuals to focus and carefully attend to the information to be learned, which by itself can enhance learning. They include strategies such as elaboration, visualization, and creating mnemonics. These are all methods that a clinician teaches a client to use when the client needs to learn and recall factual material. In these situations, *using the memory strategy* is the target of intervention; that is, the goal is for the client to demonstrate implementing the strategy and be able to do so with a variety of materials and contexts (e.g., training a client to use a concept map strategy to link and summarize new learning). This is in contrast to the rote, overlearning of discrete facts and simple routines described in Chapter 6. For rote learning, the target is the *retrieval of a specific fact* (e.g., training a client to list the colleges their grandchildren attend), and the clinician may choose to use a mnemonic as an ingredient to support the learning of that specific fact. This is an important distinction for clinicians to understand: Does the client need to learn/memorize a fact to be recalled in specific situations (e.g., home address), or does the client need to learn a strategy that they can apply to recall a range of facts in a range of contexts (e.g., applying elaboration procedures to learn information in textbooks)? Table 7.3 summarizes common examples of memory strategies that clinicians may teach their clients to apply in a range of contexts.

Internal memory strategies aim to facilitate access to stored semantic networks of information and use these networks to assist with storage and retrieval processes (West, 1995). Wilson (1995) listed the following reasons that account for successful use of internal memory strategies:

- Strategies encourage a deeper level of processing, which improves recall.
- Strategies often integrate isolated information.
- Strategies often provide built-in retrieval cues.

While the goal of training any strategy is for the client to use the strategy independently, there may be times when the severity of the client's memory impairment precludes them from doing so. However, some of these clients may still have life participation aims that require engaging in new learning (e.g., taking an academic course). In

TABLE 7.3. Examples of Cognitive Strategies for Managing Memory

Strategy	Description	Examples of how clients applied the strategy
Visual imagery	Creating a story, or using location or concept images to help remember new information.	Remembering a list of items that need to be packed each morning by picturing items in different places in the kitchen.
Rehearsal	Rote repetition of target information. Often used in conjunction with other strategies. Frequently different practice schedules (massed immediate practice vs. distributed over time) are used strategically to enhance learning.	Going over vocabulary words first with mass repetition and then adding more time between rehearsals.
Making associations	Linking information to be remembered to something meaningful.	Making an acronym (e.g., YUM) to remember three medications that start with "y," "u," and "m."
Verbal elaboration	Assigning further detail to something to be remembered.	Describing key concept from work training using own words and two details; concept mapping.
Semantic association	Relating new information to concepts that are known.	Remembering people's names by thinking of a word that rhymes with it (e.g., "Mary is hairy").

Sample categories are from O'Neil-Pirozzi, Sohlberg, and Kennedy (2016).

these circumstances, the clinician will train the pertinent everyday people (e.g., tutor, family member) to continually provide prompting to support the client in applying the memory strategy (e.g., using concept maps) to maximize the client's chances of later retrieval of the information.

Kaschel and colleagues (2002) discussed the importance of systematic instruction to ensure that memory strategies, which can be unnatural and complicated, are adequately learned and employed in everyday contexts. Results from their randomized controlled trial suggested that imagery training to enhance recall can be effective when it incorporates specific training components. Their treatment ingredients, described at the end of this chapter, followed systematic instruction principles and included a hierarchy of exercises that gave participants practice using the strategies and then helped them transfer strategy use to their everyday lives. O'Neil-Pirozzi and colleagues (2010) also conducted a controlled study evaluating the effects of teaching internal memory strategies to people with brain injury. They showed that a group therapy process that emphasized training in semantic association (i.e., categorization and clustering), semantic elaboration/chaining, and imagery (auditory and visual) resulted in significant improvements on standardized tests of semantic memory.

As part of a series of publications by the Academy of Neurologic Communication Disorders and Sciences (ANCDS) on evidence-based practice (EBP) in the clinical management of neurogenic communication disorders, an ANCDS working group completed a systematic review of evidence for using internal memory strategies (O'Neil-Pirozzi,

Kennedy, Sohlberg, 2016). Forty-six articles met inclusion/exclusion criteria and were included in the review. The authors identified eight different categories of strategies in the literature, with visual imagery the most frequently studied, in isolation or in combination with other internal strategies. Despite significant variability in research methods and outcomes across studies, the authors concluded that the evidence supported the use of internal memory strategies for individuals with brain injury. Important, however, was the authors' conclusion that future research needs to use person-centered outcome measures of effectiveness, as 80% of the studies reviewed used decontextualized, non-functional outcomes such as performance on a standardized memory test. Additionally, the authors noted that systematic instruction procedures appeared to be the optimal approach for introducing and training strategies, as studies that used systematic instruction reported the largest treatment effects.

Strategies to Improve Academic and Vocational Performance

A functional domain with a long history of being successfully supported by cognitive strategy instruction is academic performance. We note that the strategies used to improve academic performance are often the same as those applied to improve effectiveness in the workplace for tasks that require reading, writing, and learning. The study-skills strategy literature for students with developmental learning challenges is large and provides a cross-population resource for strategy use with the brain injury population; however, more work is needed specifically with students whose learning challenges are a result of ABI. Below we describe several studies conducted in the brain injury population.

One of the most common academic activities for which cognitive strategies are used is to facilitate reading comprehension and retention. A recent systematic review and meta-analysis describes the deficits in global reading ability, including reading comprehension, that result from ABI and limit functional reading (Pei & O'Brien, 2021).

A frequently used reading comprehension strategy in the ABI literature is Preview, Question, Read, State, and Test (PQRST; Ciaramelli, Neri, Marini, & Braghittoni, 2015), which has been used to support recall of text passages. Readers are taught to complete each strategy phase sequentially while reading to build meaning constructs and strengthen associations. Another group of researchers used a phase model of reading strategy and designed and evaluated a multicomponent reading comprehension strategy package specifically for people with brain injury returning to postsecondary academic settings and needing assistance reading college-level textbook material (Griffiths, Sohlberg, Kirk, Fickas, & Biancarosa, 2016). The reading strategies were designed to be completed at three different phases in the reading process: prereading, during reading, and postreading. Prereading strategies guide readers through a preview phase where they review the section headings in the target academic textbook chapter. The active reading phase guides them to select up to three key ideas per paragraph and then summarize key points in their own words. The review phase encourages testing oneself on the summary content. The results of their study indicated that the use of a three-phase reading comprehension strategy was associated with recall of more correct information units in immediate and delayed free recall tasks, more efficient recall in a delayed free recall task, and increased accuracy recognizing statements in a sentence verification task.

Butler and colleagues (2008) developed a package of cognitive strategies designed to improve general academic performance in school-age children and adolescents with attention and executive function impairments resulting from radiation and chemotherapy for cancer treatment. Just like the aforementioned reading comprehension strategy package, the authors categorized strategies in three phases according to the chronology in which they would be used: *task preparation, during a task,* and *posttask* (see Table 7.4). The strategies were applied in conjunction with attention exercises and shown to result in functional gains, but the multicomponent nature of the intervention makes it difficult to parse out the contribution of the strategies versus the attention activities.

A less commonly studied domain in the ABI literature is the use of strategies for writing. Although there is a robust writing strategy literature in the area of learning disabilities, there has been very little research in brain injury. One study provided preliminary support for writing strategy prompts during essay writing by people with brain injury (Ledbetter, Sohlberg, Fickas, Horney, & McIntosh, 2019). The strategy intervention prompted the clients with cognitive impairment following brain injury to perform certain writing functions, such as checking that their work contained a thesis statement; reviewing it to ensure that paragraphs contained a main idea and supporting details; ensuring that the essay contained a conclusion; and re-reviewing their essay before finishing it. Results of the study showed increased essay quality when strategy prompts were provided.

As previously discussed, clinical application of strategy use allows the clinician and client to collaborate to personalize a strategy that addresses functional need and helps the client manage the cognitive issues that are affecting their academics. Strategies can be used for every aspect of academic performance including studying for tests, completing assignments, and managing materials. The selection and coaching processes will be the same whether for academic or vocational tasks that require reading documents and writing reports.

TABLE 7.4. Examples of Cognitive Strategies Used at Different Task Intervals to Improve School Performance

Task preparation strategies	During-task strategies	Posttask strategies
"Magic words": Selected to increase confidence or assist with affective state.	"Talk to myself": Verbal mediation.	"Check my work": Increase self-monitoring.
"Soup breath": Relaxation technique.	"Mark my place": Assist with sustained attention.	"Ask for feedback": Increase self-monitoring.
"Game face": Approach task with confidence and minimize distraction.	"Start at top" or "Row by row": Assist with organization and attention.	"Reward myself": Increase engagement.
"World record": Increase engagement.	"Time-out": Pacing strategy.	
"Warm up my brain": Increase readiness.	"Look at floor": Increase focus during public speaking or reading tasks.	
	"Ask for a hint": Solicit support.	

Based on Butler et al. (2008).

This chapter has thus far reviewed a wide range of cognitive strategies that can be applied to assist with a myriad of cognitive challenges and applied to support any number of functional targets. There is substantial evidence to support the use of strategy instruction for people with cognitive impairments following brain injury. What is often not explicit in the research is the methods for personalizing, teaching, and evaluating strategy use (O'Neil-Pirozzi et al., 2016). The next section applies the PIE framework to strategy instruction and provides clinicians with specifics for clinical implementation.

PIE: PLANNING FOR STRATEGY INSTRUCTION

By now the reader will be familiar with the PIE framework. Chapter 5 provides a thorough description of the key elements involved in the treatment process. In this chapter, we review the elements that are specific to cognitive strategy instruction. For the sake of clarity, this chapter describes the PIE elements relevant to cognitive strategy instruction in the distinct categories of *planning*, *implementation*, and *evaluation*, and the reader is referred to Chapter 5 for a reminder of how the PIE process is actually circular and iterative. In this chapter, we review assessment and target selection under *planning*, the application of treatment ingredients under *implementation*, and the selection and administration of treatment measures under *evaluation*. In practice, however, the clinician will have selected treatment ingredients and measurement tools as part of the planning process and will be conducting ongoing evaluation and treatment modification throughout therapy. We begin with a review of the two key components in the planning phase: assessment and selection of treatment targets and aims.

Assess and Hypothesize

The clinician will first consider the abilities and needs of the individual client. Generating a profile of client characteristics relevant to strategy training will usually begin with a clinical interview of the client and relevant everyday people and may include standardized cognitive testing depending on the clinician's hypothesis about the nature of the client's cognitive challenges. Test information can be helpful for both determining whether strategy training would be effective and also assisting with the selection of a strategy. Assessment may thus include standardized testing and observation or self/family report protocols, as well as a clinical interview.

During the assessment process, the clinician will assess whether strategy training would be a good match for the client in terms of the client's preferences and abilities. The motivational interview processes described in Chapter 3 will reveal whether the client has sufficient motivation and awareness to recognize the benefits of strategy use and would consider using this approach. While facts and simple routines (Chapter 6) and the use of external aids (Chapter 8) can be trained as automatic behavioral sequences that tap into procedural memory without significant client insight, the initial use of cognitive strategies requires an understanding of when to implement the strategy and a sense of how the strategy will be helpful (Sohlberg & Mateer, 2001). Ideally, strategy implementation will become automatic over time with practice.

The interview process will also allow the clinician to answer the following questions:

1. *What is the specific need?*
2. *Where is the target environment?*
3. *When will the client implement the strategy?*

The clinician will begin the planning process by *specifying the need and associated challenge* that the strategy will address. Selecting a best-fit strategy requires conducting a systematic needs assessment that leads to hypotheses about the nature of the cognitive challenges that may be addressed by strategy training. For example, a clinician may hypothesize that the underlying issue preventing a client from completing their aim "to feel socially connected" is a limitation in self-regulation of comments during conversations, as the client makes comments that are off-putting to other people. This hypothesis suggests the potential for a conversational strategy that assists with self-regulation and self-monitoring. Alternatively, the clinician may hypothesize that the underlying challenge is due to lack of initiation, which may indicate the potential for an "ask partner a question" strategy to increase participation in conversation. Interviews, home visits if possible, and perhaps executive function assessment may assist with hypothesis testing and lead to strategy options to review and discuss with the client.

Assessing the target environment is critical to identifying a good strategy match, as environmental factors can have a critical influence strategy use. For example, training the client to use a mindfulness strategy for homework is unlikely to be effective if there is no reliable quiet space. The clinician's task is to determine which assessments will be necessary and feasible.

A needs assessment is the process by which *the clinician identifies factors unique to the client and environment that will determine the best strategy match for the client's needs*. Essentially, the clinician is conducting an ecological assessment integrating relevant client characteristics (cognitive, psychosocial, physical, and sensory abilities as well as sociocultural values) with environmental considerations, then generating possible strategy options that will address the need and be usable by the client in their environment. Figure 7.1 depicts the clinical decision-making process to help identify a good strategy match—in this case, for a client who is struggling to complete household chores (for a blank version of this form, see Form 7.1 at the end of this chapter, as well as a fillable version in the digital files accompanying this book). In some cases, it might be necessary to conduct a dynamic assessment or trial intervention period to determine which strategy will be most useful. For example, a clinician may assist the client in using two different strategies to complete a task and then encourage the client to compare the two strategies' effectiveness in helping the client achieve their target. The client will also provide input about preferences for different types of strategies (particularly if that strategy is something they would not have used premorbidly or looks conspicuous in public). The adoption of a strategy is more likely if the assessment process is collaborative and person-centered, where the client is involved in the strategy selection, has endorsed its utility, and perceives it to be useful (Frampton et al., 2017).

Clinicians and researchers at the University of Minnesota and the U.S. Department of Veteran Affairs created a program emphasizing client involvement in the selection of strategies (Ferguson, MacLennan, Cates, Rich, & Hughes, 2021). The authors provided clients with strategy options and encouraged clients to select *Just One Thing* (JOT) from the list that would help them move forward. Their goal was to simplify instructions and training by having the client commit to "just one target" that would address a priority

Strategy Selection Worksheet

DEFINE THE NEED

A. To manage processing deficits in order to complete selected goals (e.g., maintain attention; control impulsivity; remember information):	**OR**	B. To improve performance on a specific activity (e.g., reading comprehension, writing accurate work report): *Completing household chores in a timely manner (vs. abandoning part-way and having to return later and start from scratch)*

⬇   ⬇

CONSIDER KEY CLIENT & STRATEGY CHARACTERISTICS

☑ **Maximum strategy complexity** (e.g., number of steps; level of abstraction) that can be processed by client:

Abstraction not a concern for client or need; must limit # steps to 4–5 (per assessment results re working memory)

☑ **Client insight and motivation:**

Strong, no concerns; wants to do this independently (no prompting from husband)

☑ **Environmental triggers to initiate strategy use:**

Items tend to accumulate in visible locations (e.g., mail ends up on table near front door, laundry sits in laundry room)

☑ **Timing of strategy use:**

No specific timing need identified as long as chores are done each week

☑ **Opportunities to use strategy:**

Minimum 3 times per week; likely at least 5 times per week

⬇   ⬇

GENERATE OPTIONS FOR COGNITIVE STRATEGIES

1. *State "Focus" each time mind wanders from a step involved in the chore*

2. *Self-talk verbal mediation strategy to "say out loud" steps of each chore (client feels this level of detail is needed to achieve independence)*

3.

FIGURE 7.1. Matching strategy, need, and client.

area. To teach strategy use, they used systematic instruction, including a self-reflection process in which the client evaluated whether the strategy was useful.

Once the strategy is selected, the clinician, usually in collaboration with the client, will identify the steps or components involved in using the strategy in order to systematically train different behaviors. Essentially, the clinician generates a task analysis to teach and monitor progress on strategy learning. The two clinical Case Applications at the end of this chapter illustrate the systematic strategy selection and identification of strategy steps.

Define Targets, Aims, and Measures

An important part of the planning process is to identify the desired outcome or aim. The clinician must be clear on the answer to this question: *Why am I teaching this strategy?* And it should be specified as part of the planning process. At this juncture, the clinician will specify measurable targets and aims and plan for multilevel evaluation. Examples of measurement are described in the "PIE: Evaluating Outcomes of Cognitive Strategy Instruction" section.

Confirm Treatment Aims and Impact Measures

As described in Chapter 4, treatment aims, often called long-term goals, represent broader aspects of daily functioning, often involve more than one skill, and may require more than one discipline's contribution. Aims often fall into the participation level of the International Classification of Functioning, Disability and Health (ICF) model. Examples of treatment aims that lead to the selection of a strategy designed to improve retention of textbook material might be "improve grade point average" or "pass all classes." Examples of a treatment aim that lead to a goal management strategy might be "increase independence for household tasks" or "be promoted to next level at workplace." The selected strategy should be directly related to the achievement of the aim. Collaboratively identifying the aim through the assessment process will ensure that therapy goals are meaningful and functional. Impact measures associated with aims are described in the "PIE: Evaluating" section below and may include goal attainment scaling (GAS) or other impact data as detailed in Chapter 5.

Confirm Treatment Targets and Progress Measures

As described in Chapter 4, treatment targets are the specific aspects of function that is expected to change as a direct result of therapy. Ultimately, treatment targets are selected because they will lead to the client achieving their aims. In the case of strategies, they are only useful if they impact function or the selected treatment aim. There will usually be several treatment targets associated with one treatment aim.

Using the Rehabilitation Treatment Specification System (RTSS) framework outlined in Chapter 4, treatment targets for cognitive strategy training often include both representational/knowledge targets (R targets) and skill/habit targets (S targets). Strategies can be somewhat abstract given that they are internally generated and designed to help complete a specific activity or improve some aspect of daily functioning. Some clients will be able to generate their own strategy and easily learn any associated components. Their treatment targets might just involve practice (S targets) applying the strategy. Other clients will need to acquire prerequisite knowledge and/or address psychosocial factors (R targets). For example, clients must understand and remember the purpose of any steps needed to execute the target strategy. They must also have sufficient motivation to initiate strategy use. Knowledge and affective states that are prerequisite to strategy use will be addressed as R targets. Examples of R targets might be "to independently state the names and describe the purpose of each step of the PQRST strategy" or "to move to level 4 on the 'readiness' scale." S targets will relate to being able to demonstrate strategy use. A common initial S target may be "to independently demonstrate application of the five goal management strategy steps in session as applied to completing budgeting and bill-paying activities."

The clinician will identify progress measures for the established targets, which typically will include evaluating the client's understanding and ability to use the strategy or demonstrate the steps in the strategy that have been taught. Progress measures ultimately should capture whether strategy use is being generalized and maintained in the target environments and, if so, whether the strategy is addressing the identified need. The "PIE: Evaluating" section below gives samples of session data for measuring treatment progress on target acquisition as well as generalization, maintenance, and impact data.

Goal (Target and Aim) Writing

Chapter 5 outlined the components necessary for writing treatment targets and aims, including treatment approach, treatment target, objective performance measurement, criteria, level of independence, and conditions/context. See Forms 5.1 and 5.2 in Chapter 5 for target and aim writing checklists using Specific, Measurable, Attainable, Relevant, and Time-based (SMART) criteria and GAS requirements. Examples of goals are also provided in the Case Applications that appear at the end of this chapter.

The planning process will have generated a target strategy, with individual steps or behaviors that comprise the strategy, to achieve a specific treatment aim. Planning will also include identification of treatment ingredients or the components of the specific intervention to be used with individual clients. The next phase is to *implement* strategy training.

PIE: IMPLEMENTING COGNITIVE STRATEGY INSTRUCTION

The training plan for teaching a person with cognitive impairments to use strategies varies greatly depending on the client and strategy, and separate training phases may or may not be necessary. A review of compensatory memory strategy interventions reported a wide range of therapy doses ranging from a single hour used to describe and demonstrate a strategy to therapy programs that required 30 treatment hours over several weeks (West, 1995).

Effective strategy use in everyday settings requires the client to independently and usually automatically initiate strategy use in the needed context. The clinician will evaluate the following prerequisites in order to know where to start in training.

Knowledge

- The client knows the goals of the strategy and the specific procedures or steps.
- The client recognizes tasks or environments that will benefit from strategy use.
- The client knows how strategy use will meet their needs.

Affective and Motivational States

- The client believes that the strategy will be useful, the level of effort to use the strategy will be worthwhile, and they are capable of implementing the strategy.
- The client feels sufficiently motivated to use the strategy and be engaged in the process of strategy development and training.

Skills

- The client can demonstrate the strategy steps.

The sequence of steps in the training program depends on the extent to which the client meets the above prerequisites at the beginning of the training. The clinician will begin the implementation phase by assessing the client's knowledge, affective and motivational state, and relevant skills. The strategy will have been selected with input from the client using the process as shown in Figure 7.1. The clinician may have previously determined that separate R targets are required to ensure sufficient knowledge and motivation to implement the strategy. Alternatively, the clinician may identify treatment ingredients that are designed to promote engagement and motivation and embed them as part of the S target for teaching the strategy. For example, the clinician might have the client rate level of motivation or track their correct responses while they are training the strategy steps.

If the clinician has determined that there should be a separate R target for teaching the prerequisite knowledge and mindset for using the strategy before launching into strategy training, they would select ingredients such as asking questions and teaching responses based on need. Sample questions are listed below followed by an example of S target training:

Sample Questions Assessing Requisite Knowledge

1. "If you implement [the target strategy], how do you think it will help you?"
2. "What are the specific steps you would follow to apply [the target strategy]?"
3. "When do you think you would use [the target strategy]?"

Sample Questions Assessing Requisite Affective and Motivational States

1. "If our therapy time is successful in teaching you to use [the target strategy] in your everyday life, do you think it will be valuable? Why or why not?"
2. "On a scale of 1–5, where 1 is 'very easy' and 5 is 'impossible,' how hard do you think it will be to do [the target strategy]?"
3. "Do you think it will be worth trying the strategy?"

Requisite Skills

1. "Show me how you might use our strategy to do [the goal activity]."
2. "Show me what you would do if [a given circumstance or event] occurred."

(Provide scenarios for the client to demonstrate the ability to use, not use, and be able to adapt the strategy appropriately.)

If the client lacks requisite knowledge and beliefs, the acquisition phase of training will need to address teaching these concepts and information as described below. Clients with milder cognitive impairments, particularly those with relatively intact executive functions, may be able to skip the acquisition phase or may only need a short period of the S (skill) target training. These clients may see a demonstration of the strategy in their treatment session, be able to use the strategy in their home environment, and become independent in applying it to a variety of situations. Others will require formal training and planning for generalization and maintenance. Below we outline training phases with the understanding that the clinician will identify which areas need to be addressed for any given client.

Initial Acquisition Phase of Training

As described above, for some clients the initial phase of training may be used to target conceptual knowledge or motivation and will require targeted instruction. For all clients, it will be important to establish that they know how and when to use the target strategy before beginning to train the steps. Three guiding questions will help ensure clients are clear on the purpose and use of the strategy:

- The goals of this strategy are to help me _____.
- I use this strategy when _____.
- These are the steps of the strategy: _____.

If the client cannot demonstrate the requisite knowledge, the clinician may need to explicitly train this information as indicated above. Ingredients for training this information (R target) could include the clinician writing down the information and asking the client to assist in generating the answers, and then reviewing information using the errorless and spaced retrieval regimen discussed in Chapter 6 for training simple facts and concepts. Figure 7.2 is a sample data-collection sheet that can be used to monitor a client's learning of basic strategy information (also available as Form 7.2 at the end of the chapter and in the accompanying digital files). A set of four questions are asked at the beginning and end of the therapy session. Note that for clients with significant impairments in declarative memory or insight, the question wording should be varied to avoid a stimulus-bound response. Clients with severe memory impairments may learn a hyper-specific response such that a question worded the same each time triggers an automatic response that is not processed consciously. For example, the clinician may vary the phrasing of the question: "How can your strategy be useful to you?" to "Why would you want to use your strategy?" or "Share some benefits you might get from using the strategy." This will help train the concept and prevent hyperspecificity.

A second target of the initial acquisition phase is to ensure that the client can perform the strategy correctly in an optimal context (e.g., with maximum support and structure and no distractions). The clinician will usually begin by teaching the client the individual steps or components of the strategy, typically using the error minimization techniques and massed practice followed by distributed-practice methods described in

Strategy Knowledge Questions

	Date Jan 23		Date Jan 25		Date Jan 27	
	Start	End	Start	End	Start	End
What is the name of your strategy?	A	A	A	I	I	I
Describe the steps in your strategy.	M	A	A	A	A	I
What are examples of when you would use your strategy?	A	A	A	I	I	I
How can your strategy be useful to you?	M	M	A	A	A	I

M = Modeled—presented entire answer.

A = Assisted—gave partial response.

I = Independent—reasonable answer.

FIGURE 7.2. Monitoring strategy knowledge: completed form for Strategy Knowledge Questions.

Chapter 5. Hence, the therapy ingredients are systematic instruction applied to strategy implementation. Readers should review the information in Chapters 5 and 6 for the training framework that is particularly important for establishing a new behavior when a client has declarative learning impairments.

Acquisition of a strategy often requires providing explicit cues to prompt steps or components. The clinician will begin by modeling strategy use, then may introduce one of the following learning supports as the strategy is being practiced:

- Checklist of the strategy steps
- Written cue cards prompting strategy steps
- Auditory prompt (e.g., alarm) to initiate strategy
- Client stating each step or a keyword representing that step as it is implemented

Ideally, the client will internalize the steps of the strategy and these supports will be withdrawn during the mastery phase, although some clients may benefit from or require an ongoing reference such as a checklist or an auditory prompt. The clinician will demonstrate the different components of the strategy and then have the client implement the strategy. With practice, the client should be able to retain the target strategy steps over increasing time intervals. Again, this may be achieved through the use of massed practice when initially learning the steps (or when an error is made) followed by longer intervals of distributed practice using the aforementioned learning supports as determined by the clinician.

Figures 7.3 and 7.4 show sample completed therapy session and progress monitoring datasheets for recording the performance of a client learning to use a self-talk

Therapy Session Data Form—Target Acquisition, Mastery, Generalization (Strategy Use)

Client Name: Hareem **Date:** Jan 25 **Location:** Clinic **Others Present:** Amir (husband)

Target: Independently use the self-talk verbal mediation strategy for **Associated Aim:** Complete all household tasks on chore list within scheduled timeframe independently **Training Phase:** Acquisition

home chores practiced in session

Ingredients—Items:
Index card with strategy steps
Index card with steps for chores
Items required for chores
Blank progress recording sheet

Ingredients—Actions:
Reviewing strategy rationale, steps
Error control with repeated practice
Chaining of steps

Ingredients—Motivators:
Hareem will record own progress
Encouragement/praise

Measurement Plan:
steps done independently
Length of time to complete relative to anticipated time

Check-in Info and Results of Homework: Feeling frustrated and non-productive therefore very motivated to start strategy. Selected 3 priority chores (reading and sorting mail, reconciling monthly Visa to budget, preparing grocery list), prepared steps for each and brought materials for each.

Practice Data: Strategy Steps:	Retention Probe	Practice 1:	Practice 2:	Practice 3:	Practice 4:
		Mail	Mail	Mail	Mail
5. when done, fill out chore performance sheet		+	+		+
4b. say step in your head as you do it		N/A	N/A		N/A
4a. say each step/action aloud as you do it		5/5	5/5		5/5

(continued)

FIGURE 7.3. Example of completed Therapy Session Data Form—Target Acquisition, Mastery, Generalization (Strategy Use).

150

Therapy Session Data Form—Target Acquisition, Mastery, Generalization (Strategy Use) *(page 2 of 2)*

Practice Data:	Retention Probe	Practice 1:	Practice 2:	Practice 3:	Practice 4:
3. begin task		+	+	–	+
2. gather needed materials (enter #)		3/3	3/3	2/3	3/3
1. select chore, state chore and target time aloud		+	+	+	+
Comments:	No retention probe—first time working on strategy today	Model plus index cards prior to every step	Model faded but directed to index cards for every step	No supports; distracted by phone during step 2; instructed strategy steps again	Returned to directing to index cards before each step to reduce errors

Session Summary/Analysis of Progress:

Independent with index cards; did not record predicted or actual times today

Feedback and Homework Provided (task, context, ingredients, tracking):

Replicate exactly as above using index cards and only for mail sorting right now

Plan for Next Session:

Fade supports (leave chore task card visible but remove card with strategy steps); add additional chore if support fading successful

FIGURE 7.3. *(continued)*

151

Progress Monitoring Form—
Target Acquisition, Mastery, Generalization (Strategy Use)

Client Name: Hareem   **Target:** Independently use the self-talk verbal mediation strategy for home chores practiced in session   **Training Phase:** Acquisition

Select the summary measure being tracked (must use the same from each session):

☑ Retention probe result from start of each session

☐ Average of each session's practice trial results

☐ Other:

	Summary Measure			
	Jan 28	Feb 1	Feb 4	Feb 8
Strategy Steps:	Mail Sorting	Mail Sorting	Mail Sorting	Mail Sorting
5. when done, fill out chore performance sheet			+	+
4b. say step in your head as you do it			N/A	N/A
4a. say each step/action aloud as you do it	–	3/5	5/5	5/5
3. begin task	+	+	+	+
2. gather needed materials (enter #)	3/3	3/3	+	+
1. select chore, state chore and target time aloud	+	+	+	+
Ingredients:				
Prompts and Supports:	Retention Probe: -index card provided for needed materials and steps involved in chore but not for strategy steps	Retention Probe: -index card provided for needed materials and steps involved in chore but not for strategy steps; completed first 3	Retention Probe: -index card provided for needed materials and steps involved in chore but not for strategy steps	Retention Probe: -no index cards provided at all! Practice Trials: -added Grocery List for 1 practice trial (used index card

(continued)

FIGURE 7.4. Example of completed Progress Monitoring Form—Target Acquisition, Mastery, Generalization (Strategy Use).

	Practice Trials: -required massed practice of step 4, chaining to step 3 and adding spoken "let's start" to step 3 to help initiate self-talk in step 4	chore steps using out loud self talk before getting distracted Practice Trials: -independently achieved all 5 steps in final practice trial	Practice Trials: -independently achieved all 5 strategy steps in final practice trial without referring to chore task cards!	for tasks involved in chore but no card required for strategy steps) –same level of success -will continue task generalization and start moving toward distributed practice
Motivational:	-Records own progress -Encouragement and praise	-Records own progress -Encouragement and praise	-Records own progress -Encouragement and praise	-Records own progress -Encouragement and praise
Other Measures:				
	9 min to complete final practice trial, had estimated 5, ratio = 1.8	Time ratio in final practice trial = 1.5	Time ratio in retention probe = 1.6	Time ratio in retention probe = 1.3

FIGURE 7.4. *(continued)*

strategy (see Forms 7.3 and 7.4 at the end of the chapter for blank versions of these forms, as well as fillable versions in the digital files accompanying this book). The data were taken early in the acquisition phase. This sample client would have already demonstrated knowledge of the strategy and understanding of the benefits and application and will have moved on to practicing the strategy during a structured therapy session. Once the client can independently demonstrate use of the strategy on target tasks in the clinic, training will move on to the generalization phase. There may be instances when the strategy can be trained directly on the ultimate target from the beginning. For example, a clinician may work with a client in their home or workplace where targets occur, or the target may be completely replicable in the clinical setting (e.g., via role-playing or in interactions with an attending family member).

Mastery and Generalization Phase of Training

The mastery phase occurs when knowledge about the strategy purpose and ability to follow the basic strategy steps has been acquired, but strategy implementation is not consistent and has not generalized to the natural environment. For clients who have executive function impairments but relatively intact declarative memory, moving to the mastery and generalization phase may occur after a single session. Clients with moderate to severe declarative learning impairments may require more practice and review to learn the basic strategy steps. Information about when to implement the strategy also may need to be formally taught. Failure to generalize treatment gains to everyday life is the hallmark of executive function impairments, so these clients will require specific attention to generalization as a part of their training process as discussed below.

The goal of the mastery and generalization phase of training is to increase the fluency and automaticity with which the client implements the strategy in everyday life. In many cases, targeting generalization may occur in tandem with the acquisition phase and might not represent a sequential set of targets. Generalization targets are achieved by attending to four aspects of training:

1. **Fading learning supports.** This refers to the progressive withdrawal of supports such as clinician prompts and cues, and also internalization of the strategies. For example, if the client is saying each step aloud as it is completed, this can be faded to inner speech ("say it in your head"). Similarly, the client may go from physically checking off each step on a checklist to using the list as a written reference when needed. Some clients may always depend on external cues and prompts to use their strategies, particularly clients who have severe memory or executive function impairments and those who need to use the strategy in an unpredictable context. If an external cue or prompt is effective, efficient, and preferred by the client, there is no *a priori* reason to remove it.

2. **Lengthening the distributed practice.** The clinician will increase the interval between practice trials to reinforce independent strategy use over increasingly longer periods of time. When the retention probe administered at the beginning of the session indicates sufficient fluency with the strategy steps, the clinician can start varying training contexts to promote generalization.

3. **Incorporating or increasing stimulus variability.** For many clients, unless their cognitive impairments are very mild, generalization or transfer of learning will need to be planned and trained explicitly. A main goal of this stage is to identify triggers that will facilitate the *initiation of strategy use* in the *target context*. These will have been identified in the planning process and then incorporated during this phase of training. Examples of generalization training methods include:

- Varying training stimuli so the strategy can be triggered by a variety of environmental cues
- Involving people in the natural environment who will serve as "cues" in everyday life
- Training strategy use in the target everyday context
- Creating a home program for practicing strategy use in collaboration with client and home supports
- Providing the client with everyday reminders to implement the strategy between therapy session; using cues such as voicemail, text messages, or email

4. **Increasing or maintaining engagement.** It may be difficult for the client to maintain motivation and interest in using the strategy beyond the clinic, particularly if it is difficult to use. While this was addressed earlier in training by collaborating with the client in strategy selection, it also is important to consider strategies to maintain client motivation and engagement after discharge. As discussed in Chapter 3, these factors are important predictors of long-term treatment adherence. Ingredients to increase enthusiasm and commitment for implementing strategy include:

- Creating a customized log to help the client and/or support people record strategy use and impact to provide a concrete record of improved functioning with strategy use
- Conducting motivational interviewing (see Chapter 3; Miller & Rollnick, 1991), where you ask questions that encourage the client to explore ambivalence about using the strategy, such as asking about situations when the strategy would have been useful, even if the client was not able to implement it
- Collaborating with the client to identify potential benefits and barriers to strategy use in daily living, and developing alternative plans
- Developing record sheet showing benefit of strategy use (e.g., time saved, number or type of goals completed, improvements in task accuracy, duration of time devoted to target task)
- Developing a formal plan for maintaining strategy use, such as the client setting future reminders in their calendar

Maintenance Phase

As described in earlier chapters, the maintenance phase refers to therapy methods that increase the likelihood that a rehabilitation target will be retained after therapy ends. The clinician should actively plan how to avoid abandonment of strategy use once therapeutic support is no longer available. For a strategy to be maintained, it must become automatic and internalized. The primary methods to promote ongoing implementation of a strategy are the *incorporation of natural supports* and *cumulative review* (see Chapter 5). The techniques listed above for increasing metacognitive engagement facilitate the involvement of natural supports and provide a mechanism for checking in on strategy use. The use of diaries, logs, and "check-ins" can be very helpful for maintaining strategy use particularly during the phase when therapy supports are withdrawn.

In terms of long-term strategy use, it is important to acknowledge that contexts and situations change; mechanisms need to be in place for reevaluating strategy effectiveness. Depending on the service delivery model, context, and strategy complexity, the client may benefit from follow-up visits and phone support to maintain or modify strategy use over time.

PIE: EVALUATING OUTCOMES OF COGNITIVE STRATEGY TRAINING

Previous chapters have emphasized the importance of multilevel outcome evaluation. As noted, the planning process results in selection of *targets* or short-term objectives addressed in therapy sessions leading to *aims* or long-term, functional outcomes. The different types of evaluation needed to direct intervention include three progress measures: *target acquisition data*, *generalization probe data*, and *maintenance data* in addition to *impact data* selected to evaluate functional outcome. Examples of the different types of data needed are shown in Table 7.5 and provided in the Case Applications at the end of the chapter. Chapter 5 contains a thorough review of measurement selection and outcome evaluation requirements.

Acquisition data measures progress in both knowledge and motivation (R targets) and also skills in using the strategy (S targets). For strategy training in the acquisition phase, data may be used to evaluate R targets such as accuracy of the client's response

TABLE 7.5. Examples of Strategy Measurement

Type of data	Examples	Purpose
Target acquisition data	• Ability to independently list and describe each step in the strategy • Ability to independently state purpose and benefit of strategy • Number of possible applications client able to generate for using strategy during their week • Number of strategy steps demonstrated in clinic session with no prompting • Longest time interval client retained and demonstrated the entire strategy	• Measure knowledge and skills to carry out strategy. • Guide decisions about progress toward short-term objectives and indicate when to move on or provide more review.
Generalization probes	• Number of entries in strategy diary • Number of teacher observations of independent strategy use • Number of strategy checklists completed during the week • Spouse or client ratings of "helpfulness" in strategy log • Number of times lost place during reading session • Number of reminders to return to task	• Measure use of strategy in intended context. • Measure perception of effectiveness.
Maintenance probes	• Number of times strategy used weekly according to entries in the strategy log for initial 2 months following cessation of treatment • Number of strategy checklists turned in to teacher during weeks 2 and 3 after therapy	• Measure implementation of strategy over time.
Impact data	• Grades on weekly history quizzes • Number of items on "to do" list completed independently • Ability to greet church-group members by name as reported by spouse • Caregiver burden rating for spouse reminders • Improvements on the Inattention Rating Scale	• Measure whether implementation of strategy is meeting identified need.

to knowledge questions about the components of the strategy and when and where to use the strategy. Motivation or engagement may be measured by using a "readiness to use strategy" self-rating. Acquisition data may be used to measure S targets such as the number of strategy steps the client demonstrates independently on a practice activity. Skills training will require practice scenarios to facilitate strategy practice. Acquisition data may also be used to evaluate fluency or efficiency of strategy use (e.g., number of steps initiated without hesitation) in addition to accuracy. These data will guide therapy and tell the clinician when to move forward in therapy or back up and provide additional support or training. As strategy implementation becomes consistent, strategy use will be measured under different conditions, including application in everyday environments. These are the generalization and maintenance data.

Generalization and maintenance data will often address both S and R targets and capture initiation of strategy use in naturalistic contexts, amount of support required, and perceived helpfulness and satisfaction with the strategy. Self-report logs, as well as other types of logs and questionnaires, may be used to gather these data. Again, these data will tell the clinician whether they need to decrease or add supports.

It is necessary to measure the impact of strategy use and determine whether the strategy achieved the desired functional impact in the client's everyday life. This may be in the form of a GAS scale that uses an overall functional goal broken into five potential levels of progress (see goal attainment scaling in Chapter 5). For example, the GAS aim might be to "greet sewing club members by first name," to be achieved by training the client to use the strategy of reading members' nametags before greeting them. A confidant in the group could track the number of correct names used in two different meetings after the strategy had been learned, which would provide a GAS score that could be used as the impact measure.

An alternative measurement example might be used with a client who had learned a goal-completion strategy and was implementing it in the target environments. The clinician could measure whether the strategy resulted in improved task completion on a task log kept by the spouse.

USE OF STRATEGIES FOLLOWING MILD TRAUMATIC BRAIN INJURY/CONCUSSION

One group for whom strategy use is particularly helpful are individuals recovering from mild traumatic brain injury (mTBI; aka concussion). There is good evidence of benefits of psychoeducation on recovery and prevention of persistent symptoms after mTBI, including education on strategies to manage symptoms, for both children (McNally et al., 2018) and adults (Mittenberg, Tremont, Zielinski, Fichera, & Rayls, 1996; Vanderploeg, Belanger, Curtiss, Bowles, & Cooper, 2019). Compared with a control group, Mittenberg and colleagues (1996) demonstrated that providing adult clients with mTBI in the emergency room with information on expectations for recovery and strategies for managing symptoms reduced overall symptom duration time. When learning declarative information is the target, one well-validated ingredient for typical adults is the *teach-back method*, which focuses on the communication and delivery of information between the clinician and the client (Talevski et al., 2020). Teach-back involves asking clients to explain in their own words what a health provider has just told them. Any misunderstandings are then clarified by the health provider and understanding is checked again. This process continues until the client can correctly recall the information that was given. The teach-back method is "not a test of the person's knowledge as much as an exploration of how well the information has been taught and what needs to be clarified or reviewed" (Talevski et al., 2020).

When clients may be coming for one or two visits to receive education and symptom management strategies that they will independently implement, it may be helpful to use the teach-back method. Figure 7.5 depicts a flowchart showing the process of implementing teach-back, termed *Team-Ed* (Selven & Batts, 2021). Implementation is illustrated by the script in Figure 7.6, which addresses sleep hygiene, a very common area of strategy management that aims to prevent cognitive symptoms associated with poor sleep (Chesnutt, 2021). Note that while clients with mTBI might not require systematic instruction techniques to *learn* strategies, they may need structured intervention to acquire the habit of *using* those strategies. At minimum, when habitual strategy use is

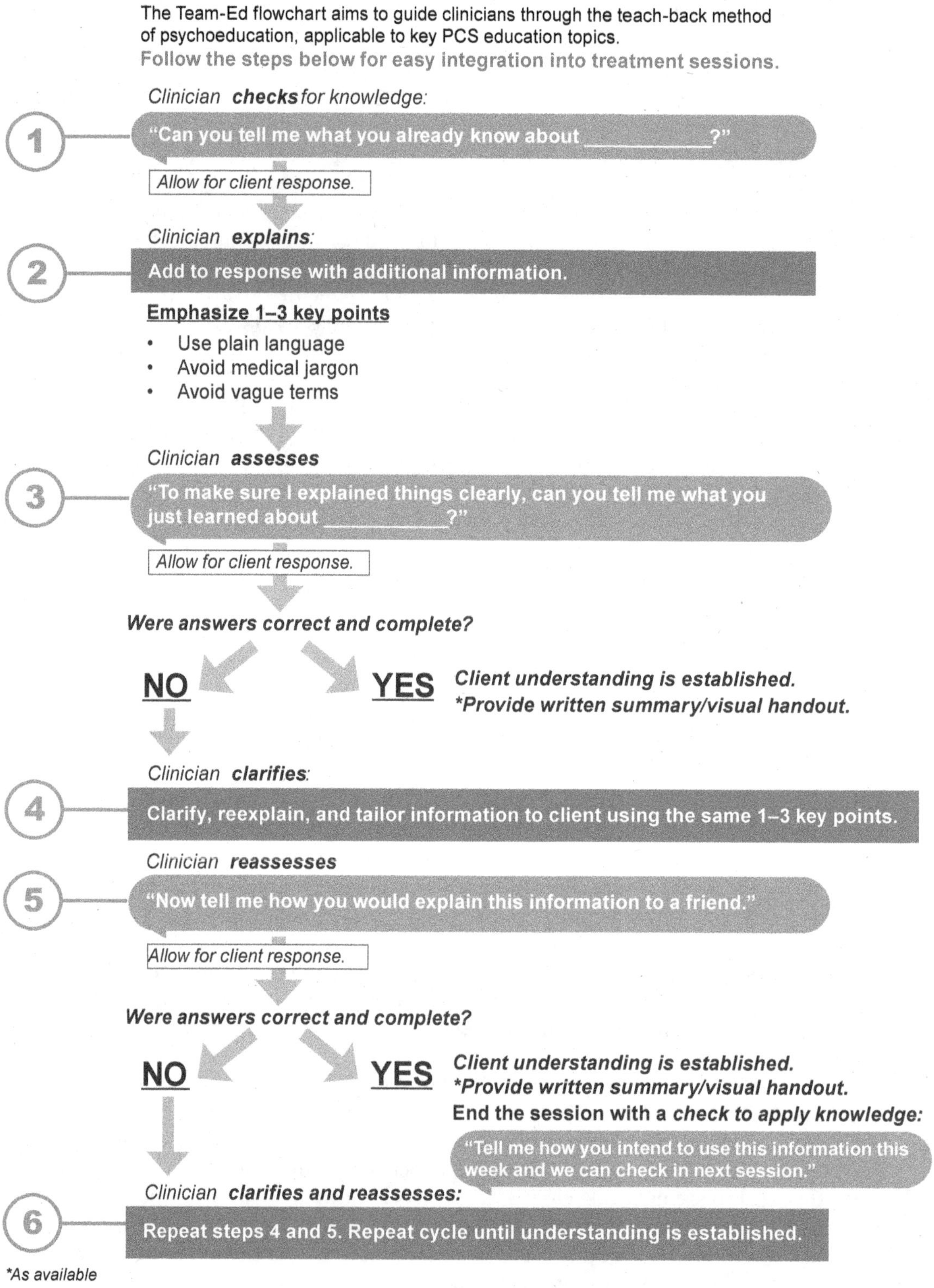

The Team-Ed flowchart aims to guide clinicians through the teach-back method of psychoeducation, applicable to key PCS education topics.
Follow the steps below for easy integration into treatment sessions.

Clinician **checks** for knowledge:

1 "Can you tell me what you already know about _____?"

Allow for client response.

Clinician **explains**:

2 Add to response with additional information.

Emphasize 1–3 key points
- Use plain language
- Avoid medical jargon
- Avoid vague terms

Clinician **assesses**

3 "To make sure I explained things clearly, can you tell me what you just learned about _____?"

Allow for client response.

Were answers correct and complete?

NO   **YES**   Client understanding is established.
Provide written summary/visual handout.

Clinician **clarifies**:

4 Clarify, reexplain, and tailor information to client using the same 1–3 key points.

Clinician **reassesses**

5 "Now tell me how you would explain this information to a friend."

Allow for client response.

Were answers correct and complete?

NO   **YES**   *Client understanding is established.*
Provide written summary/visual handout.
End the session with a *check to apply knowledge*:

"Tell me how you intend to use this information this week and we can check in next session."

Clinician **clarifies and reassesses**:

6 Repeat steps 4 and 5. Repeat cycle until understanding is established.

*As available

FIGURE 7.5. The teach-back method of education (Team-Ed) flowchart for persistent concussion symptoms (PCS). Adapted by permission from Amy Selven and Betsy Batts.

PCS psychoeducation topic: Sleep Hygiene

This script provides an example scenario between clinician and client during a treatment session. The clinician uses the teach-back method of education to discuss the topic of sleep hygiene with the client. The *italicized* text highlights the teach-back prompts from the Team-Ed flowchart.

Clinician: *Can you tell me what you know about sleep hygiene?*

Client: I don't really know what sleep hygiene is. I guess it means that sleep is important—try to get 8 hours?

Clinician: Good, let me add on some information. Sleep hygiene refers to healthy sleeping habits. There are several ways to help improve your sleep including reducing caffeine and alcohol, setting a regular bedtime and routine, and creating a comfortable and quiet sleeping space. By getting enough quality sleep, you can help your brain recover and help minimize the effects that things like anxiety, or memory and attention issues have on your day.

Clinician: *To make sure I explained things clearly, can you tell me what you just learned about sleep hygiene?*

Client: Sure. So, sleep hygiene is healthy sleeping habits. Some things like caffeine and alcohol are not good for sleep. By getting better sleep, it can help me get better faster.

Clinician: Great! Let me clarify a few things. There are some other ways that you can also improve your sleep—things like getting a consistent bedtime and a quiet space to sleep so that you can feel well-rested and give your brain a chance to recover. You're right that it can help you get better faster, but it can also help minimize anxiety, memory and attention issues in your day-to-day activities.

Clinician: *Now, tell me how you would explain sleep hygiene and ways to improve sleep to a friend.*

Client: Okay, I would tell them that sleep hygiene is good sleeping habits. Some ways to do this are, not having caffeine or alcohol, going to bed at the same time every night, and having a quiet place to sleep. This will help my concussion recovery and lower the impact of other things like memory/attention problems and anxiety.

Clinician: Excellent, you covered all the main points! *Before you go, tell me how you intend to use this information this week and we can check in on it next week.*

Client: I usually get up at 7 am for work, so I'm going to use the bedtime reminder on my phone to help me go to bed at 10 pm. That way I can set up a routine.

Clinician: That's a great plan! Next session, I'm going to ask about how that went. *Also, here's a handout covering the information we talked about today. If you have any questions, write them down and we can talk about it next week.*

FIGURE 7.6. Team-Ed example script. Adapted by permission from Amy Selven and Betsy Batts.

the target, then intervention must include ingredients to increase the client's motivation and likelihood of generalizing a strategy to everyday life (see the discussion of motivation ingredients in Chapters 3 and 4).

SUMMARY

This chapter has provided an overview of cognitive strategy training as an approach to manage cognitive impairments. A summary of the clinical sequence and procedures for selecting and training the use of cognitive strategies is as follows:

PLAN

- Interview the client to learn who they are; determine possible treatment aims that reflect sociocultural lived experiences, beliefs, values, and identities; and select assessment tools and procedures to determine if strategy training is the optimal treatment approach.
- Administer assessment tools and procedures to evaluate hypotheses about cognitive challenges interfering with functional aims and determine whether the client has the prerequisite abilities to effectively use cognitive strategies.
- Conduct a needs assessment that integrates relevant client characteristics (cognitive, psychosocial, physical, and sensory abilities as well as sociocultural values) with environmental considerations and then generate possible strategy options.
- Select a strategy to train in therapy that addresses functional needs and conduct a task analysis to identify the steps or components of the strategy.
- Define functional and meaningful treatment aims and associated impact measures.
- Determine whether the client will need motivational or knowledge targets (R targets) and, if so, develop the corresponding targets and measures.
- Develop skill/habit targets (S targets) that operationalize the steps or components of the strategy that will be trained and define associated progress measures.
- Use SMART and/or GAS formatting for aims and targets (see Forms 5.1 and 5.2 in Chapter 5).
- Identify the phase of learning (acquisition, mastery/generalization, or maintenance) and select ingredients that are appropriate for the target group (e.g., distributed practice for S targets, self-reflection or knowledge questions for R targets) as well as the client's skills, values, and psychological status.

IMPLEMENT

- Prepare session data and progress monitoring forms (see Forms 7.3 and 7.4).
- In the initial treatment session, train the strategy steps in an optimal context with all required supports for that client (e.g., checklist of strategy steps, cue cards, prompts).
- In each subsequent session:
  o Review strategy application homework results.
  o Conduct a retention probe to determine recall of strategy steps since the prior session.
  o Conduct practice trials, starting at the level indicated by the retention probe.

- o At the generalization phase of learning, alter strategy training ingredients to support generalization (e.g., fading supports, increasing distributed practice intervals, increasing stimulus variability, ensuring sustained motivation).
- o At the maintenance phase of learning, alter ingredients to maximize natural supports and sustain motivation and accountability (e.g., diaries, check-ins).
- o Document results and prescribe homework.

EVALUATE

- • After each session, analyze progress to guide advancement to the next phase of learning.
- • In the generalization and/or maintenance phases, obtain impact measures to evaluate the achievement of treatment aims and guide the continuance or discontinuation of intervention.

PUTTING IT ALL TOGETHER: CASE APPLICATIONS

In the remainder of the chapter, we provide examples to show the integration of the PIE framework for strategy training with actual clients. We begin by detailing two examples of strategy training taken from the research literature that illustrate and support key components of the PIE framework. We selected the imagery strategy training described by Kaschel and colleagues (2002), as it used a rigorous experimental design with detailed description of the training process and reported positive outcomes. We also summarize the strategy training curriculum evaluated in a pilot study by Novakovic-Agopian and colleagues (2018) that evaluated strategy training to address challenges related to executive dysfunction. The research examples are followed by the description of two Case Applications that represent composite clients from our own practices. In the first Case Application, we support the reader in working through the stages of applying the information in a structured manner, making use of the various forms presented in this book, and supply sample completed forms. In the second Case Application, we provide similar structured guidance, but instead of supplying sample completed forms, we encourage the reader to complete the procedures independently.

Two Examples from the Literature

Research Example 1

Kaschel and colleagues (2002) completed a randomized controlled trial comparing visual imagery strategy training to "pragmatic memory training" (i.e., usual care) for adults with memory impairments after acquired brain injury (primarily TBI or stroke). The goal of the imagery strategy was to enable clients to rapidly generate simple but distinct images of nonvisual information (e.g., conversations, text, prospective actions to be completed) and use the images as retrieval cues for target verbal information or carrying out intended tasks (prospective memory tasks). The training program included two training phases, and treatment efficacy was measured by comparing recall in clients who received the training to that of clients receiving other types of memory treatment.

The first training phase in the imagery group, analogous to the acquisition phase of implementation in the PIE framework, taught participants the basic skill of quickly generating images. It contained three components: (1) motivation for imagery training, in which participants were shown how generation of autobiographical images enhanced their recall; (2) practice with rapid generation of images of simple objects; and (3) practice with generation and retrieval of images of simple actions. The acquisition of the basic skill of generating images was hierarchically organized and systematically increased in difficulty. Initially, objects and actions were presented visually using video. Gradually, the screen was withdrawn and object and action names were read to the participants with no visual cues. In addition, the rate of stimulus presentation was gradually increased as clients became more adept at generating and recalling images. In the final step of the acquisition phase, participants recalled several objects and three complex actions. Once a participant could recall three complex actions using self-generated pictures during a filled retention interval of 90 seconds, they were considered to have met the learning criteria for the acquisition phase. Acquisition criteria were established for each level of difficulty and, if failures occurred, training continued at the same level until criteria were reached. As such, this procedure followed the instructional principles described throughout this manual of aiming for high rates of correct practice and using distributed practice.

The second phase of training, the individualized transfer period, was analogous to the generalization and mastery phases of the PIE framework. The researchers selected individualized verbal targets and prospective memory tasks that were relevant to each participant (e.g., books related to the participant's job, newspapers that they read, or their own appointments or tasks). Participants were taught to identify the target information to be remembered, consider how imagery could be used to remember this information, and then practice using the imagery. Each participant's recall was recorded.

The researchers described multiple types of evaluation, another component of the PIE framework. The authors collected session data on the accuracy of recall using imagery during the acquisition and transfer phases of learning and used these data to determine when the participant could advance to the next level of difficulty. Efficacy of the intervention was evaluated using standardized neuropsychological tests, including a story recall test and an "appointments" test. Generalization was measured using relatives' ratings of frequency of memory problems. The researchers also collected control data on neuropsychological functions not expected to improve (e.g., selective attention). Maintenance data were collected at a 3-month follow-up visit. Results showed that clients with mild memory impairments learned to generate distinct images rapidly and use these images successfully to remember either information they had read or actions they intended to carry out. There was specific improvement on neuropsychological tests related to verbal recall and prospective memory and not on tests of selective attention. Relatives reported a decreased frequency of memory failures in everyday life, and all of these effects were maintained over 3 months.

In summary, a cognitive strategy, visual imagery, was shown to be highly efficacious when training was systematic and incorporated motivation, skill acquisition, generalization, and maintenance. This program provides a training model for any type of metacognitive strategy.

Research Example 2

Novakovic-Agopian and colleagues (2018) reported results of an executive function intervention for veterans with chronic challenges after brain injury. The intervention was

Goal-Oriented Attention Self-Regulation (GOALS), a training program that taught participants mindfulness-based attention regulation and goal management strategies and how to apply them to participant-selected real-life goals. GOALS training emphasized training regulation of distractibility by teaching participants to use a cognitive strategy (Stop-Relax-Refocus) to stop activity when distracted, anxious, and/or overwhelmed; relax; and then refocus attention on the current primary goal. Consistent with the PIE framework of moving from acquisition to generalization and maintenance, participants were taught to apply the strategies to simple information-processing tasks and then progressed to applying them to more challenging low-structure situations occurring in their own lives. Generalization training was provided by asking participants to identify personally relevant and feasible functional goals (e.g., finding an apartment, looking for a job, writing a school term paper) and applying the goal management strategies to the functional task(s) of their choice.

Results showed that training resulted in increased likelihood for competitive employment and long-term improvement in daily functioning. The study provides support for systematic training that moves from acquisition, to mastery, to maintenance.

Two Case Applications

Below we provide two case examples where strategy training was applied to help clients achieve their aims. For Case Application 1, as we describe the stages of intervention, we direct the reader to practice applying the information in a structured manner, making use of the various forms presented in this book (fillable forms for each item are included in the digital files accompanying this book). Completed Case Application Sample Answers are included at the end of this chapter. For Case Application 2, we offer the reader an opportunity to practice and apply the principles and procedures reviewed in this chapter and demonstrated in Case Application 1. Sample answers are not provided for this case. Rather, this case provides an opportunity for readers to practice their skill in following a structured approach in planning, implementing, and evaluating the intervention.

CASE APPLICATION 1—ESTHER

Description of Client

The client, Esther, was a 54-year-old Pacific Islander who was seen for therapy 2 years after surgical resection, chemotherapy, and radiation to treat cancer. While medical treatment had been successful in treating Esther's cancer, it had left her with cognitive impairments. She was receiving outpatient services because she complained of not being able to organize and complete tasks. She ran a small bookkeeping business from her home and reported difficulty meeting deadlines. Although she sat down at her computer at 9 a.m. most weekdays, when she opened her bookkeeping program, the current- and past-due task reminder widget seemed to have even more items than the day before. She also described frustration about the messy state of her home office, not to mention other areas in the home. She lived with her husband, who was retired, and had two grown children who lived out of state. Esther was authorized for an assessment and five outpatient visits.

Planning

The speech-language pathologist initiated a needs assessment, including an interview with the client and her husband as well as supplementary cognitive testing to evaluate memory, attention, and executive functions. The assessment revealed the following client profile:

Sociocultural values. Esther greatly valued independence and ensuring that others perceived her as highly effective and efficient. Microaggressions had been ever-present throughout her lifetime of social, academic, and vocational experiences, and she was proud of having succeeded despite them.

Cognitive findings. Esther's scores on standardized memory and attention tests were within normal limits. Scores on tests of executive function were in the moderately impaired range, particularly on tests requiring self-regulation and the ability to monitor completion of multiple tasks. She was observed to respond impulsively on some tests. Regarding daily cognition, Esther's prior learning and knowledge of bookkeeping tasks as well as other work and home-management tasks (e.g., knowledge of her husband's food allergies) remained intact. She was proficient in using a computer and in using multiple applications on her cell phone.

Physical and sensory functions. Esther reported no concerns.

Psychosocial functioning. Esther reported that she was frustrated by negative changes in her own performance on home-management and work tasks, and she appeared highly motivated to improve her situation. Her husband stated that while Esther was self-aware and frustrated by her difficulties, this awareness tended to occur after a task or activity had not gone well. She tended to be overly optimistic and dive into tasks with limited self-regulation and not use her prior negative experiences to guide future behavior. He said that Esther became resentful if he tried to assist.

Environmental variables. Esther's husband kept the home environment organized and tended to clean up when Esther had started but not completed multiple projects. Esther had hired an assistant to help with office organization tasks for an hour or so each week. Esther valued this support, but also found it stressful knowing that someone was coming into her home every week.

Esther's aim was to improve task completion for home and work activities and eliminate the problem of "multiple things started and nothing completed." The results of the interview and testing revealed a need for a strategy that would provide structure for Esther and help her control impulsivity and improve task persistence.

Application Practice

Fill out Form 7.1: Strategy Selection Worksheet using the information provided above. Once complete, compare to completed Case Application Sample Answer: Form 7.1 at the end of this chapter.

Form 7.1 allowed the clinician to synthesize the key information gathered, document the important variables to consider when selecting a strategy, and then present options for goal completion strategies to Esther and her husband. Two strategies were of most interest to them: (1) goal management strategy (Levine et al., 2000) and (2) a customized self-monitoring, task-persistence strategy. After discussion, it was decided that the most useful approach would be a customized strategy that helped Esther set goals, monitor time and progress, and reflect on performance. It was felt that this would provide more structure and accountability than a goal management strategy that might not address her difficulty in straying from the target task and beginning a new task. Esther and her husband collaborated with the therapist to design a strategy that would build on her strengths, which included motivation and fluency with a cell phone and apps, and compensate for her difficulties with self-monitoring and task persistence. They defined the steps of the strategy and piloted it in the clinic together before finalizing the plan. It was important for Esther to have a strategy that emphasized self-affirmation and reflection. The following were the agreed-upon steps of the strategy:

1. Esther would identify the activity she wanted to engage in and set her phone alarm for 10-minute increments for a total duration of 30 minutes.
2. When the alarm went off, she would reflect on her performance:
   - If she had stayed on the target task, she would verbally reinforce herself.
   - If she had gone off-task, she would redirect herself back to the target activity.
3. After the 30-minute interval was complete, Esther would rate her level of distractedness during the task on her Notes app.

Application Practice

Document the aim, target, ingredients, and strategy steps on Form 7.3: Therapy Session Data Form. Target acquisition, generalization, and maintenance will be measured by independence in carrying out the strategy steps in increasingly varied contexts, but additional measures could *also* be included. Based on the information provided above, brainstorm ideas for other measures that could be meaningful to Esther. Add this measurement plan to Form 7.3. Copy the target, training phase, and strategy steps onto Form 7.4: Progress Monitoring Form. Compare your forms to the Case Application Sample Answer: Form 7.3, Session 1 and Case Application Sample Answer: Form 7.4, at the end of the chapter, but don't peek at the data sections yet!

In addition to measures of performance in session, Esther and her husband developed a "task journal" to document the ultimate impact of the new strategy on the number of home and work tasks completed each week. They planned to document the tasks that had been started and completed as intended, any interfering tasks that Esther started that interrupted the completion of the target task, and their respective frustration levels.

Application Practice

Based on the information above and using the checklist in Form 5.2 in Chapter 5, create three GAS scales to measure the ultimate impact of strategy training in Esther's day-to-day life. Compare your scales with the Case Application Sample Answer: Rating and Attainment Scales at the end of the chapter.

Implementation

The acquisition phase of training initially focused on R targets relating to motivational variables and increasing Esther's knowledge of how her self-monitoring strategy might help address some of the problems identified in the "task journal." Following the template in Form 7.2: Strategy Knowledge Questions, Esther was able to describe how her strategy might allow her to complete discrete bookkeeping tasks. For example, she described how the strategy would help her continue inputting account data and resisting checking email, as not doing that had resulted in her not inputting target account data in the past. Esther was able to verbalize the steps of the strategy after several demonstrations and made herself a small cue card to post at her computer. She also prepared a list of self-affirming statements to select from when successful so that she could provide herself with specific feedback instead of the generic "good work" that she thought she might default to.

Esther then moved to the S target of becoming independent in implementing the strategy. In addition to the previously defined steps, as an error-prevention method Esther agreed to begin by having the clinician gently prompt her to look at her cue card or cell phone at the 5-minute mark if she appeared to be getting distracted. She practiced using the strategy in the clinic for bookkeeping tasks identified in her task journal (e.g., entering expense receipts for a client). Because of the length of the strategy practice (30 minutes for each trial), the prepractice retention probe focused on Esther verbally explaining the steps of the strategy (the R target) instead of demonstrating them (the S target), and the clinician decided to use the final practice trial at each session as the summary measure to monitor session-to-session performance.

In the first practice trial at the first session, Esther independently selected an expense receipt task and set the timer. In both the first and second 10-minute periods, the clinician noticed that Esther's attention appeared to be wandering and therefore used the agreed-upon error-prevention method of prompting her to look at her cue card at the 5-minute mark. When the timer went off at the 10-minute mark in both the first and second segments, Esther redirected herself. About a minute into the final 10-minute segment, Esther closed her laptop and said she needed a break. When she returned, the clinician began a second practice trial, and Esther completed the first two steps of the strategy independently (including using a self-affirming statement for staying on task for 10 minutes) and completed steps 2b and 2c with prompts at the 5-minute mark. Esther forgot to complete the distraction rating, so the clinician had to remind her and she gave herself a 4 on her scale of 5 (highly distracted) to 0 (not distracted at all). The clinician recommended that Esther replicate this task at home the next day with another expense receipt activity. In spite of not wanting to rely on her husband for support, Esther agreed to have him provide a prompt at the 5-minute mark if needed during practice completed in this first week of intervention.

Application Practice

Document the practice results from Session 1 on Form 7.3 and document the summative measure for this first session on Form 7.4. Compare your forms to the Case Application Sample Answer: Form 7.3, Session 1 and Case Application Sample Answer: Form 7.4, at the end of the chapter.

In Session 2 on August 12, Esther reported following through with the strategy practice at home the prior day. She did not document her results, but her husband reported that he had to prompt her at the midpoint of each of the 10-minute segments, which resulted in an argument in the third segment. Esther reported that she no longer wished to complete this practice with her husband's help. She also indicated that she had decided to turn off email notifications until she became more effective in carrying out the strategy. During the retention probe at the beginning of the session, Esther demonstrated 100% accuracy in describing setting the alarm on her cell phone, self-evaluating her task performance each time the alarm came and then continuing her task, and entering her "temptation to stray from task" rating on her Notes application on her cell phone. In both practice trials in Session 2, Esther demonstrated all five steps of the strategy without the error-prevention prompting while completing her computer bookkeeping tasks in the clinic. In the first trial, she used a self-affirming statement in step 2a but had to redirect herself for the other steps. In the second practice trial, she was able to use self-affirming statements in steps 2a and 2c. She rated her temptation to stray as a 3 in both trials. Esther was encouraged to replicate this practice at home the next day, still focusing on expense receipts, but remembering to document her results this time. If Esther continued with this level of success, the clinician planned to expand the range of bookkeeping tasks to include revenue receipt entry.

Application Practice

Create a new Form 7.3 to document this session's results and add the summative information to Form 7.4. Compare your forms to the Case Application Sample Answer: Form 7.3, Session 2 and Case Application Sample Answer: Form 7.4, at the end of the chapter.

The generalization phase of training focused on increasing the range of tasks that Esther practiced in the clinic and reinforcing her use of the strategy at home through the task journal. In Session 3 on August 14, the clinician added a different type of bookkeeping task (revenue receipts), and in Session 4 a week later (the clinician increased the length of time between sessions), Esther agreed to include home bill payments. She independently completed each step of the strategy on all four trials completed across these two sessions. Although she still needed to redirect herself at the 10-minute mark about one-third of the time, she was always successful in doing so and even rated herself as a 2 on her distraction rating scale on the last home payment activity. In Session 4, Esther was also able to move the cue card off to the side rather than having it in her immediate line of sight: she reported feeling optimistic that she could soon put it away altogether.

Esther's husband had been documenting her performance in their task journal, but when Esther identified feeling sensitive about him overseeing her performance, they decided that she would complete the performance logs in the task journal, and he would just add comments from his perspective. Esther was using the strategy successfully according to the performance logs brought to the fourth session.

Application Practice

You may skip generating additional session data forms but add the summative measures from Sessions 3 and 4 to Form 7.4 along with other key highlights from these sessions. Compare your form with Case Application Sample Answer: Form 7.4.

Evaluation

The initial evaluation included target acquisition data tracking the number of strategy steps completed independently for the tasks completed in therapy sessions, the percentage of 10-minute segments that required redirection versus reward, and the distraction rating. Generalization data used the same metric for tasks of increasing variety completed in the clinic as well as similar tasks completed at home and documented in the performance logs.

The fifth and last treatment session was used both as a maintenance/follow-up session and to administer impact measures. It was scheduled 4 weeks after the fourth session. Esther and her husband brought in the performance logs and reported that the strategy was working well. The performance logs showed that Esther continued to implement the strategy independently over the 4-week maintenance period. She continued to vary in needing to redirect versus reward herself when the alarm went off, but she reported not being very concerned with that because of other successes. For example, the logs showed that she successfully completed 10 to 12 target tasks per week. These were mostly bookkeeping-related, but she was consistent with home bill payments and usually consistent with laundry folding. She rarely recorded a "temptation to stray" rating of greater than 1. The couple had made one adjustment to the strategy: Esther decided to set the alarm for 20-minute rather than 10-minute intervals as she was now able to stick to the task at hand for this amount of time, and a longer task interval allowed her to make more progress and feel reinforced for her persistence. Esther no longer needed to hire external help to stay on top of her work duties, and this helped bring her overall stress down to an "acceptable" level on her scale. She reported being hopeful that she might achieve the "optimal" level as she continued to internalize and generalize the strategy further.

Application Practice

Compare your scales with the Case Application Sample Answer: Achieved Rating and Attainment Scales at the end of the chapter.

CASE APPLICATION 2—ANDERS

Description of Client

The client, Anders, was a 24-year-old veteran of mixed racial background who was seen for outpatient therapy services for impairments due to an mTBI as a result of repeated blast injuries incurred during 3 years of combat duty. He was also diagnosed with posttraumatic stress disorder (PTSD). Anders had completed high school and had no previous learning difficulties, although he reported being unmotivated in school as an adolescent, mostly receiving C's and D's. At the time of therapy, he was enrolled in several general studies courses at the local community college in preparation to transfer to the university to pursue a teaching credential. He was living independently with his girlfriend. Anders was receiving counseling to manage anxiety symptoms and was then referred for cognitive rehabilitation due to difficulties with recalling what he read in his textbooks. During the initial interview, Anders reported that he completely understood his textbook assignments while he was reading, but later could not recall the information sufficiently to answer questions on a quiz. He had tried to use extensive repetition and note taking, but this had not improved his performance and seemed to be worsening his fatigue levels each day.

Planning

The clinician initiated a needs assessment including an interview with Anders and review of his recent neuropsychological test results. The following key findings were revealed:

Sociocultural values. Anders reported that, as an adolescent, he had lacked purpose and direction, but the military had instilled in him a deep respect for self-discipline and a "can do" attitude. His mother was proud of him for having followed in her family's history of military service.

Cognitive findings. Anders's IQ was within normal limits. Testing showed a moderate impairment in working memory, mild impairment in new learning and immediate recall for verbal information, and moderate impairment in delayed verbal recall. A reading assessment revealed that comprehension of paragraph-length material was within normal limits.

Physical and sensory functions. Anders described experiencing headaches when working in brightly lit rooms and also a "shields up" phenomenon where he suddenly couldn't process any incoming information.

Psychosocial functioning. Anders described episodes of significant anxiety symptoms, including profuse sweating, rapid heart rate, and a sense of needing to urgently relocate. These episodes often occurred when he was studying, and once his anxiety began it would escalate and he would need to cease the study session. Anders also reported struggling to adapt to structuring his own days after a number of years of highly regimented routines. He reported that being self-disciplined was easier when each day's events were structured for him, and admitted to being worried that he was becoming "lazy" again. He was very motivated to perform well in his classes and was eager to pursue a teaching career. Anders's descriptions of his difficulties suggested good self-awareness and insight.

Environmental variables. Anders described difficulty concentrating if he was near a window or in fluorescent lighting, if someone approached his study table or desk, or if he heard ambient noise.

Results of the interview and testing revealed the need for a reading strategy that would help Anders to more deeply process new information and connect it to existing semantic knowledge to compensate for impairments in working memory and verbal learning. It was also clear that the strategy would need to help him organize his study environment in order to manage anxiety. Using Form 7.1 to guide the process, the clinician was able to propose options for several different reading strategies, including use of a graphic organizer that facilitated mapping main ideas and supporting facts and the SQ3R (Survey, Question, Read, Recite, Review) strategy that facilitated preview, active reading, and review. The clinician had Anders try both strategies using a dynamic assessment. The latter strategy was clearly superior at helping him retain content using a reading passage from one of his textbooks. Anders and the clinician therefore agreed upon the following steps for his study strategy:

Space: Anders would survey the environment to select a location that would minimize the chance for anxiety symptoms to occur and where he could integrate the anxiety management breathing strategies he had been taught in counseling. Key characteristics of a good study environment included quiet, low traffic, no windows, and no fluorescent lighting. Some study rooms at the library met these criteria, as did the loft in his apartment. This step of the strategy required Anders to ensure he was in a conducive study space before embarking on the SQ3R strategy that follows.

Survey: Anders would skim the material to make note of the main topics and ideas.

Question: Anders would generate questions to guide his reading of the material, grouped into sections based on his initial survey of the chapter.

Read: Anders would then use the structure provided from the prior two steps to read the material.

Recite: After each section of the chapter, Anders would ask himself the questions he generated earlier and try to answer them from memory, and if he could not, look back in the text to find the correct information.

Review: At the conclusion of the chapter, Anders would re-review the questions for the entire chapter, try to first answer from memory, and if not possible, check back in the text.

The six steps were written out with detailed instructions on a piece of paper and then copied in short form (Space, Survey, Question, Read, Recite, Review) onto a small cue card. The evaluation plan was to collect: (1) acquisition data to measure Anders's learning of the steps of the strategy; (2) strategy generalization/maintenance by having Anders bring in homework agendas that he used to record where he studied and what he accomplished; and (3) impact data by having Anders report his performance on class quizzes.

Application Practice

Document the aim, target, ingredients, strategy steps, and measurement plan on Form 7.3: Therapy Session Data Form. Where information has not been specifically provided above, brainstorm options that would work for Anders. Copy the pertinent items onto Form 7.4: Progress Monitoring Form. Referring to Form 5.3 in Chapter 5, generate a progression plan to systematically increase the complexity of reading tasks. Using the checklist in Form 5.2 in Chapter 5, create one or two GAS scales to measure the ultimate impact of strategy training in Anders's day-to-day life. No sample answers are provided; instead, complete this task independently to practice application of the principles in the planning stage.

Implementation

The acquisition phase of training initially focused on teaching Anders to describe (R target) and demonstrate (S target) each of the six steps of his reading strategy. Given Anders's strong insight and motivation, the clinician quickly determined that there was no need to conduct monitoring of his strategy knowledge and instead moved from the R target into practice with the S target. Anders brought in his textbooks, and the clinician selected different chapters to use as training stimuli in conjunction with the homework agenda form that had been created. Initially, Anders demonstrated each step by reading aloud the full description of the step and then completing it. This was then faded to just using the short forms on the cue card. As session data, the clinician recorded the percentage of time Anders could describe and complete each step with just the written cue list. Within three sessions over 2 weeks, Anders was independent in implementing his strategy for selected passages. While there continued to be no need to provide training on motivational factors or strategy knowledge, Anders did require an additional target relating to recognizing when he was approaching the "shields up" phenomenon so that he could plan for a break, rather than suddenly abandoning the task at hand. A new strategy plan was made to integrate this target into the overall intervention plan.

The generalization phase of training was concurrent with the acquisition phase as Anders was asked to bring in his homework agendas from the very beginning of strategy instruction. Strategy successes and difficulties were reviewed using the homework agendas. As Anders became more efficient and independent in using his reading strategy during the therapy session, the clinician used the progression plan to select reading passages that were longer and more complex. As Anders began to successfully use his reading strategy, therapy was reduced to once every 2 weeks. Maintenance probes evaluating strategy use were taken by counting the number of times the strategy was used as reported on the homework agenda.

Application Practice

Brainstorm hypothetical results from each training session, based on the information provided above. Document these training results on Forms 7.3 and 7.4. Once again, no sample answers are provided; instead, generate responses and then compare with the principles in the implementation stage.

Evaluation

The initial evaluation included the target acquisition/generalization data tracking the number of strategy steps completed independently as well as homework logs showing what was accomplished each day. The ultimate impact of strategy training was evaluated by examining Anders's performance on his class reading quizzes. He had received a C or D on all of his quizzes prior to his midterm (the first 2 weeks of therapy). He began to demonstrate independent, accurate use of his strategy during Week 3 of therapy, and his quiz average improved. He received three B's and one C during the subsequent weeks of the term. Interestingly, while still experiencing headaches, Anders reported that his anxiety symptoms occurring during study periods had greatly diminished. He shared that he no longer needed to be as rigid about selecting study spaces and was able to focus without anxiety when sitting at different study desks throughout the library. He felt that the self-regulation imposed by the reading strategy process provided him with a sense of control, and his improved reading performance helped mitigate anxiety. Anders's new reading and study strategies provided additional structure to his day, and he began feel as if his self-discipline was returning. Finally, Anders reported less fatigue and less time redoing previously studied material due to recognizing signs of when the "shields up" phenomenon would occur and therefore wrapping up his study time in advance.

Application Practice

Using the information above, generate one or two additional GAS scales that could have been used to measure the ultimate impact of strategy training in Anders's day-to-day life. Make sure that there are five equidistant, unidimensional, measurable levels of progress, with baseline performance being a –1.

Strategy Selection Worksheet

DEFINE THE NEED

A. To manage processing deficits in order to complete selected goals (e.g., maintain attention; control impulsivity; remember information):	OR B. To improve performance on a specific activity (e.g., reading comprehension, writing accurate work report): *Reduced impulsivity and improved task persistence for home and work tasks—starting with bookkeeping*

⬇ ⬇

CONSIDER KEY CLIENT & STRATEGY CHARACTERISTICS

☑ Maximum strategy complexity (e.g., number of steps; level of abstraction) that can be processed by client:

No issues with attn, memory, comprehension; impulsivity and poor self-regulation during multi-step tasks—need emphasis on task persistence

☑ Client insight and motivation:

Motivation is high but insight is low pre-task initiation (tends to be overly optimistic)

☑ Environmental triggers to initiate strategy use:

When bookkeeping program is started on computer, a widget showing reminders for current and old items opens automatically

☑ Timing of strategy use:

9am on weekdays (when Esther sits down at the computer to start her workday)

☑ Opportunities to use strategy:

For bookkeeping—4 mornings/week (Wednesdays will be "off" days for mental rest); once expanded to other tasks, many more opportunities

⬇ ⬇

GENERATE OPTIONS FOR COGNITIVE STRATEGIES

1. *Goal management strategy*
2. *Customized self-monitoring, task persistence strategy*
3.

Therapy Session Data Form—Target Acquisition, Mastery, Generalization (Strategy Use)

Client Name: Esther   **Date:** Aug 10   **Location:** Clinic   **Others Present:** Joseph (husband)   **Training Phase:** Acquisition

Target: Independently use the "time, remind, reflect" strategy twice per day, 4 days per week

Associated Aim: Complete all bookkeeping tasks on time with no outside support required

Ingredients—Items:
Timer and Notes app on phone
Cue card with strategy steps
Laptop with bookkeeping program
Blank progress recording sheet

Ingredients—Actions:
Reviewing strategy rationale, steps
Prompting to look at cue card or phone when she appears to be distracted (to promote errorless completion)

Ingredients—Motivators:
Esther records own progress
Encouragement/praise
List of self-affirming statements

Measurement Plan:
steps done independently
self-affirms vs redirects
Distraction rating

Check-in Info and Results of Homework: Esther brought all required materials with her, including a list of 5 different self-affirming statements.

Practice Data:	Retention Probe	Practice 1:	Practice 2:	Practice 3:	Practice 4:
Strategy Steps:		Expense Receipts	Expense Receipts		
3. rate overall level of distractedness during task			− Needed reminder Rating = 4		
2c. self-affirm or redirect after third 10 min		D/C Requested break	+ Prompt at 5 min mark Self-redirect		
2b. self-affirm or redirect after second 10 min		+ Prompt at 5 min mark Self-redirect	+ Prompt at 5 min mark Self-redirect		

(continued)

Practice Data:	Retention Probe	Practice 1:	Practice 2:	Practice 3:	Practice 4:
2a. self-affirm or redirect after first 10 min		+ Prompt at 5 min mark Self-redirect	+ No prompt Self-affirm		
1. select task, set timer for 10 min x 3		+	+		
Comments:	Esther verbally described steps 100% (no time for full probe)	++distractible (looking around room, sighing) even before 5 min mark	Retained focus well for first 10 min segment		

Session Summary/Analysis of Progress:

No difficulties using apps, understands steps and value of strategy, needs support to stay engaged with task

Feedback and Homework Provided (task, context, ingredients, tracking):

Repeat task at home tomorrow—OK for Joseph to provide prompt at 5 min mark if needed (Esther agreed to this when reviewing her session results)

Plan for Next Session:

Continue with expense receipts task but see if 5 min prompt can be faded

Esther's Goal Attainment Scales—To Be Achieved in 5–6 Weeks

1. Esther no longer needs outside help for work tasks.

2. GAS results:

Tasks Completed in Past Week

-2 Much less than expected	-1 Less than expected (baseline)	0 Expected outcome	+1 Better than expected	+2 Much better than expected
Does not complete any tasks without help.	Completes 1–2 tasks per week without help.	Completes 3–5 tasks per week without help.	Completes 6–10 tasks per week without help.	Completes 10 or more tasks per week without help.

Stress Level in Past Week

-2 Much less than expected	-1 Less than expected (baseline)	0 Expected outcome	+1 Better than expected	+2 Much better than expected
Stress level reported as extreme.	Stress level reported as high.	Stress level reported as moderate.	Stress level reported as mild or acceptable.	Stress level reported as optimal.

Distraction Level in Past Week

-2 Much less than expected	-1 Less than expected (baseline)	0 Expected outcome	+1 Better than expected	+2 Much better than expected
Average temptation to stray rating = 3–5.	Average temptation to stray rating = 2–3.	Average daily temptation to stray rating = 1–2.	Average temptation to stray rating = 0–1.	Average temptation to stray rating = 0.

Therapy Impact Data for Esther

Tasks Completed in Past Week

−2	−1	0	+1	+2
Much less than expected	**Less than expected (baseline)**	**Expected outcome**	**Better than expected**	**Much better than expected**
Does not complete any tasks without help.	Completes 1–2 tasks per week without help.	Completes 3–5 tasks per week without help.	Completes 6–10 tasks per week without help.	Completes 10 or more tasks per week without help.

Stress Level in Past Week

−2	−1	0	+1	+2
Much less than expected	**Less than expected (baseline)**	**Expected outcome**	**Better than expected**	**Much better than expected**
Stress level reported as extreme.	Stress level reported as high.	Stress level reported as moderate.	Stress level reported as mild or acceptable.	Stress level reported as optimal.

Distraction Level in Past Week

−2	−1	0	+1	+2
Much less than expected	**Less than expected (baseline)**	**Expected outcome**	**Better than expected**	**Much better than expected**
Average temptation to stray rating = 3–5.	Average temptation to stray rating = 2–3.	Average daily temptation to stray rating = 1–2.	Average temptation to stray rating = 0–1.	Average temptation to stray rating = 0.

Therapy Session Data Form—Target Acquisition, Mastery, Generalization (Strategy Use)

Client Name: Esther   **Date:** Aug 12   **Location:** Clinic   **Others Present:** Joseph (husband)   **Training Phase:** Acquisition

Target: Independently use the "time, remind, reflect" strategy twice per day, 4 days per week on time with no outside support required

Associated Aim: Complete all bookkeeping tasks on time with no outside support required

Ingredients—Items:
Timer and Notes app on phone
Cue card with strategy steps
Laptop with bookkeeping program
Blank progress recording sheet

Ingredients—Actions:
Reviewing strategy rationale, steps
Frequent practice

Ingredients—Motivators:
Esther records own progress
Encouragement/praise
List of self-affirming statements

Measurement Plan:
steps done independently
self-affirms vs redirects
Distraction rating

Check-in Info and Results of Homework: Hmwk completed but not documented, Joseph had to prompt at 5 min mark—Esther would prefer not to involve him going forward as it strains relationship

Practice Data:	Retention Probe	Practice 1:	Practice 2:	Practice 3:	Practice 4:
Strategy Steps:		Expense Receipts	Expense Receipts		
3. rate overall level of distractedness during task		+ Rating = 3	+ Rating = 3		
2c. self-affirm or redirect after third 10 min		+ Self-redirect	+ Self-affirm		
2b. self-affirm or redirect after second 10 min		+ Self-redirect	+ Self-redirect		

(continued)

Therapy Session Data Form—Target Acquisition, Mastery, Generalization (Strategy Use) *(page 2 of 2)*

Practice Data:	Retention Probe	Practice 1:	Practice 2:	Practice 3:	Practice 4:
2a. self-affirm or redirect after first 10 min		+ Self-affirm	+ Self-affirm		
1. select task, set timer for 10 min x 3		+	+		
Comments:	Esther verbally described steps 100% (no time for full probe)	No clinician prompting	No clinician prompting		

Session Summary/Analysis of Progress:

Successful fading of 5 min prompt; Esther completing tasks but still reporting strong temptation to stray—keeps cue card in direct line of sight to assist with maintaining focus (would like to not have to use this eventually); decided to keep email notifications turned off for now

Feedback and Homework Provided (task, context, ingredients, tracking):

Repeat task at home tomorrow with no support from Joseph—remember to document

Plan for Next Session:

Expand to other bookkeeping tasks

Progress Monitoring Form—
Target Acquisition, Mastery, Generalization (Strategy Use)

Client Name: Esther **Target:** Independently use the "time, remind, reflect" strategy twice per day, 4 days per week **Training Phase:** Acquisition-Generalization

Select the summary measure being tracked (must use the same from each session):

☐ Retention probe result from start of each session

☐ Average of each session's practice trial results

☑ Other: Final practice trial results (due to available time in each session)

	Summary Measure			
	Aug 10	Aug 12	Aug 14	Aug 21
Strategy Steps:	Expenses	Expenses	Expenses/Revenue	Exp/Rev/Bills
3. rate overall level of distractedness during task	−	+	+	+
2c. self-affirm or redirect after third 10 min	Prompt at 5 min Self-redirect	+ self-affirm	+ self-redirect	+ self-affirm
2b. self-affirm or redirect after second 10 min	Prompt at 5 min Self-redirect	+ self-redirect	+ self-affirm	+ self-redirect
2a. self-affirm or redirect after first 10 min	+ self-affirm	+ self-affirm	+ self-affirm	+ self-affirm
1. select task, set timer for 10 min x 3	+	+	+	+
Ingredients:				
Prompts and Supports:	-cue card and timer -clinician prompt initiated at 5 min mark anytime Esther appeared distracted (not required for 2a)	-cue card and timer with cue card in immediate line of sight (clinician prompting no longer required!)	-cue card and timer with cue card in immediate line of sight	-cue card and timer -moved cue card off to the side and still successful!
Motivational:	-Records own progress -Encouragement and praise -Own list of self-affirming stmts	-Records own progress -Encouragement and praise -Own list of self-affirming stmts	-Records own progress -Encouragement and praise -Own list of self-affirming stmts	-Records own progress -Encouragement and praise -Own list of self-affirming stmts
Other Measures:				
	Distraction rating = 4 33% self-affirms, 67% self-redirects	Distraction rating = 3 67% self-affirms	Distraction rating = 3 67% self-affirms	Distraction rating = 2 67% self-affirms (similar level of success reported for home practice)

Strategy Selection Worksheet

DEFINE THE NEED

A. To manage processing deficits in order to complete selected goals (e.g., maintain attention; control impulsivity; remember information):	OR	B. To improve performance on a specific activity (e.g., reading comprehension, writing accurate work report):

⬇   ⬇

CONSIDER KEY CLIENT & STRATEGY CHARACTERISTICS

☐ Maximum strategy complexity (e.g., number of steps; level of abstraction) that can be processed by client:

☐ Client insight and motivation:

☐ Environmental triggers to initiate strategy use:

☐ Timing of strategy use:

☐ Opportunities to use strategy:

⬇   ⬇

GENERATE OPTIONS FOR COGNITIVE STRATEGIES

1.

2.

3.

FORM 7.2
Strategy Knowledge Questions

	Date:		Date:		Date:	
	Start	End	Start	End	Start	End
What is the name of your strategy?						
Describe the steps in your strategy.						
What are examples of when you would use your strategy?						
How can your strategy be useful to you?						

M = Modeled—presented entire answer.

A = Assisted—gave partial response.

I = Independent—reasonable answer.

Therapy Session Data Form—Target Acquisition, Mastery, Generalization (Strategy Use)

Client Name: **Date:**   **Location:**   **Others Present:**

Target: **Associated Aim:**   **Training Phase:**

Ingredients—Items: **Ingredients—Actions:**   **Ingredients—Motivators:**   **Measurement Plan:**

Check-in Info and Results of Homework:

Practice Data:	Retention Probe	Practice 1:	Practice 2:	Practice 3:	Practice 4:
Strategy Steps:					

(continued)

Therapy Session Data Form—Target Acquisition, Mastery, Generalization (Strategy Use) *(page 2 of 2)*

Practice Data:	Retention Probe	Practice 1:	Practice 2:	Practice 3:	Practice 4:
Comments:					

Session Summary/Analysis of Progress:

Feedback and Homework Provided (task, context, ingredients, tracking):

Plan for Next Session:

Progress Monitoring Form—
Target Acquisition, Mastery, Generalization (Strategy Use)

Client Name: **Target:**   **Training Phase:**

Select the summary measure being tracked (must use the same from each session):

☐ Retention probe result from start of each session

☐ Average of each session's practice trial results

☐ Other:

	Summary Measure			
	Date 1:	Date 2:	Date 3:	Date 4:
Strategy Steps:				
Ingredients:				
Prompts and Supports:				
Motivational:				
Other Measures:				

CHAPTER 8

External Cognitive Aid Instruction

External cognitive aids support cognitive function by facilitating clients' ability to engage in or complete desired tasks or activities. A vast array of tools or devices can help people compensate for cognitive impairments by either (1) limiting the load on their cognitive processing (e.g., providing electronic reminders to reduce demands on memory or executive functions) or (2) modifying the target task or environment (e.g., using text readers that bypass reading). The overall purpose of an external aid is to capitalize on a person's residual abilities, substitute alternative methods for activity completion, and/ or provide external support to complete a desired task (LoPresti, Mihailidis, & Kirsch, 2004).

A number of different labels have been used to refer to external cognitive aids, including "cognitive orthoses" and "cognitive prosthetics" (Cole, 1999; Kirsch, Levine, Fallon-Krueger, & Jaros, 1987). More recently, terms such as *assistive technology for cognition* (ATC; Scherer & Federici, 2015) and *cognitive support technologies* (CST; Jacobs et al., 2017) have been adopted in the literature to describe the range of aids that are available to support everyday cognition in people with cognitive impairments. In this chapter, we use the broad term *external cognitive aids* because it is most consistent with terminology used by clinicians and encompasses all peripheral cognitive supports, including high- and low-tech devices, tools, or programs, as well as those specifically designed for rehabilitative purposes and those developed for mainstream users.

This chapter focuses on the use of external cognitive aids as a cognitive rehabilitation intervention option. However, as reviewed in Chapter 7, most cognitive rehabilitation programs integrate and combine different intervention approaches. Lambez and Vakil (2021) conducted a systematic review and meta-analysis examining the effectiveness of a wide variety of memory interventions including internal cognitive aids (e.g., memory strategies) and external cognitive aids. They found that intervention using both internal strategies and external tools had the greatest effectiveness. Their review highlights the need to personalize the selection of an approach for individual clients.

Given the explosion of technology in every realm of societal functioning, from work productivity to social interaction, the options for external supports for people with cognitive impairments are endless. The increased availability of technology to help individuals compensate for cognitive impairments is one of the most notable advances in neuropsychological rehabilitation. Clinicians working in cognitive rehabilitation must be knowledgeable about options that may be useful to their clients. This can be challenging given the pace at which platforms and tools are evolving. For example, personal digital assistants (PDAs), previously mainstream electronic memory tools, were shown to be efficacious for individuals with memory impairments (Svoboda, Richards, Leach, & Mertens, 2012), and then that technology was replaced by cell phones and then smartphones with a never-ending supply of downloadable software applications requiring clinicians to continually evolve their clinical practice (Vasquez, Lloyd-Kuzik, & Moscovitch, 2021).

The benefits of external cognitive aids are self-evident. They can support the completion of functional activities in naturalistic settings and reduce caregiver burden and stress by helping individuals with cognitive impairments function more independently. The successful use of external aid technology to improve functional memory, organization, and specific task completion has been demonstrated by numerous studies and systematic reviews (Charters, Gillett, & Simpson, 2015; de Joode, van Heugten, Verhey, & van Boxtel, 2010; Ferguson, Friedland, & Woodberry, 2015; Sohlberg et al., 2007). One meta-analysis revealed that "prosthetic technology" improved performance on everyday tasks requiring memory, with a large effect size of $d = 1.27$ (Jamieson, Cullen, McGee-Lennon, Brewster, & Evans, 2014). Overall, the literature examining the efficacy of external tools is favorable. What is missing, however, is key information about best practice for selecting aids, training clients to use them, and ensuring they continue to use their aids after training.

Leopold, Lourie, Petras, and Elias (2015) conducted a comprehensive systematic review to evaluate the effectiveness of ATC as an everyday compensatory tool for cognitive impairments following traumatic brain injury (TBI). Most studies were case studies or quasi-experimental studies with small sample sizes. Results showed a positive association between the use of ATCs and participants' ability to complete target tasks, regardless of age, severity of injury, and time post onset. However, results suggested that most individuals abandoned devices after using them for a short time or after support was no longer present because the devices did not meet the user's functional needs or preferences or because they were not efficient or easily implemented.

USER PERSPECTIVES

The most important influence on an individual's use of an external cognitive aid is how well it serves that person. The degree to which the aid supports desired task completion or goal attainment, matches a person's routines and preferences, and does not cause stress and frustration will determine whether the individual continues to use a tool (Scherer & Federici, 2015). Hence, it is critical that clinicians pay attention to clients' perspectives on use of external cognitive aids. Several studies have examined attitudes and perspectives of people with acquired brain injury toward the use of external cognitive aids, beginning with the introduction of PDAs. Hart and colleagues (Hart,

Buchhofer, & Vaccaro, 2004) surveyed attitudes toward portable electronic devices such as PDAs, handheld computers, and digital voice recorders in participants with TBI. While less than one-third of participants had experience using devices, researchers found simplicity of use, availability of technical support, and long-lasting battery power were the key attributes most valued by users who did use devices.

De Joode and colleagues (2010) reported similar findings in their investigation of attitudes among adults with ABI toward ATC, including mobile phones and PDAs. At that time, still only a minority were currently using devices, with major barriers being cost and lack of familiarity; however, most clients, caregivers, and professionals were positive about the option to use external aids. A similar study also found that participants with brain injury felt positive about using technology as long as it was affordable, reliable, and they could receive adequate training and support in using the device (Chu, Brown, Harniss, Kautz, & Johnson, 2014). Evald (2015) interviewed 13 people with brain injury about their experiences using smartphones as part of an intervention study and found that audible and visual reminders and the all-in-one nature of smartphones were the commonly reported advantages, while battery life, usability, and concern about loss or failure of the device were the reported disadvantages. These results show that participants' perceptions of barriers to and preferences for using technology have been consistent over time, regardless of the changing technology.

In more recent years, there has been an increase in the use of external aids by people with brain injury. A comparison study showed that the percent of people using smartphones is similar between those with and without brain injury (Wong, Sinclair, Seabrook, McKay, & Ponsford, 2017). Interestingly, participants with brain injury in that study mostly had severe injuries, suggesting that smartphones are an accessible form of external aid. Both injured and noninjured groups cited their main uses of the smartphone as being for communication (e.g., calls, text messages); to assist with memory and organization (e.g., calendars, alarm reminders, notes); and for Internet access. Unsurprisingly, when asked about the main benefit of using a smartphone, both groups listed multifunctionality, portability and convenience, and easy access to the Internet (Wong et al., 2017). Importantly, participants with brain injury rated the most important features of a smartphone as being simple to learn how to use; having a long-lasting battery; and having large, easy-to-see displays, while these characteristics were rated as less essential among the non-brain-injured comparison group.

Findings from studies evaluating clients' usage and preference for external aids have the following implications for cognitive rehabilitation (Scherer & Federici, 2015; Wong et al., 2017):

- Smartphones are accessible, acceptable, convenient for most people with brain injury, and are favorably perceived for supporting memory and organization as well as other specific activities. It is critical to note, however, that many people lack the resources to purchase smartphones or Wi-Fi access, so they are clearly not a solution for all.
- Selection of external cognitive aids should carefully consider the preferences, attitudes, and needs of individual clients.
- Dedicated instruction or training in the use of external cognitive aids is important to ensure ongoing use.
- Developers of apps and tools designed for people with brain injury should prioritize simplicity, large displays, and accessibility of technical support.

Readiness and Self-Awareness

Research findings are consistent in the need to match client profiles and preferences to the selected external aid. What is not clear, however, is the level of self-awareness necessary for a client to effectively engage in the selection process. As described in Chapters 2 and 3, diminished self-awareness is a common challenge following brain injury and can result from multiple sources, including damage to the brain networks and structures that allow us to understand disabilities (anosognosia) as well as psychological states where clients are not able to endorse changes in function because it is too emotionally painful (denial). Most clients will need a certain amount of awareness of their disability in order to engage in training and adopt a tool. Typically, the level of self-awareness will be assessed during a clinical interview, possibly using a tool such as the Self-Awareness of Deficits Interview (Fleming et al., 1996). If a client does not have adequate self-awareness to move forward with selection of and training in use of an external aid, they may benefit from some initial therapy directed at increasing self-awareness (an R target). Evidence for addressing self-awareness deficits supports the use of experiential exercises with structured feedback related to the target cognitive domain or activity for which the client lacks insight. For example, Schmidt and colleagues (2013) showed that when clients with diminished self-awareness following brain injury were provided with video feedback and facilitated reflection with a clinician during a meal preparation task, they were able to increase their awareness and understanding of their cognitive deficits. Improved insight and self-awareness may need to be targeted prior to selecting and training in use of an external aid.

As will be described, the PIE framework is consistent with the research findings that emphasize careful matching of an external cognitive aid to the individual client profile and the use of systematic instruction focused on ensuring sustained use in order to promote engagement in desired tasks and activities in the relevant everyday contexts.

Types of External Aids[1]

The process of selecting an external cognitive aid is a critical clinical skill and begins with a clinician being familiar with the range of assistive options to help clients compensate for their impairments. If the match is not ideal from the standpoint of the consumer, the technology may not be used, or will not be used optimally. Scherer and Federici (2015) offer the following categories to illustrate the range of possible outcomes when clients are provided with and taught to use an external aid:

1. Optimal use under all recommended conditions and situations
2. Partial use, where it is used in some situations but not others or part of the time
3. Nonuse, where the technology is initially used but is set aside because it is no longer needed
4. Avoidance of use, where use is not even considered
5. Reluctant use, where the individual uses it but does so with displeasure
6. Abandonment or permanently giving up use usually out of frustration or annoyance

---

[1] Much of the material in this subsection was based on a 2018 webinar produced by the American Speech–Language–Hearing Association (ASHA): "Beyond Workbooks: Functional Cognitive Rehabilitation for Traumatic Brain Injuries" by Don MacLennan and McKay Moore Sohlberg.

Items 1–3 can be considered successful outcomes of the process if the individual reports a benefit from using or having used the technology. Items 4–6, however, indicate a failure of the process to serve that individual well. Indeed, the overall abandonment rate has been approximately 30% for the past 30 years (Scherer & Federici, 2015). Matching the technology to the client profile is critical.

With the ever-changing landscape of technology, most clinicians do not have the time to research and learn all the available options in order to select the perfect match for an external aid. This is particularly true with regard to knowledge of the vast number of apps. There are over 1 million apps in the major app stores, rendering it impossible for any clinician to keep current. That said, knowledge and familiarity with categories of options and resources to investigate apps and tools are critical. Table 8.1 gives examples of app categories associated with specific functional tasks that are common tasks clients want to perform. There are different apps available for each of the app categories, which requires knowing the usability, price, complexity, compatibility including the specific device, and features for each of the apps.

A common clinical mistake is for clinicians to make recommendations for external cognitive aids by considering the overall tool without knowledge of its particular functions and features. Like all consumers, clinicians are vulnerable to trends, marketing, and peer behavior. What should be avoided is the hunt for "best brain injury apps" as the matching of an app to an individual is key. When it comes to selecting an app, the clinician should ask two key questions:

1. What cognitive domain(s) does the external cognitive aid support?
2. What are the target activities or tasks that the external cognitive aid(s) could support?

For clinicians who do not have reimbursable time to research tools outside of treatment, one strategy is to explore options with clients during the session. As described in Chapter 3, motivation and empowerment are critical to optimizing the buy-in and

TABLE 8.1. Examples of Functional Tasks Associated with Different App Categories

App categories	Sample functional tasks
Contacts	Finding phone/numbers
Calendars	Remembering birthdays that are important to me
Calendars	Tracking my appointments
Calendars	Following my daily schedule
Shopping/cooking	Making a grocery list for a recipe
Task learning	Following the procedures for operating a machine at work
Task management	Completing my to do list
Money management	Sticking to my budget
Medication reminder	Taking my pills at the correct time

efficacy of cognitive rehabilitation. Having clients read app or product reviews and conduct their own reviews as part of their therapy can increase engagement in aid selection and help ensure the optimal tool is chosen. Form 8.1 at the end of this chapter and in the digital files accompanying this book is a sample app review that can be completed by a client to help them engage in the selection process. The form can be adapted to provide more or less support.

The Internet can be very useful for identifying options for external cognitive aids, with the caveat that clinicians need to engage in a systematic process of matching the aid to the person, as described above. There are brain-injury-specific websites that provide efficient means to research external aid options. One resource is *https://bestconnections.org*; it provides free and low-cost technology webinars for people with brain injury to teach them about apps designed to help people with tasks affected by cognitive impairments following brain injury. The site also offers trainings for professionals who want to learn the fundamentals of smart technology or how best to train people with brain injury. Staff TBI Skill Builder (*https://cbirt.org/research/current-projects/stafftbi-skill-builder*) is another provider training option and consists of a 14-module, online training program to teach professionals new to ABI the skills needed to assist people with brain injury. The training includes information on effective methods for teaching the use of memory aids. Preliminary experimental evaluation suggested that the training increased key knowledge for staff newly working with people who have cognitive impairments following brain injury (Powell et al., 2021).

YouTube is another vehicle to view videos of specific tools that might be a potential match for clients. Often, a clinician will be familiar with the overall function of a particular app but not know details about features that may be key to their client's adoption. For example, when considering the use of a calendar app, it may be important to know specific features such as those listed in Table 8.2 to determine if that app should be offered as an option.

TABLE 8.2. Examples of Features to Consider during External Cognitive Aid Selection

Possible features to consider for calendar app or device	Additional features to consider for task management app or device
Notification and reminder systems	Organization options
Alarm features (loudness, snooze, nag, location, repeat, pop up)	• Categorize tasks • Prioritize tasks • Subtasks, checklists, notes
Input: speech to text; SIRI	Synch to calendar
Universal application (iPhone, iPad, Apple Watch; Facebook)	
Recurring events	
Multiple views (day, week, month year)	
Multiple calendars (family, work etc.)	
File sharing (synch with other people's calendars)	
Customizing events	
Synch mechanism: native calendar, Google calendar	

Table 8.3 maps the cognitive domains that external cognitive aids commonly support onto examples of aid and app features. Mapping cognitive needs to particular activities can help guide the selection of external cognitive aids. For example, if a client has difficulty with retrospective episodic memory, that client might benefit from supports for recall of events, tasks, or conversations. If a client has difficulty with prospective memory, they might benefit from supports that help schedule and prompt upcoming events.

Current smartphone technology additionally includes speech-to-text, text-to-speech, quick-fire entries, multidevice/app synching, and accessibility features, all of which permit additional customization to client needs.

The remainder of the chapter describes the clinical processes corresponding to the Planning, Implementation, and Evaluation (PIE) of external cognitive aids as a treatment approach.

TABLE 8.3. Cognitive Domains Mapped Onto Examples of Different Aid and App Features

Cognitive domain	Description	Examples of aid/app features
Attention	Holding and processing information in mind	• Alarms • Recurring alarms to maintain focus • Periodic alarms to take breaks • Checklists to stay on task
Episodic memory	Remembering daily events and experiences	• Notes • Pictures • Speech to text • Voice recording • Geotracking • Synching to other apps/devices/cloud
Semantic memory	Remembering facts and knowledge-based information	• Calendars • Notes • Internet search
Prospective memory	Remembering to initiate future intentions	• Pre-alarms for time management • Snooze, nag alarms for people who lose intention quickly • Repeating events/tasks for people who need cues for routine • Synching to other apps/devices/cloud
Procedural memory	Remembering procedures and steps	• Notes • Checklists
New learning	Ability/rate of learning new information	• Rehearsal • Distributed practice • Text to speech
Executive functions	Initiation, planning, organization, problem solving, self-monitoring	• Alarms • Categorize tasks, events • Prioritize tasks, events • Subtasks, checklists, notes • Set goals, monitor progress

PIE: PLANNING FOR USE OF EXTERNAL AIDS

By now the reader will be familiar with the PIE framework. Chapter 5 provides a thorough description of the key elements involved in the treatment process. In this chapter, we review the elements that are specific to training use of external cognitive aids. This chapter describes the PIE elements relevant to external aid training under the distinct categories of planning, implementation, and evaluation. The reader is referred to Chapter 5 for a reminder of how the PIE process is actually circular and iterative. In this chapter, we review assessment and target selection under *planning*, the application of treatment ingredients under *implementation*, and the selection and administration of treatment measures under *evaluation*. In practice, however, the clinician will have selected treatment ingredients and measurement tools as part of the planning process and will be conducting ongoing evaluation and treatment modification throughout therapy. We begin with a review of the two key components in the planning phase: assessment and selection of treatment targets and aims.

PIE: PLANNING THERAPY FOR EXTERNAL COGNITIVE AIDS

Assess and Hypothesize

The clinician will complete an initial file review and collaborative clinical interview with the individual and relevant stakeholders to develop hypotheses about what cognitive areas may be affected and what desired activities are disrupted as a result of cognitive challenges. This may involve administering formal and informal cognitive assessments, and/or talking to significant others to test hypotheses about the source of cognitive impairments, which will be important for matching possible external aids. The collaborative clinical interview will be key to identifying whether external cognitive aids are a good option for a client. If the client and clinician decide to investigate this intervention approach, one of the primary assessment tasks will be to gather information that will result in a good match between the client and the external aid.

A seminal clinical process to guide identification of an external tool that is a good fit for a client is the Matching Person & Technology (MPT) assessment process (Scherer & Craddock, 2005; Scherer & Federici, 2015). The goal of this collaborative assessment is to identify a tool *for a specific user, for a specific purpose, in a specific environment*. This process may be completed using any number of available questionnaires embedded in the interview process.

Form 8.2 at the end of this chapter provides a tool to help structure the collaborative interview matching process following the MPT framework. The form is also in the digital files accompanying this book. The External Aid Needs Assessment protocol shown in Form 8.2 is designed to help a clinician and client collaboratively select an external aid that will be well matched to the individual client (Sohlberg & Mateer, 2001). This protocol facilitates the collection of information in three broad areas: (1) client priorities and needs, (2) organic factors (cognitive/learning profile and physical profile), and (3) personal factors (past/current use of external aids, preferences, and supports). It can be used as an interview guide to help the clinician conduct a comprehensive needs assessment, which will help the clinician identify the external aid most likely to be adopted and specify relevant targets and aims. Clients or care providers with sufficient background may complete the needs assessment independently.

The importance of matching a user to a device via a thorough, comprehensive assessment process is emphasized in the external aid literature and in clinical practice. It is also important to recognize that the alignment of a client's needs and abilities with device features *changes over time*, particularly at critical transition points (e.g., at discharge from hospital to home or from rehabilitation to community living, with developmental changes in executive functions, with improvements in awareness or acceptance of disability). One of the biggest challenges is that transition points are typically accompanied by a transition to a new set of clinical or education providers. Anticipating these junctures is important in the selection process.

Define Targets, Aims, and Measures

An important part of the planning process is to identify the desired outcome or aim that the external aid will support. This will be integrated with the assessment process. The clinician needs to be clear on the following:

- *Why am I teaching the use of this aid?* (leads to development of treatment aim)
- *What are the steps and key contextual variables that are involved in using the aid?* (leads to development of treatment targets)

These two questions will help the clinician specify measurable targets and aims and plan for multilevel evaluation. Examples of measurement are described under "PIE: Evaluating Outcomes When Training External Cognitive Aids."

Confirm Treatment Aims and Impact Measures

Treatment *aims* represent the functional outcome or goal that the client hopes to achieve. The aim is usually an activity, task, or state of mind that has been negatively impacted by particular cognitive challenges that the clinician has identified in their assessment. Examples might include performance of specific tasks, such as *read and remember newspaper articles* or *independently cook dinner* or *initiate more social outings*. Aims can also be broad, such as *increase daily productivity* or *feel more socially connected* or *improve school performance*. Aims can be linked to quantitative indices (e.g., number of tasks completed on a to-do list) or worked into goal attainment scales (e.g., levels of satisfaction with social interaction). The selected external aid should directly support and facilitate achievement of the aim. Collaboratively identifying the aim through the assessment process will ensure that therapy goals are meaningful and functional for that person.

Confirm Treatment Targets and Progress Measures

Treatment targets, sometimes called short-term goals, represent a specific aspect of function that is expected to change as a direct result of the treatment activities delivered during the therapy session. The treatment targets are selected because they will lead to achievement of the aim or functional outcome. External aids are only useful if they impact function or the selected treatment aim. There will usually be several treatment targets associated with learning to use and implement an external aid.

To develop treatment targets for teaching the use of external aids, clinicians will usually generate a task analysis for the external aid that lists the specific steps needed to use that particular aid in the desired contexts. Constructing a task analysis helps the clinician specify training targets for teaching the steps to use the device, considering contextual variables that may support or impede use of the device. Examples of targets are provided in the "PIE: Evaluating Outcomes" section.

Teaching the steps to use a particular aid involves S (skill) targets. If it is necessary to focus specifically on helping a client become ready to embrace the use of an aid or engage in the therapy, before training begins, then the clinician could specify a separate readiness or engagement R (representation) target. Otherwise, teaching of S targets will always incorporate clinical ingredients that facilitate motivation and self-efficacy.

Goal (Target and Aim) Writing

Chapter 5 outlined the components necessary for writing treatment targets and aims, including treatment approach, treatment target, objective performance measurement, criteria, level of independence, and conditions/context. See Forms 5.1 and 5.2 in Chapter 5 for target- and aim-writing checklists using SMART and goal attainment scaling (GAS) requirements. Examples of targets are also provided in the Case Applications that appear at the end of this chapter.

The planning process will result in a selected external aid and individual steps or behaviors to operationalize use of the aid to achieve a specific treatment aim. Planning will also include identification of treatment ingredients to be used with individual clients. The next phase is to *implement* training to teach the steps or behaviors that will lead to effective use of the external aid.

PIE: IMPLEMENTING USE OF EXTERNAL AIDS

Teaching the use of an external aid is often best conceptualized as two sets of activities: (1) teaching the *mechanics* of using the aid (the S targets), and (2) identifying the *supports and reinforcements* necessary for using an aid in the *target contexts*.

As discussed throughout this text, it is useful to think of instruction for people with cognitive impairments as having three phases: acquisition, mastery and generalization, and maintenance. Acquisition refers to the initial phase of laying down a concept, behavior, or procedure. It is comprised of the processes needed to establish new learning or relearning. Mastery and generalization are achieved when learning becomes more fluent and automatic and is extended to new contexts or tasks in some way. Maintenance is the continued use or demonstration of the learning in the target contexts. During the assessment process, which includes evaluating the client's cognitive profile, the clinician will have determined whether there is a need for structured training to use the external aid *or* whether the client already knows the mechanics for tool use and just needs training to establish the habit of using the aid. For example, if a client has a significant declarative memory impairment that affects their ability to learn new information or procedures, they may need very structured, errorless practice using massed practice followed by distributed practice (the acquisition stage of training) to learn steps related to device use. However, if they have previously used the tool and the targets are focused on consistency or use in particular contexts, the client may not need acquisition training and training can focus on mastery and generalization. The following sections describe the procedures used in each phase when training the use of external aids.

Initial Acquisition Phase of Training

The purpose of therapy at this phase is to establish the procedures and motivation for using the selected external aid. It is critical from the outset to ensure that there is buy-in from the client. A vital predictor of the adoption of an external aid and determiner of long-term use is a person's *initial reaction*, including perceptions of the relative advantages or disadvantages of the device in terms of usability and impact on quality of life (Scherer & Federici, 2015). Hence, a person's introductory experience using the tool is important. If the client has a positive initial experience and sees advantages to using the device, their intention to use the device is reinforced. Five important clinical actions will maximize the likelihood of initial positive experiences leading to adoption and continued use of the external aid:

1. Selection of the tool is based on a comprehensive needs assessment with attention to key contextual and client factors.
2. The selection process is collaborative: the client participates in the decision making for choosing and customizing the device.
3. The tool and procedures for using it are tailored to the individual and their environment.
4. Initial training of device use (for those who need instruction in the procedures) is set up to ensure success: systematic instruction is used to teach each step in an efficient manner so the client is able to use the device as quickly as possible.
5. Training examples are relevant to and valued by the client and thus are reinforcing from the outset. This helps clients to understand the benefits of the tool from the start of training.

The first two training considerations will have been met during the selection process that was reviewed under assessment. The next three will be ensured by following the systematic instruction process for the acquisition phase reviewed in Chapter 5.

Session 1 of the training will begin with a baseline probe to determine the step at which to begin teaching use of the aid. The prompt for the probe might be "Show me how you would use your camera to take a photo of where you parked your car." As shown in Figure 8.1, for a client learning to take photos to remember parking locations, the clinician will record the correct and incorrect responses, and any prompts used to determine at what step the training process should begin (for a blank form for clinical use, see Form 8.3: Baseline Probe for External Aid Use at the end of the chapter and in the digital files accompanying this book).

If the initial probe reveals that the client is unable to demonstrate the sequence of steps in the task analysis for using the device, the clinician might then model an individual step and have the client "show what you would do next," to determine if the sequence of steps was learned as a single procedure. This will help the clinician know if steps can be bundled together and identify the amount of practice that might be needed.

Baseline Probe for External Aid Use

Prompt: Show me how you use your camera to take a photo of where you parked your car.		
Context where probe obtained: Went out into parking lot outside clinic		

Steps Recalled Independently:

Steps	Correct?	Comments
1. Open smartphone	✓	Completed quickly and easily
2. Touch camera icon	✓	Quick and easy—can combine steps 1–2
3. Take photo of car location in parking lot	✗	Took photo of car but didn't include any location markers in the image
4. Save photo in Parking Lot album	✓	Saved photo no problem
5. Add caption if location marker in photo may be insufficient (Optional)	✗	Did not add caption

Other Comments/Observations:
- Completed all steps quickly
- When asked to open photo of car, he opened the correct photo album without support and selected the correct photo without support by using date stamp (but only 1 other photo in this album today)
- After opening today's photo, when asked to describe how helpful the image would be, did not appear to be aware that there were no clues as to the car's location within the parking lot
- Upon discussion, decided that renaming photo album to Parking Location Hints would help remind him to check if location markers were present in the image, and if they weren't, he could retake the photo or add a caption—will therefore add a step to review photo and make decision

FIGURE 8.1. Completed Baseline Probe for External Aid Use.

The type of prompting that should be used during the training process (if any) will be determined in this baseline probe. In some cases, the clinician may elect to do a dynamic assessment to see what types of prompts are most effective. Ultimately, the clinician will fade prompts as the client acquires the steps; thus, it will be important to identify what type of prompting is facilitative. Examples of prompts include:

- Checklist of the steps in using the aid
- Written cue cards prompting use of the steps
- Auditory prompt (e.g., alarm) to initiate use of the aid
- Client states each step or a keyword representing that step as it is implemented

Each subsequent session will begin with a retention probe, which follows the same format as the baseline probe without the use of any identified prompts. The purpose of the retention probe is to evaluate recall from previous sessions and indicate the step where training in the current session should begin. After the probe, training begins with the clinician modeling or prompting the step that the client has successfully completed and then adding it to the next new step so that the client is chaining and practicing the new step in conjunction with the prior step that is already firm. Training will usually call for the client to mass practice the two steps. Periodically, the clinician will have the client start from the initial step to make sure all the steps are integrated. With practice, the client should be able to retain the target steps over increasing time intervals. Fundamental to the initial acquisition phase is to *minimize the client's errors, move from a massed to distributed practice schedule,* and *provide sufficient opportunities for practice and repetition.*

Figures 8.2 and 8.3 are sample completed therapy session and progress monitoring datasheets for recording the performance of a client learning to take photos of parking lot locations (see Forms 8.4 and 8.5 at the end of the chapter for blank versions of these forms, as well as fillable versions in the digital files accompanying this book). The data were collected early in the acquisition phase, but with the client learning to use the aid quickly, generalization (incorporating varied stimuli) was built in right away.

To review, the following constitutes the acquisition training sequence:

- A probe is taken at the beginning of each session. This session probe tells the clinician where to begin in therapy.
- Treatment ingredients during the session include:
  - Ingredients to minimize errors during practice (clinician demonstration, fading of prompts).
  - High rates of repetition with intensive massed practice in the acquisition phase to establish the skill, if needed.
  - Chaining newly learned steps with previously learned steps.
  - Distributing or spacing practice once the steps are learned.
  - Quickly correcting any errors and providing additional repeated practice on that step or sequence, before fading prompts. When an error is made, the clinician will isolate a step that the client is not performing accurately and provide intensive practice until that step is mastered, then chain it back to the routine (i.e., have the client practice the step multiple times and then complete the preceding step and the difficult-to-learn step together before moving to longer practice intervals).
  - Ingredients to increase motivation and adherence (e.g., anticipation of difficult steps, charting own data, reinforcement).

Mastery and Generalization Phase of Training

The goal of the mastery and generalization phase of training is to increase the fluency and automaticity with which the client uses the external aid in everyday life. In many cases, training for generalization may occur in tandem with the acquisition phase and might not represent a separate set of targets. Generalization targets are achieved by attending to three categories of treatment ingredients:

1. **Fading learning supports.** This refers to the progressive withdrawal of supports such as clinician prompts and cues, and also internalization of the steps involved in using

Therapy Session Data Form—Target Acquisition, Mastery, Generalization (External Aid Use)

Client Name: Scott   **Date:** Oct 8   **Location:** Clinic   **Others Present:** N/A   **Training Phase:** Acquisition

Target: Independently use camera and album apps to record **Associated Aim:** Locate car in parking lot in less than 10 specific location of car in familiar parking lots   minutes when leaving a mall or office

Ingredients—Items:
Large monitor with Google Street View open
Index card with list of steps
Blank progress recording sheet

Ingredients—Actions:
Reviewing steps, highlighting key items
Massed practice with error control
Chaining of steps

Ingredients—Motivators:
Scott will record own progress
Encouragement/praise

Measurement Plan:
steps done ind. without index card
1–5 rating of helpfulness of location cues in photo or caption

Check-in Info and Results of Homework: Reported getting lost again earlier this week after attending Brain Injury Assoc meeting at the grocery store that donates their community room to the group. Scott brought a list of the common locations he visits that have large parking lots (grocery store, hospital, this clinic, Cotton Factory where he takes woodturning lessons, mall, spouse's office building). Scott had renamed album to Parking Location Hints.

Practice Data:	Retention Probe	Practice 1:		Practice 2:		Practice 3:		Practice 4:	
External Aid Steps:		Grocery Store		Grocery Store		Grocery Store		Grocery Store	
5. if detail is insufficient, retake or add caption		N/A : Sufficient detail				+ : caption		+ : retake	
4. decide if photo detail is sufficient or not	–	+		– : MCCC++		+		+	

FIGURE 8.2. Example of completed Therapy Session Data Form—Target Acquisition, Mastery, Generalization (External Aid Use).

(continued)

Therapy Session Data Form—Target Acquisition, Mastery, Generalization (External Aid Use) (page 2 of 2)

Practice Data:	Retention Probe	Practice 1:	Practice 2:	Practice 3:	Practice 4:
3. save photo in Parking Location Hints album	+	+	+ +	+	+
2. take photo of car location in parking lot	+	+	+	N/A	N/A
1. open phone and touch camera icon	+	+	+	N/A	N/A
Comments:	Insufficient info but Scott closed app before evaluating; modeled and re-instructed	Directed to index card prior to each step	Removed card; massed practice of step 4 after error, chained to step 3 (M = model, C = cue card)	No card; steps 1–2 mastered, so started at step 3	No card; started at step 3 again

Session Summary/Analysis of Progress:

Independent with cue card; massed practice plus chaining supported fading of cue card (will store in phone pocket just in case)

Feedback and Homework Provided (task, context, ingredients, tracking):

Use cue card when picking up spouse from work this afternoon and when attending Cotton Factory on Monday (set alarms to remind); complete 2–3 practice trials with Google Maps at home each day with spouse

Plan for Next Session:

Increase variety of locations on Google Maps, ? practice in clinic parking lot, implement 1–5 rating at step 4

FIGURE 8.2. (continued)

Progress Monitoring—Target Acquisition, Mastery, Generalization (External Aid Use)

Client Name: Scott   **Target:** Independently use camera and album apps to record specific location of car in familiar parking lots   **Training Phase:** Acquisition-Mastery-Generalization

Select the summary measure being tracked (must use the same from each session):

☑ Retention probe result from start of each session
☐ Average of each session's practice trial results
☐ Other:

	Summary Measure			
	Oct 8	Oct 12	Oct 15	Oct 22
External Aid Steps:	Grocery (Google)	Office (Google)	Office (Google)	Clinic (Actual)
5. if detail is insufficient, retake or add caption			+ retake	
4. decide if photo detail is sufficient or not	−	−	+	−
3. save photo in Parking Location Hints album	+	+	+	+
2. take photo of car location in parking lot	+	+	+	+
1. open phone and touch camera icon	+	+	+	+
Ingredients:				
Prompts and Supports:	No supports or prompts used during any retention probes			
	During practice trials after retention probe: -Index card for initial practice but then faded, required massed practice to support success on step 4 initially but then independent except photos required extra detail each time	Changed location to Office for probe and trials During practice trials after probe: -No card used but required massed practice for step 4 again (new location) -Remaining trials done ind. but photos still needed extra detail	During practice trials after retention probe: -Ind. without index card for all steps -Photo specificity improved over trials -Did last trial in clinic parking lot	Did retention probe and all practice trials in clinic lot (distracted during retention probe) During practice trials after retention probe: -Ind. for steps 1-3, needed massed practice for step 4 with chaining to step 3 in this distracting environment
Motivational:	-Records own progress -Encouragement and praise	-Records own progress -Encouragement and praise	-Records own progress -Encouragement and praise	-Records own progress -Encouragement and praise
Other Measures:				
	N/A	-Photo specificity rating averaged 2/5	Photo specificity rating was 2/5 in first trial but 4/5 in final 2 trials	-Photo specificity ranged from 3–4/5

FIGURE 8.3. Example of completed Progress Monitoring Form—Target Acquisition, Mastery, Generalization (External Aid Use).

the aid. For example, if the client is saying each step aloud as it is completed, this can be faded to inner speech ("say it in your head"). Similarly, the client may go from physically checking off each step on a checklist to using the list as a written reference when needed. Some clients may *always* depend on external cues and prompts to use their aid, particularly clients who have severe memory or executive function impairments and those who need to use the aid in an unpredictable context. If an external cue or prompt is effective, efficient, and preferred by the client, there is no *a priori* reason to remove it.

2. **Lengthening the distributed practice.** The clinician will increase the interval between practice trials to reinforce independent tool use over increasingly longer periods of time. When the session probe administered at the beginning of the session indicates sufficient fluency with the steps, the clinician can start varying training contexts to promote generalization.

3. **Incorporating or increasing stimulus variability.** For many clients, unless their cognitive impairments are very mild, generalization or transfer of learning will need to be planned and trained explicitly. A main goal of this stage is to identify triggers that will facilitate the *initiation of external aid use* in the *target context*. These will have been identified in the planning process and then incorporated during this phase of training. Examples of generalization training methods include:

- Varying training stimuli so use of the aid can be triggered by a variety of environmental cues
- Involving people in the natural environment who will serve as "cues" in everyday life
- Training use of the aid in the target everyday context
- Outlining a home program for practicing using the aid, in collaboration with client and home supports
- Providing the client with everyday reminders to implement the external aid between therapy sessions, using cues such as voicemail, text messages, email, or reminders/alarms within the aid itself

4. **Increasing or maintaining engagement.** It may be difficult for the client to maintain motivation and interest in using the aid beyond the clinic, particularly if it is difficult to use. While this was addressed earlier in training by collaborating with the client in selecting the aid, it also is important to consider strategies to maintain client motivation and engagement after discharge. As discussed in Chapter 3, these factors are important predictors of long-term treatment adherence. Methods to increase enthusiasm and commitment for implementing use of the aid include:

- Creating a customized log to help client and/or support people record aid use and impact to provide a concrete record of improved functioning with aid use
- Conducting motivational interviewing (MI, see Chapter 3; Miller & Rollnick, 2012) where you ask questions that encourage the client to explore ambivalence about using the aid, such as asking about situations when the aid would have been useful even if the client was not able to implement it
- Collaborating with the client to identify potential benefits and barriers to using the external aid in daily living and developing alternative plans

Maintenance Phase

As described in earlier chapters, the maintenance phase refers to therapy methods that increase the likelihood that a rehabilitation target will be retained after therapy ends. The clinician should actively plan how to avoid abandonment of external aid use once therapeutic support is no longer available. Many devices end up in a closet gathering dust, and many apps are never opened after being downloaded. The best insurance against device abandonment has already been detailed in the preceding sections; it includes (1) selecting a device that meets the needs of the client, (2) effectively training the use of the device, and (3) setting up ongoing reinforcement and support for device implementation. If possible, it may be helpful to increase the time interval between therapy sessions as therapy progresses, or schedule follow-up visits to promote generalization and make any needed adjustments to the plan for using the device.

For use of an aid to be maintained, it must become automatic and internalized. The primary methods to promote ongoing implementation of an aid are the *incorporation of natural supports* and *cumulative review* (see Chapter 5). The techniques listed above for increasing metacognitive engagement facilitate the involvement of natural supports and provide a mechanism for monitoring aid use. The use of diaries, logs, and "check-ins" can be very helpful for maintaining use of an aid, particularly during the phase when therapy supports are withdrawn.

In terms of long-term use of an external aid, it is important to acknowledge that contexts and situations change and so does technology; mechanisms need to be in place for reevaluating the effectiveness of the aid. Depending on the service delivery model and complexity of the aid, the client may need follow-up visits or phone support to maintain effective use of an aid over time.

PIE: EVALUATING OUTCOMES WHEN TRAINING EXTERNAL COGNITIVE AIDS

Previous chapters in this text have emphasized the importance of multilevel outcome evaluation. The clinician will need methods to measure (1) whether the client learns *how to use* the device, (2) whether the client *initiates using the device in the target contexts*, and (3) the *effect or impact of using the device*. These are not binary measures, as there are degrees of learning, initiation, and impact as explained in this section.

As noted, the planning process results in selection of *targets* addressed in therapy sessions leading to *aims* or functional outcomes. The types of evaluation needed to direct intervention include three progress measures: *target acquisition data*, *generalization probe data*, and *maintenance data*, in addition to *impact data* selected to evaluate functional outcome. Examples of different types of evaluation data are shown in Table 8.4 and provided in the Case Applications at the end of the chapter. Chapter 5 also contains a thorough review of measurement selection and outcome evaluation requirements.

Acquisition data will primarily measure skill in using the aid (S targets). For example, as shown in Table 8.4, acquisition data may be used to measure S targets such as number of steps client demonstrates independently on a practice activity. Skills training will require having scenarios to facilitate practicing using the aid. These data will

TABLE 8.4. Examples of Different Types of Data for External Aids

Sample external aid targets	Sample target acquisition data	Sample target mastery/ generalization data	Sample target maintenance data	Sample impact data (used to measure aims or outcome)
Independent use of pill box reminder system (S target)	# of task analysis steps completed with no prompts for one pill	# of task analysis steps completed with no prompts when all five pills are in the box (generalization to using with multiple pills)	Caregiver report on level of independence for using reminder system	# of evenings all pills taken at correct time with no prompting
Use Google Calendar to enter and access to do list (S target)	# of task analysis steps completed with no prompts	Average time to enter/access three items on to do list within calendar (fluency)	# of items in calendar at 2-month follow-up visit	Percent of to do items independently completed weekly as listed on Goal Attainment Scale
Independent use of homework assignment app (S target)	# of homework assignments independently entered during session	# of homework assignments independently entered between sessions (generalization to home)	Teacher report of frequency of app use and homework completion rate at IEP meeting	# of missing assignments on electronic grading system
Use of Google Maps with Siri for navigating in neighborhood on daily walks (S target)	# of cues given during session to put in location and start Siri for practice walks	# of cues given by spouse to put in location and start Siri on the two established practice walks (generalization to neighborhood)	Client report of satisfaction level of device use during daily walks	Spouse confidence ratings for letting client take walks solo
Increase motivation to use reminder app on iPhone (R target)	Ratings on confidence and readiness scales	Read and report on app reviews	N/A	Request to try out reminder app

be used in the session for progress monitoring. As reviewed in the "PIE: Implementing Use" section, Forms 8.4 and 8.5 allow probing and tracking the number of steps or components in order to direct treatment. For external aid training in the acquisition phase, data may be used to evaluate R targets such as motivation or engagement, which can be measured using a "perceived usefulness" rating that is added to a form once the client is familiar with it. Acquisition data may also be used to evaluate fluency or efficiency of aid use in addition to accuracy. These data will guide therapy and tell the clinician when to move forward in therapy or back up and provide additional support or training. As implementation of the aid becomes consistent, use will be measured under different conditions, including application in everyday environments. These are the generalization and maintenance data.

Mastery and generalization data will often address both S and R targets and will capture fluency or efficiency of aid use (e.g., number of steps initiated without hesitation or the amount of time to enter information in an aid), initiation of aid use in naturalistic contexts, the amount of support required, and helpfulness/satisfaction ratings. Self-report logs, as well as other types of report logs and questionnaires, may be used to gather these data. Again, such data can direct the need to decrease or add supports. Maintenance data will examine sustained use or impact as shown in Table 8.4.

It is also important to measure impact of external aid use and determine whether using the aid achieved the desired functional impact in the client's everyday life. This may be in the form of a GAS scale that uses an overall functional goal broken into five potential levels of progress [see Goal Attainment Scaling (GAS) in Chapter 5]. In the table below, we give an example of an aim from Table 8.4 that uses GAS to measure the impact of the external aid training. The associated targets and intervention components are also listed.

Aim

Improve home productivity by attaining Level 1 on Goal Attainment Scale.

Cognitive domain being addressed: Executive functions

Functional domain: Productivity

Intervention approach: Use of Google Calendar for keeping a to-do list

Intervention ingredients: Systematic instruction components (error minimization, massed practice moving to distributed practice on task analysis, use of practice scenarios with desired task)

Target 1: Independently and accurately complete all 10 steps for using the calendar system

Target 2: Enter and access data for three items in less than 3 minutes

Goal Attainment Scale

Level 2 (much more than expected): Completes 80–100% of items on the weekly to-do list

Level 1 (more than expected): Completes 60–79% of items on the weekly to-do list

Level 0 (expected): Completes 40–59% of items on the weekly to-do list

Level –1 (baseline): Completes 20–39% (not using a system, but just remembers it)

Level –2 (below expected): Completes less than 20%

(Note that the levels are equidistant, unidimensional, directly related to the use of the tool, and functional for the client. See Chapter 5 for a description of Goal Attainment Scales.)

There are many options for measuring outcomes that can be translated into objective aims either through the generation of GAS scales or with SMART formulation:

• **Frequency of device or app use** (e.g., Ownsworth & McFarland, 1999; Schmitter-Edgecombe, Fahy, Whelan, & Long, 1995; Wright, 2020). Some external aids display usage data. For example, if a client is being trained to use a medication chart to record time, date, and dose, the clinician can document the number of recordings. Similarly, a clinician may count the number of entries in a diary or journal for a client using this aid for psychosocial or memory goals.

- **Performance on structured tasks designed to probe naturalistic use of an app.** A clinician can structure an assessment to determine if the aid is used successfully. For example, to measure the outcome of training a client to use a calendar function in a cell phone, the clinician might set up a probe and alter the session time and measure whether the client initiated and accurately used the calendar function to enter the scheduling information.

- **Retrospective questionnaires assessing performance in the domain facilitated by the external aid.** The clinician can design or use existing tools that measure potential change in the domain that the target aid was selected to assist. For example, memory questionnaires, quality-of-life scales, mood scales, and coping questionnaires may be used as relevant and appropriate for the target. Examples are the Everyday Memory Questionnaire (EMQ; Sunderland, Harris, & Baddeley, 1983), Cognitive Failures Questionnaire (Broadbent, Cooper, FitzGerald, & Parkes, 1982), Subjective Memory Questionnaire (Davis, Cockburn, Wade, & Smith, 1995), and Traumatic Brain Injury Quality-of-Life (TBI-QOL; Tulsky et al., 2016).

- **Performance on the tasks cued by the aid** (e.g., Kirsch et al., 1987; Wade & Troy, 2001; Wright & Sohlberg, 2021). A useful way to measure outcome is to determine whether the client is carrying out the target tasks the aid is designed to support. For example, if a client is using a navigation device such as a GPS system, an outcome measurement strategy might be to document the number of trips completed successfully in a 1-week period. Similarly, to measure outcomes for a client learning to use a checklist system for completing vocational tasks, the clinician may ask the client's employer to record the number of tasks completed without cueing.

- **Ratings of participant preference, satisfaction, or perception of improved performance** (Kim, Burke, Dowds, Boone, & Park, 2000; Ownsworth & McFarland, 1999; Schmitter-Edgecombe et al., 1995; Wright et al., 2001). Rating systems can be established to solicit and measure a client's perceptions about factors related to usability and impact.

The above measures offer options for documenting the impact of training the use of external aids. Depending on the type of training and the aid, and the specific type of outcome to be measured, the clinician can select the measures most appropriate to the client.

SUMMARY

Technology advances over the past decade have created abundant options for external aids that can help clients with cognitive impairments live more fully and independently. Below we provide a summary of the clinical processes for matching technology to individuals, developing goals and implementing training designed to promote sustained adoption and effective use of tools.

PLAN

- Interview to learn who the client is; determine possible treatment aims that reflect their sociocultural lived experiences, beliefs, values, and identities; and select assessment tools and procedures to determine if training use of an external aid may be a useful treatment approach.
- Administer assessment tools and procedures to evaluate hypotheses about cognitive challenges interfering with functional aims and determine whether the client has prerequisite abilities to effectively use an external aid.
- Conduct a needs assessment that uses a Matching Person & Technology (MPT) process and evaluates relevant client characteristics (cognitive, psychosocial, physical, and sensory abilities as well as sociocultural values) with environmental considerations. Consider using a tool such as the External Aid Needs Assessment interview (Form 8.2) to help identify aims and targets and select an aid.
- Generate a task analysis listing the steps involved in using the aid.
- Define functional and meaningful treatment aims and associated impact measures.
- Determine whether the client will need motivational or knowledge targets (R targets) and, if so, develop the corresponding targets and measures.
- Develop skill/habit (S) targets that operationalize the steps that will be trained to use the aid and define associated progress measures.
- Use SMART and/or GAS formatting for aims and targets (see Forms 5.1 and 5.2 in Chapter 5).
- Identify the phase of learning (acquisition, mastery/generalization, or maintenance) and select ingredients that are appropriate for the target group (e.g., distributed practice for S targets, self-reflection or knowledge questions for R targets) as well as the client's skills, values, and psychological status.

IMPLEMENT

- In the initial treatment session, obtain a baseline probe to determine where in the list of steps for training use of the external aid should begin (see Form 8.3) and which ingredients will be most effective in training during the acquisition phase. Important ingredients for this phase of learning include:
  - Ingredients to minimize client errors during practice (clinician demonstration, fading of prompts).
  - High rates of repetition with intensive massed practice in the acquisition phase to establish the skill, if necessary.
  - Chaining newly learned steps with previously learned steps.
  - Distributing or spacing practice once the steps are learned.
  - Quickly correcting any errors and providing additional repeated practice on that step or sequence, before fading prompts. When an error is made, the clinician will isolate a step that the client is not performing accurately and provide intensive practice until that step is mastered, then chain it back to the routine (i.e., have the client practice the step multiple times and then complete the preceding step and the difficult-to-learn step together before moving to longer practice intervals).
  - Ingredients to increase motivation and adherence (e.g., anticipation of difficult steps, charting own data, reinforcement).

- Prepare session data and progress monitoring forms (see Forms 8.4 and 8.5).
- In each subsequent session:
  - Review external aid homework results.
  - Conduct a retention probe to determine recall of steps involved in using the aid since prior session and the continuing need for any prompts or supports.
  - Conduct practice trials, starting at the level indicated by the retention probe.
  - At the generalization phase of learning, alter external aid ingredients to support generalization (e.g., fading supports, increasing distributed practice intervals, increasing stimulus variability, ensuring sustained motivation).
  - At the maintenance phase of learning, alter ingredients to maximize natural supports and sustain motivation and accountability (e.g., diaries, check-ins).
  - Document results and prescribe homework.

EVALUATE

- After each session, analyze progress to guide advancement to the next phase of learning (for examples, see the earlier Table 8.4).
- In the generalization and/or maintenance phases, obtain impact measures to evaluate the achievement of treatment aims and guide the continuance or discontinuation of intervention (e.g., frequency of app/aid use, satisfaction with app/aid, level of success achieved on functional tasks).

PUTTING IT ALL TOGETHER: CASE APPLICATIONS

In the remainder of the chapter, we provide examples to demonstrate the integration of the PIE framework for training use of external aids with actual clients. We begin by detailing an example of external aid training taken from the research literature (Svoboda & Richards, 2009) that illustrates and supports key components of the PIE framework. This case highlights attending to both acquisition and generalization and the implementation of error minimization to instruct an individual with severe memory impairments in the steps to use an external aid. The research example is followed by a description of two Case Applications that represent composite clients from our own practices. In the first Case Application, we support the reader in working through the stages of applying the information in a structured manner, making use of the various forms presented in this book, and we also supply sample completed forms. In the second Case Application, we provide similar structured guidance, but instead of supplying sample completed forms, we encourage the reader to complete the procedures independently.

A Case Example from the Literature

A single-case experiment evaluated the outcome of training a client with severe anterograde amnesia to use a smartphone to compensate for a declarative memory impairment that limited the client's ability to perform prospective tasks and recall recent events (Svoboda & Richards, 2009). The training was consistent with the principles of the PIE framework described in this chapter. Smartphone training consisted of two phases: basic skill acquisition and real-life generalization. The first phase used principles of errorless learning (EL) to teach content and procedures required for use of target applications on the smartphone. Each application was broken into its component steps. Performance on each component step was measured using a cueing hierarchy. The criterion for moving to the next stage of training was 98% correct on all steps within a single training session. The client successfully acquired all three calendar functions that were targeted in eight 1-hour training sessions.

In the generalization stage, the clinician introduced novel applications using the same EL approach and gave take-home assignments to use the phone for increasingly complex tasks. The client successfully and rapidly acquired the skills for using the address book, camera, camcorder, voice recorder, and other functions of the phone. In addition to session data measuring number of trials to criterion, outcome was measured as the percent of five assigned phone calls successfully completed by the client each week. Impact was measured by a standardized memory questionnaire that involved rating the frequency of occurrence of common memory mistakes and an assessment of smartphone use.

Results showed that the client demonstrated consistent and creative generalization of smartphone skills across a broad range of real-life memory-demanding circumstances. The authors suggested that theory-driven, systematic, hierarchically organized training can allow individuals with severe memory impairment to exploit commercially available tools to successfully support memory.

Two Case Applications

Below we provide two case examples where external aid training was applied to help clients achieve their aims. For Case Application 1, as we describe the stages of intervention, we direct the reader to practice applying the information in a structured manner, making use of the various forms presented in this book (fillable forms for each item are included in the digital files accompanying this book). Completed Case Application Sample Answers are included at the end of this chapter. For Case Application 2, we offer the reader an opportunity to practice and apply the principles and procedures reviewed in this chapter and demonstrated in Case Application 1. Sample answers are not provided for this case. What is most important is to follow a structured approach in planning, implementing, and evaluating the intervention.

CASE APPLICATION 1—HAP

Description of Client

The client, named Henry ("Hap"), was a 45-year-old male who had been a long-haul trucker. Hap's wife Sondra, a nurse, was supportive and involved in her husband's rehabilitation. The couple had a 7-year-old son Cole. Hap was 1 year post severe brain injury from an accident that occurred while truck driving for a large company. He had fallen asleep while driving overtime. He received a large settlement from his company, which maintained contact and provided ongoing support. Following his accident, Hap received intensive inpatient rehabilitation followed by 3-month-long treatment in a residential brain injury program, where he participated in a comprehensive, integrated program, receiving services from an occupational therapist (OT), a physical therapist (PT), psychiatrist, and speech-language pathologist (SLP). Hap made good progress in self-care skills, walking, speech and language, and self-awareness and acceptance. While in the program, the team embedded their discipline-specific goals using the development of a manual for trucker safety training. For example, Hap worked on his language goals while writing portions of the manual and on his social cognition goals by taking the perspective of truck drivers who would read the manual. Hap's company was committed to using the manual, which featured his story. This project had helped Hap find renewed meaning in his life. Following completion of the residential program, Hap returned home to live with his family and began outpatient cognitive rehabilitation.

Planning

The clinician reviewed the records on file, conducted a clinical interview with Hap and Sondra, and readministered several cognitive assessments to evaluate recovery. Based on the clinical interview and stated goals and needs, the clinician conducted the External Aids Needs Assessment interview (Form 8.2). The assessment process revealed the following client profile:

Sociocultural values. Hap indicated that while Sondra had always taken on more of the child-rearing duties in the family, he greatly valued how his son looked up to him for being strong, fearless, and adventurous. Before his father's accident, Cole had often been overheard telling friends that his dad was a "world explorer," just like the truck drivers they watched on TV. It was important to Hap that his son continue to view him in these ways, but he worried that the loss of his truck-driving identity would alter this perception. The External Aid Needs Assessment interview revealed that Hap had previously been fluent in using his smartphone for communication (calling and texting), FaceTime, map navigation, and conducting Internet searches, but he did not use it for scheduling or managing task completion. Since being discharged home, he hadn't used his phone, but while in the residential program, he had received support for relearning to use it for communication and map navigation.

Cognitive findings. Hap's test results showed severe declarative recall and new learning deficits and moderate to severe attention deficits. No impulsivity was observed, but frustration was apparent on tasks that Hap perceived should be easy.

Physical and sensory functions. Hap stated that he was experiencing some reduced sensation and fine motor coordination in his right hand, and that being left-handed had allowed him to compensate. His gait was adequate for many daily activities, but he needed to pay extra attention if higher levels of coordination, speed, or balance were required. He continued to work with both an OT and a PT to address these areas.

Psychosocial functioning. Hap reported that he was aware of the large volume of household and child-rearing tasks that Sondra had taken on since his injury, in addition to working almost full-time shifts. While Sondra was accustomed to this in short stints due to the nature of Hap's job, the constant demands of managing their son, their household, and Hap's medical and rehabilitation needs were starting to take their toll. Sondra shared that Hap had recently begun expressing frustration with her in the moment if she hadn't managed a given task to his satisfaction, but later during quiet conversation after their son had gone to bed, he would acknowledge that he knew how much she was trying to juggle. Hap reported feelings of guilt for the changes his accident had imposed on his family. Hap and Sondra were able to describe grief related to changes in Hap's ability, while also acknowledging gratitude for his survival and recovery. The couple appeared resilient and to benefit from opportunities to acknowledge loss and progress.

Environmental variables. Hap's half-ton pickup truck was in the garage, and Sondra kept the keys with her at all times as Hap was not permitted to drive. With Hap's medical and social appointments and their son's increasing involvement in sports activities, Sondra's role as the sole driver in the family was challenging. She identified transportation as one of her biggest caregiving burdens, and Hap identified his lack of independence in terms of transportation as one of his primary concerns.

During the clinical interview, Hap clearly identified that his aim was to contribute to managing household demands, starting with a resumption of driving to appointments and social get-togethers. Knowing that he would not get medical clearance to resume driving in the short term, the clinician applied motivational interviewing techniques, and Hap decided that he would adjust his plan from driving to managing his transportation needs via other means. The External Aids Needs Assessment interview provided evidence that using an app to access a ride-share program would be a good match for Hap's needs, interests, and abilities (he particularly liked the mapping and address recall features of using an app vs. simply phoning the company). Using the app review sheet in Form 8.1, Hap was able to compare two apps from large ride-share companies and one from a local company that was designed for seniors and people with disabilities. Although Hap wasn't keen on being considered either a senior or someone with a disability, his analysis suggested that the features associated with the local ride-share app would be much better suited to his needs. A task analysis revealed that the following steps would be required to use the app:

1. Press the car icon on the phone to open the app.
2. Press "My Locations" in the app.
3. Choose the desired location from the drop-down menu.
4. Press the phone icon and wait for a "thumbs up" confirmation.
5. Press the alarm clock icon.
6. Walk outside to meet the car when the alarm goes off.

A baseline probe was completed as part of the assessment on June 2, which showed that Hap could easily locate the ride-share icon on the main screen of his phone (step 1) and because he selected a horn-honking alarm sound, he immediately recognized that it was time to go meet the car when the alarm went off (step 6). However, he needed prompts or visual cues to complete steps 2–5.

Application Practice

Use the information above to complete Form 8.3: Baseline Probe for External Aid Use and compare it with the Case Application Sample Answer: Form 8.3 at the end of the chapter.

The first target was for Hap to independently complete all steps of the ride-share app without having to refer to instructions. In addition to measuring his accuracy in completing the steps, Hap also wanted to tally how many rides he booked to appointments each week as he believed that this would help increase his motivation to keep practicing with the app.

Application Practice

Document the aim, target, ingredients, and steps for using the app on Form 8.4: Therapy Session Data Form. Target acquisition, generalization, and maintenance will be measured by independence in using the app in increasingly varied contexts, but Hap's additional requested measure of target success should also be included. Add this measurement plan to Form 8.4. Copy the target, training phase, and app steps onto Form 8.5: Progress Monitoring Form to be ready for the "at a glance" summary of Hap's session-to-session progress. Compare your forms to the Case Application Sample Answers at the end of the chapter (Form 8.4, Session 1, and Form 8.5), but don't peek at the data sections yet!

Beyond measuring independent app use in session and the number of rides booked each week, Hap and Sondra wanted measures to evaluate the ultimate impact that independent use of the app would have on key pressure points in their daily lives: a reduced caregiver burden for Sondra and an improved sense of contribution to the household for Hap. They decided to complete their ratings after Cole had gone to bed each night and make notes of anything that could further support continued improvement in their ratings.

Application Practice

Based on the information above and referring to the checklists in Forms 5.1 and 5.2 in Chapter 5, create a rating scale for Sondra to measure caregiver burden and a GAS scale for Hap to measure his perception of contribution to the household. Compare your scales with the Case Application Sample Answer: Rating and Attainment Scales at the end of the chapter.

Implementation

Hap did not require any training on R targets relating to motivation, as he was very focused on managing his own transportation needs to regain a small part of his prior identity. However, there was a risk of him shifting focus to driving himself instead of using the ride-share service, so motivational interviewing techniques were built in as an ingredient in his app training as needed and the clinician was prepared to add an R target related to understanding the rationale for not driving if that became necessary.

To support acquisition phase learning of the S target of independent use of the app, the clinician created a double-sided cue card with screenshots of each of the six steps. The card was designed to fit into a pocket in Hap's cell phone case. In addition, the app developers had built in a "learning mode" whereby the steps could be practiced without actually hailing a ride, so the clinician set the app to learning mode and then asked Hap and Sondra to work together to enter the medical/rehabilitation appointment locations he attended, along with his home address for the return trips.

In the first therapy session on June 9, the clinician administered a retention probe to see what Hap recalled from when they first reviewed the steps to using the app. Hap could easily find the ride-share app on his phone but hesitated when looking for the "My Locations" section and instead randomly pressed a range of different icons in the app and became frustrated. Before moving on to the practice trials, the clinician reinstructed and modeled how to access the "My Locations" icon on the app. Hap and Sondra did report that they had together entered all of the required locations in the app.

The clinician began practice trials in this first therapy session by retrieving the cue card from the smartphone case and placing it directly on the table in front of Hap. They selected the physiotherapy clinic as the target location because Hap went there almost every day for therapy or exercise classes, and the appointments often occurred after his in-home cognitive rehabilitation session was completed. Prior to every step of the first practice trial, the clinician modeled the response and also pointed to that step on the cue card. With these error minimization techniques, Hap successfully finished all six steps. He didn't require any supports for step 6 as he immediately recognized that the horn-honking alarm meant he needed to go meet the car. The clinician began the second practice trial at step 2 because step 1 appeared to be established and automatic. The model was faded for this practice trial, and the clinician instead just pointed to the cue card prior to every step. Hap was once again successful on all steps and once again did not need the cue card for the final one. In the third practice round, the clinician decided to start at step 2 again but this time removed the cue card. Hap completed steps 2–3 quickly and accurately but "drew a blank" for step 4. The clinician therefore completed massed practice with step 4: two repetitions with modeling, two repetitions with the cue card, and then two repetitions without supports, chained to step 3. In the fourth and final practice trial of the session, the clinician started at step 3 given that Hap hadn't had any trouble with steps 1–2 in the prior practice trials. Hap was successful at recalling step 4 this time but "froze" with step 5, so the clinician again implemented massed practice: two repetitions with modeling, two repetitions with the cue card, and then two repetitions without supports, chained to step 4.

Application Practice

Document the practice results from Session 1 on Form 8.4 and document the summative measure for this first session (prepractice retention probe) on Form 8.5. Generate ideas for home practice to assign for Hap and Sondra, based on the results obtained in session, and document this information on Form 8.4. Compare your forms to the Case Application Sample Answers at the end of the chapter (Form 8.4, Session 1, and Form 8.5).

In Session 2 on June 13, Sondra reported that she and Hap had practiced with the app 2 to 3 times each evening using the cue card, and Hap was successful with all steps each time. Hap additionally reported that Sondra had phoned to remind him to have his cue card out to help with booking rides twice since the last session, and he successfully completed both bookings. In the retention probe at the start of the session, Hap was fully independent on steps 1–3 but was unable to recall what to do after selecting the location, so the clinician completed reinstruction and modeling, focusing on step 4 and the preceding step 3, before starting practice trials. Now that Hap was independent with steps 1–3, the clinician began practice trials on step 3. In order to ensure errorless performance for the first trial, Hap was asked to refer to the cue card prior to completing each step, and he was successful on all steps. The clinician then faded this cue for the second practice trial and asked Hap to complete the steps without supports. Steps 3–4 were completed accurately and quickly, but Hap thought he was done after waiting for the thumbs up icon and closed the app. The clinician therefore did massed practice with step 5: with one round of modeling, two rounds using the cue card, then three rounds without supports but chaining to step 4. Hap then successfully completed all six steps without supports in the third practice trial. For the final practice trial of the session, Hap asked to book a real trip to the physiotherapy clinic, as he was heading there next. The clinician therefore started Hap at step 1, and Hap was able to complete all six steps independently and accurately. While waiting for the ride to arrive, Hap asked if perhaps driving himself would be a good option to save having to wait, so the clinician implemented MI techniques that helped reinforce Hap's original decision and rationale to use the ride-share company for now.

Application Practice

Create a new Form 8.4 to document results from the second session and add the summative information to Form 8.5. Generate home practice suggestions for Hap and Sondra based on the session's results. Compare your forms to the Case Application Sample Answers at the end of the chapter (Form 8.4, Session 2, and Form 8.5).

When the clinician arrived for Session 3 on June 20, Hap was excited to share his ride-booking log, where he had documented successfully booking five rides since the last session without using the cue card for any of them. Sondra added that they had done one practice run with the cue card and one or two without it prior to booking each ride, and Hap was successful in each attempt. He kept the cue card in the pocket of his phone case as backup but hadn't needed it that week. During the retention probe, Hap was successful with steps 1–4 but once again forgot to activate the alarm icon before shutting down the app, so the clinician completed reinstruction before moving on to practice trials. They started practice trial 1 at step 4, given Hap's repeated success with steps 1–3, and Hap was fully independent with all remaining steps. The clinician decided to advance Hap to the mastery and generalization phase by integrating distributed practice. With this new level of difficulty, they started practice trial 2 at step 3 to build on chaining before tackling the more challenging steps and they implemented a 20-second delay after each step. Hap was successful on all steps. The clinician then completed round 3 with a 30-second delay between steps and additionally changed the location from the physio clinic to the return trip home.

Because of the change in location, they started this practice trial from step 1. Hap was once again accurate in his actions and independent with all steps. For the final practice trial, Hap booked a real trip to the physiotherapy clinic for his exercise class after the cognitive rehabilitation session. The clinician again inserted a 30-second delay between steps, which Hap reported as "nerve-wracking" when booking a real trip, but he succeeded once more.

Application Practice

Create a third Form 8.4 to document results of this session and add the summative information to Form 8.5. Generate home practice suggestions for Hap and Sondra based on the session's results. Compare your forms to the Case Application Sample Answers at the end of the chapter (Form 8.4, Session 3, and Form 8.5).

Session 4 occurred on June 24, and Hap reported that he had booked six trips since the last session, including three return trips home after an appointment. The trips to the clinic were booked without supports, and the trips to return home were done using the cue card due to increased "nerves" using the app in the waiting room of the physio clinic. For the retention probe, the clinician chose the "Home" location, and Hap performed the same as he did in the last session when using the physio clinic as the location. The clinician continued to advance Hap through the mastery and generalization phase by maintaining the 30-second delay between steps, adding a 2-minute delay between practice trials and a third location (psychology clinic) to the practice trials. Hap again raised the possibility of driving himself to appointments, so the clinician used MI to refocus him on his current goal and prior rationale. Sondra joined this session via FaceTime and reported that their evening self-ratings and discussions generally continued to go well (there were occasional disagreements, but they were always resolved before the couple went to bed), and the two had begun to document some ideas to further increase Hap's independent performance of household tasks.

Application Practice

You may skip completing a fourth Form 8.4 but add the summative measure (retention probe results) from Session 4 to Form 8.5 along with other key highlights from this session. Compare your form with the Case Application Sample Answer: Form 8.5 at the end of the chapter.

Evaluation

The initial evaluation included the target acquisition data tracking the number of steps in using the app that were completed independently, as well as the number of rides booked between sessions. Generalization data used the same metrics for varied locations completed in learning mode and in operational mode, both within sessions and between sessions. Because of the good gains being seen, the clinician chose to document preliminary impact results at the beginning of the fourth week of therapy. Sondra shared that she was most typically rating her caregiver burden as a 3 (compared to 1–2 prior to therapy). She reported that it seemed unlikely that she could ever reach a 5 on her scale, but she was committed to finding ways for Hap to take on a greater workload around the house. Hap reported that he had achieved his expected outcome level and believed that he might even be able to achieve level +1 by the 6-week mark. Both Hap and Sondra agreed that the daily rating scales were helping to keep them accountable to the therapy targets and aims. Hap reported that he would like to start brainstorming ideas for a new goal relating to greater involvement in being a role model for his son, including perhaps becoming responsible for taking him to twice-weekly lacrosse practice that would be starting in a couple of months.

Application Practice

Document the impact data on Sondra's rating scale and Hap's Goal Attainment Scale and compare your information with the Case Application Sample Answer: Achieved at the end of the chapter.

CASE APPLICATION 2—MADISON

Description of Client

The client, Madison, was a 29-year-old female, second-year graduate student in business. She was returning to courses after taking off a term to recover from a concussion resulting from a bicycle accident. Madison lived with a roommate who was also a grad student. Madison had thought she was mostly healed except for periodic headaches and occasional sleep disturbances, but when she tried to go back to classes, she felt as if she was "dropping balls." She reported challenges prioritizing reading and assignments and juggling class projects, finding that she would spend too long on one project and not have time for another. At the end of the semester, Madison was scheduled to take one of the required 48-hour group take-home case exams, and she was very worried about how to manage working within a group to complete the full business case analysis required for the exam in that restricted time frame. Madison's family provided financial support for her to seek help from a private clinic specializing in post-concussion rehabilitation.

Planning

During the clinical interview, the SLP asked Madison to describe a typical day and specify her successes and frustrations. The interview revealed that Madison had the skills and knowledge to complete the academic work, but had trouble switching tasks, monitoring her time, and prioritizing what needed to be done. Additional information obtained during the assessment included:

Sociocultural values. Madison reported coming from a family with a strong history of entrepreneurship. Her parents and aunt and uncle owned two restaurants, and their succession plan included bringing her in as an owner. Madison wasn't sure this was what she wanted to do—she had seen firsthand how much hard work was involved—but she had decided to pursue an MBA in order to keep open a range of options for herself. If she was going to follow the path her family hoped she would pursue, she wanted to ensure that she was fully prepared; and if she chose a different path, she thought the MBA would still prove useful.

Cognitive findings. Madison reported that formal testing completed 2 months earlier revealed her cognitive performance to be within normal limits, but she stated that she was most definitely not back to "normal." Her self-ratings on the Behavior Rating Inventory of Executive Function (BRIEF; Goia et al., 2000) showed low scores on the Plan/Organize Scales that were part of the Cognitive Regulation Index. These scores were consistent with Madison's subjective reports of difficulty with task management.

Physical and sensory functions. Madison stated that her sleep problems and headaches had improved over the first few months post-accident, but they seemed to be worsening since her return to school. She reported that the referring occupational therapist had educated her about the impact of sleep disturbance and headaches on cognitive functions and initiated training in sleep hygiene.

Psychosocial functioning. Madison reported no psychosocial concerns. She stated that she was worried about not being able to juggle everything but had always been a hard worker and rarely let anything get to her.

Environmental variables. Madison's roommate was in a different class in the same program, so she understood the high demands, but they didn't work together on any projects. The roommate was quiet and tended to keep to herself, but she had been the one who picked up Madison from the emergency room the day of the accident. She had told Madison that she was happy to make any adjustments to their apartment to help Madison complete her schoolwork effectively.

Madison told the SLP that her goal was to "decrease the number of balls dropped" each week and regain some of her prior productivity/efficiency. The External Aid Needs Assessment interview (Form 8.2) suggested that a personalized task management system, using existing features on her desktop computer and smartphone such as the to-do list on Google Calendar tied to the alarm on her phone, would be the best solution for her. Madison was very comfortable with these aids and believed that audio alerts would be optimal for her. She also liked that the systems were synched between her phone and desktop computer, so she didn't have to always refer to the small screen on her phone. The SLP and Madison jointly decided on the following steps for using the aids:

1. Each morning, review/refine the to-do list and put its items in order of importance.
2. Assign the estimated or desired time to work on each item based on her daily schedule.
3. Set alarms for when to start each item.
4. When the alarm goes off, get the materials for that task or, if needed, reschedule the task to later in the day or another day.
5. Before starting the task, set a new (different tone) alarm for how long she will work on the task based on her original estimate.
6. When the alarm goes off, reflect on progress made, review the to-do list, and make any needed adjustments.

A baseline probe was not completed, as none of the items in the task analysis for using the aids involved new learning. The list of six steps was then typed up and laminated with columns to allow Madison to check off with a marker when each step was completed for each of the required tasks. She then rinsed off the list for use again the next day. Madison's target was to complete all six steps at least 5 days per week. For the target acquisition measure, she was asked to take a photograph of the completed task page before rinsing it off for the next day. Impact measures included a 1–10 productivity rating completed at the end of each day and a percentage tally of all the balls she successfully juggled that day (putting a "+" next to each item on her to-do list that she attended to and then calculating the percentage of "balls dropped").

Application Practice:

Document the aim, target, ingredients, steps in using the aids, and measurement plan on Form 8.4: Therapy Session Data. Where information has not been specifically provided above, brainstorm options that would work for Madison. Copy the pertinent items onto Form 8.5: Progress Monitoring. To measure the ultimate impact of implementing external aids in Madison's life, use the checklist in Form 5.1 in Chapter 5 to create a SMART-formulated aim to reflect the percentage of balls dropped and use the checklist in Form 5.2 to create a GAS scale to show changes on the productivity scale. No sample answers are provided; instead, complete this task independently to practice application of the principles in the planning stage.

Implementation

Madison agreed to an intervention plan involving six sessions. Sessions were completed virtually so that Madison could work in her own environment and not lose valuable time while traveling to and from the SLP clinic. Each "session" was divided into two or three 15- to 20-minute segments, spread out over the course of a day. This scheduling format was used at the private concussion clinic in order to provide more support at the acquisition phase and decrease intervention time during the mastery phase. At the beginning of the day, the SLP practiced steps 1–3 with Madison (and also discussed her ratings from the night before), and at the middle and/or end of the day, the SLP reviewed her performance on steps 4–6.

The acquisition phase for Madison lasted two sessions. Her progress was augmented by her strong preexisting knowledge and skills and high motivation. On the first day, Madison had her laminated list of steps ready in front of her along with several notebooks and sticky notes with coursework requirements jotted down. She required specific direction and modeling to decide on how to allocate priorities, when to start tasks, and how much time to assign to tasks. The clinician also specifically directed Madison to write down how she came to each decision so that she could refer to this information for future decisions. At the midday check-in, Madison showed her laminated page to the SLP. The page documented that she had rescheduled one task to the end of the day but completed the other task as planned. At the end-of-day check-in, Madison's laminated page showed that she had followed the allocated time/task parameters for a total of three tasks (one from the morning, two from the afternoon), forgotten about one task (turned off the alarm and then became distracted), and ended up having to reschedule the morning task again to the next day. Madison reported that steps 1–3 presented her with the most challenge, while steps 4–6 generally "seemed more manageable." She had created an online repository that both she and the SLP could access, and she uploaded the photograph of what she now called her PASS, "Planning and Accountability System and Sheet."

The second session in the acquisition phase occurred the following day. That morning, Madison reported that the night before she had given herself a productivity rating of 5/10 and recorded 40% balls dropped (she gave herself credit for the three tasks completed as planned, no credit for the missed item, and also no credit for the rescheduled item because she decided that rescheduling once would be acceptable, but not twice). The SLP used a general reminder question ("What did you do yesterday when you were making prioritization decisions?") to encourage Madison to retrieve her notes on how she prioritized and allocated time for yesterday's tasks. These notes acted as written instructions for Madison, and when referring to them, she was able to independently prioritize all six tasks in her app for the day. The clinician continued with general reminder questions (vs. the specific instruction and modeling used in the first session) for Madison to complete steps 2–3. Madison requested that the midday check-in be canceled, so the SLP just checked in at the end of the day. Madison had rescheduled one task to the next day, had missed another task due to turning off the alarm and forgetting, but completed the other four tasks as planned. Having turned off alarms without completing the required procedures on two consecutive days, the SLP referred to the data to identify the problem and then used collaborative problem solving to find a solution: altering step 4 to include a "snooze" feature after 3 minutes. With this change to the protocol, Madison's success level suggested she was ready to move to the generalization phase.

In Sessions 3–5 (two sessions in Week 2 followed by one session in Week 3), Madison demonstrated and reported consistently using her PASS for an increasing variety of tasks each day; most of the work in this generalization phase was occurring outside of the therapy sessions. The snooze function had immediately solved the initial challenge with step 4. The clinician was able to discontinue use of guided prompts and instead asked, "And what next?" Madison gradually became independent and proficient with steps 1–3, regardless of the variety of tasks scheduled and regardless of which device she was using. While she never failed to complete step 5, she wasn't always happy with her decision for the length of time allocated, and this affected how she rated herself on the productivity scale. She demonstrated full independence with step 6 for a variety of tasks and in more complex situations (e.g., with her roommate present) by the fifth session, with the only ingredient offered by the clinician being praise for progress, including a graph visually reinforcing the gains made. Madison was ready to move to the maintenance phase, and a maintenance session was booked for 3 weeks later.

Application Practice

Document the ingredients and results from the acquisition phase sessions on Form 8.4 and brainstorm hypothetical results from each generalization session, based on the information provided above. Transfer summative measures to Form 8.5. Once again, no sample answers are provided; instead, generate responses and then compare with the principles in the implementation stage.

To support the transition to maintenance, Madison agreed to have her roommate help encourage her motivation and accountability. The roommate joined the maintenance session so that Madison could demonstrate her system and both Madison and the SLP could answer any questions. Madison demonstrated or explained all steps independently and accurately. Together, Madison and her roommate then prepared a plan for how the roommate would encourage Madison to maintain her diligence in carrying out the PASS. Madison also shared contexts where she thought she might falter, and the triad brainstormed ideas to prepare for these situations. Three weeks after this session, the clinician completed a short check-in and Madison and her roommate reported on what had gone well, what difficulties they had encountered, and how they had managed them. The roommate reported that it really didn't take much effort on her part to keep Madison motivated but she was happy to continue providing encouragement as needed.

Evaluation

As described above, initial acquisition and generalization data focused on the number of steps Madison completed independently in using her aids, as well as measures of productivity and percentage of balls dropped. Productivity and percentage of balls dropped were also used as impact measures. At the time of the maintenance session, Madison reported an average productivity rating of 7/10, and had recorded a range of 0–40% balls dropped per day in the prior 3 weeks. During the final check-in session, the balls dropped figure ranged from 0 to 30% over the prior 3 weeks, and Madison said she was close to giving herself a productivity rating of 8/10 but was going to "stick with" 7.5 until she saw how she performed on the 48-hour exam coming up in a couple of weeks. Madison also reported improvement in sleep hygiene practices, and while she still experienced headaches from time to time, the frequency had returned to where it had been before she started to attend classes again. In addition to improved productivity, Madison indicated that she had begun scheduling some "me" time at least twice per week and so was now attending yoga or going for walks. She wondered if it might be helpful to increase the "me" time to 4–5 times per week.

Application Practice

Using the information above, generate one or two additional Goal Attainment Scales that could have been utilized to measure the ultimate impact of Madison's use of the external aids. Make sure that there are five equidistant, unidimensional, measurable levels of progress, with baseline performance being zero.

Baseline Probe for External Aid Use

Client: Hap	Date: June 2

Prompt:

Show me how you use the app to book a ride to the physio clinic.

Context where probe obtained:

In client home at dining table where he works

Steps Recalled Independently:

Steps	Correct?	Comments
1. Press car icon on phone to open app	✓	Completed quickly (only a few apps on main screen)
2. Press "my locations" in the app	✗	Pressed a few different icons; prompted to look at cue card and then found correct icon
3. Choose the desired location from the dropdown menu	✗	Was flustered from step 2 and forgot where he was supposed to be going, so had to prompt
4. Press the phone icon and wait for a "thumbs up" confirmation	✗	Pressed a few different icons; prompted to look at cue card and then found correct icon
5. Press the alarm clock icon	✗	Thought he was done, had to prompt to cue card
6. Go outside to meet the car when the alarm goes off	✓	Alarm sounds like a car horn—easy to recognize and associate

Other Comments/Observations:

Tended to work quickly and had a more impulsive than methodical method of looking for icons

CASE APPLICATION SAMPLE ANSWER: FORM 8.4, SESSION 1

Therapy Session Data Form—Target Acquisition, Mastery, Generalization (External Aid Use)

Client Name: Hap **Date:** June 9 **Location:** Client Home **Others Present:** Sondra (wife)

Target: Independently complete all 6 steps on app without external supports

Associated Aim: Increased contribution to managing household demands

Training Phase: Acquisition

Ingredients—Items:
Ride share app with learning mode
Cue card with list of icons/actions
Blank progress recording sheet

Ingredients—Actions:
Reviewing steps
Massed practice with error control
Chaining of steps

Ingredients—Motivators:
Hap will record own progress
Encouragement/praise
MI if driving comes up

Measurement Plan:
steps done ind. without cue card
rides booked each week

Check-in Info and Results of Homework: Hap and Sondra reported entering all of the required appointment locations in the app and also their home address for the return trips. Have not attempted to use the app yet, preferring to wait until today.

Practice Data:	Retention Probe	Practice 1:	Practice 2:	Practice 3:	Practice 4:
External Aid Steps:		Physio Clinic	Physio Clinic	Physio Clinic	Physio Clinic
6. go outside when alarm goes off		+ ind	+ ind		
5. press alarm clock icon		+	+		- MMCC ++
4. press phone icon and wait for thumbs up		+	+	- MMCC ++	++

(continued)

Therapy Session Data Form—Target Acquisition, Mastery, Generalization (External Aid Use) *(page 2 of 2)*

Practice Data:	Retention Probe	Practice 1:	Practice 2:	Practice 3:	Practice 4:
3. *select destination*		+	+	+ / ++	+
2. *press "my locations"*	–	+	+	+	N/A
1. *open phone and touch car icon*	+	+	N/A	N/A	N/A
Comments:	*After error, modeled and described step 2*	*Model + cue card prior to each response except step 6—no support needed*	*Cue card alone (no model) prior to each response except step 6—independent*	*No supports; massed practice of step 4 after error, chained to step 3 (M = model, C = cue card)*	*No supports; massed practice of step 5 after error, chained to step 4 (M = model, C = cue card)*

Session Summary/Analysis of Progress:

Excellent performance with cue card visible; massed practice plus chaining supported fading of cue card

Feedback and Homework Provided (task, context, ingredients, tracking):

Sondra to direct to cue card for each step when booking transportation between now and next session—errorless practice is key at home; do additional practice in learning mode if time; track # rides booked while using cue card.

Plan for Next Session:

Fade cue card quickly, see if possible to integrate distributed practice

Progress Monitoring Form—
Target Acquisition, Mastery, Generalization (External Aid Use)

Client Name: Hap   **Target:** Independently completely all 6 steps on app without   **Training Phase:** Acquisition-external supports Mastery-Generalization

Select the summary measure being tracked (must use the same from each session):

☑ Retention probe result from start of each session

☐ Average of each session's practice trial results

☐ Other:

	Summary Measure			
	Jun 9	Jun 13	Jun 20	Jun 24
External Aid Steps:	To Physio	To Physio	To Physio	To Home
6. go outside when alarm goes off				
5. press alarm clock icon			−	−
4. press phone icon and wait for thumbs up		−	+	+
3. select destination		+	+	+
2. press "my locations"	−	+	+	+
1. open phone and touch car icon	+	+	+	+
Ingredients:				
Prompts and Supports:	No supports or prompts used during any retention probes			
	During practice trials after retention probe: −Model + cue card for initial practice but then faded model −Began fading cue card in final trials but required massed practice to support success on steps 4–5	During practice trials after retention probe: −Cue card faded after 1st practice trial; required massed practice for step 5 in 2nd trial −Final 2 trials were done without supports	During practice trials after retention probe: −No supports −Added 20–30 sec delay in between each step −Added 1 new location (home) to practice	During practice trials after retention probe: −Used Home for retention trial −No supports −30 sec delay in between each step −2 min delay in between each trial −Added 2nd new location (Psych) to practice trials
Motivational:	−Records own progress on performance sheet −Encouragement and praise	−Records own progress −Encouragement and praise −MI re driving	−Records own progress −Encouragement and praise	−Records own progress −Encouragement and praise −MI re driving
Other Measures:				
	N/A	−Booked 2 rides to PT since last session, referring to cue card	−Booked 5 rides to PT since last session without cue card visible	−Booked 6 trips, including 3 to come home from PT (used cue card for the return trips)

Sondra's Caregiver Burden Rating Scale

1	2	3	4	5
Daily demands exceeded my capacity to manage, and I had to withdraw and let things drop.	Daily demands felt "crushing,"as if I wouldn't be able to manage everything much longer.	Daily demands were high, but I largely kept up and therefore didn't feel as hopeless.	Daily demands were moderate to high, but I kept up and usually felt OK about the situation.	Daily demands were moderate and I kept up, felt OK about the situation, and even found some true relaxation time.

Hap's Goal Attainment Scale—To Be Achieved within 6 weeks

−2 Much less than expected	−1 Less than expected (baseline)	0 Expected outcome	+1 Better than expected	+2 Much better than expected
I am not helping with daily household demands, and my behavior frequently adds to the demands. I feel like a burden.	I am not helping with daily household demands. I feel as if I lack purpose.	I am helping with or managing an average of 1 daily household demand. I feel as if I am starting to contribute again.	I am helping with or managing an average of 2 daily household demands. I feel as if I am actually contributing.	I am helping with or managing an average of 3 daily household demands. I feel as if I am making a difference.

Therapy Session Data Form—Target Acquisition, Mastery, Generalization (External Aid Use)

Client Name: Hap **Date:** June 13 **Location:** Client Home **Others Present:** Sondra (wife)

Target: Independently complete all 6 steps on app without external supports **Associated Aim:** Increased contribution to managing household demands **Training Phase:** Acquisition

Ingredients—Items:
Ride share app with learning mode
Cue card with list of icons/actions
Blank progress recording sheet

Ingredients—Actions:
Massed practice with error control
Chaining of steps
Fading cue card

Ingredients—Motivators:
Hap will record own progress
Encouragement/praise
MI if driving comes up

Measurement Plan:
steps done ind. without cue card
rides booked each week

Check-in Info and Results of Homework: Hap and Sondra did 2–3 practice runs using the cue card each evening and all were done accurately. Hap also booked 2 rides to the physio clinic since last session (Sondra phoned to remind him to have the cue card in front of him each time). They are feeling optimistic!

Practice Data: External Aid Steps:	Retention Probe	Practice 1: Physio Clinic	Practice 2: Physio Clinic	Practice 3: Physio Clinic	Practice 4: Physio Clinic
6. go outside when alarm goes off		+ ind	+	+	+
5. press alarm clock icon		+	– MMCC +++	+	+
4. press phone icon and wait for thumbs up	–	+	+++	+	+

(continued)

Therapy Session Data Form—Target Acquisition, Mastery, Generalization (External Aid Use) *(page 2 of 2)*

Practice Data:	Retention Probe	Practice 1:	Practice 2:	Practice 3:	Practice 4:
3. select destination	+	+	+	+	+
2. press "my locations"	+	N/A	N/A	N/A	+
1. open phone and touch car icon	+	N/A	N/A	N/A	+
Comments:	After error, modeled and described step 4	Directed to cue card prior to each response, except step 6—no support needed	No supports; massed practice of step 5 after error, chained to step 3 (M = model, C = cue card)	No supports for any step	No supports; booked real trip on this sequence!

Session Summary/Analysis of Progress:

Massed practice continued to support fading of cue card (cue card is good backup if needed—storing in pocket of phone case); while waiting for ride to arrive, Hap inquired about driving himself—used MI to redirect back to current targets

Feedback and Homework Provided (task, context, ingredients, tracking):

For each trip between now and next session, Sondra to do one practice sequence directing to cue card, a 2nd practice sequence without card, then final sequence to book trip without card; additional learning mode practice if time; track # rides booked

Plan for Next Session:

Move to distributed practice

227

Therapy Session Data Form—Target Acquisition, Mastery, Generalization (External Aid Use)

Client Name: Hap

Date: June 20

Location: Client Home

Others Present: Sondra (wife)

Training Phase: Mastery/Generalization

Target: Independently complete all 6 steps on app without external supports

Associated Aim: Increased contribution to managing household demands

Ingredients—Items:
Ride share app with learning mode
Cue card with list of icons/actions
Blank progress recording sheet

Ingredients—Actions:
Distributed practice
Vary locations
Massed practice if needed

Ingredients—Motivators:
Hap will record own progress
Encouragement/praise
MI if driving comes up

Measurement Plan:
steps done ind. without cue card
rides booked each week

Check-in Info and Results of Homework: Hap and Sondra did 1 practice run with cue card and 1–2 without prior to booking each trip—100% on all of these; Hap successfully booked 5 trips since last session! Cue card remains in phone pocket as back up but hasn't been used.

Practice Data:	Retention Probe	Practice 1:	Practice 2:	Practice 3:	Practice 4:
External Aid Steps:		Physio Clinic	Physio Clinic	Physio Clinic	Physio Clinic
6. go outside when alarm goes off		+	+	+	+
5. press alarm clock icon	–	+	+	+	+
4. press phone icon and wait for thumbs up	+	+	+	+	+

(continued)

Therapy Session Data Form—Target Acquisition, Mastery, Generalization (External Aid Use) *(page 2 of 2)*

Practice Data:	Retention Probe	Practice 1:	Practice 2:	Practice 3:	Practice 4:
3. select destination	+	N/A	+	+	+
2. press "my locations"	+	N/A	N/A	+	+
1. open phone and touch car icon	+	N/A	N/A	+	+
Comments:	After error, modeled and described step 5 (seemed nervous for retention probe)	Independent with all steps	No supports for any step; added 20 sec delay after each step	No supports; changed location to Home; increased to 30 sec delay per step	No supports; 30 sec delay; booked real trip to PT clinic (Hap was nervous but successful!)

Session Summary/Analysis of Progress:

Cue card fully faded (in phone case as back up); maintaining performance with 30 sec delays and change of location

Feedback and Homework Provided (task, context, ingredients, tracking):

Same as before for sessions booked from home; have Hap additionally book return sessions from Physio—Sondra to remind to use cue card given potential distraction from new location; track # rides booked

Plan for Next Session:

Advance distributed practice (add in delays between full practice trials); build on generalization (add Psych clinic to practice)

Therapy Impact after 4 Weeks

Sondra's Caregiver Burden Rating Scale

1	2	3	4	5
Daily demands exceeded my capacity to manage, and I had to withdraw and let things drop.	Daily demands felt "crushing," like I wouldn't be able to manage everything much longer.	Daily demands were high, but I largely kept up and therefore didn't feel as hopeless.	Daily demands were moderate-to-high, but I kept up and usually felt OK about the situation.	Daily demands were moderate and I kept up, felt OK about the situation, and even found some true relaxation time.

Hap's Goal Attainment Scale—to be achieved within 6 weeks

−2 Much less than expected	−1 Less than expected (baseline)	0 Expected outcome	+1 Better than expected	+2 Much better than expected
I am not helping with daily household demands, and my behavior frequently adds to the demands. I feel like a burden.	I am not helping with daily household demands. I feel as if I lack purpose.	I am helping with or managing an average of 1 daily household demand. I feel as if I am starting to contribute again.	I am helping with or managing an average of 2 daily household demands. I feel as if I am actually contributing.	I am helping with or managing an average of 3 daily household demands. I feel as if I am making a difference.

App Review Sheet for Client to Fill Out with Clinician

App name:	Cost:

Operating system: ☐ Apple iOS   ☐ Android   ☐ Windows   ☐ Other:

Purpose:

Description/features:

Rating on app store (e.g., Apple App Store, Google Play):

Number of raters:

Highlights from recent user reviews:

Personal Trial:

Design/layout (How easy is it to navigate? Can you easily find what you need? Are there so many things going on, it's too distracting to use?):

Effectiveness (Did it work for you or not? What did work well? What didn't work well?):

Will you use this app after today? Why?

External Aid Needs Assessment

Client Name: Date:

Assessment Format: a) Interview with (list all present):

OR b) Form filled out by:

I. Independence Screen for Life Participation Roles

Role (add any additional items on blank lines)	1–5 Rating 1 = unable to do 5 = able to do as well as before or N/A	Comments (place checkmark by any that are very important to you/client)	
HOME AND COMMUNITY			
Managing finances			
Planning social arrangements			
Participating in social events			
Shopping			
Planning and preparing meals			
Cleaning, doing laundry			
Arranging transportation			
Completing personal care			
Caring for children, others			
SCHOOL AND/OR WORK			
Attending class/work			
Completing homework			
Taking tests, exams			
Doing presentations			
Organizing meetings			
Writing essays, reports			
Participating in social events			
Managing correspondence			

(continued)

II. Functional Screen for Cognitive Contributing Factors

Factor (add any additional items on blank lines)	1–5 Rating 1 = not a problem 5 = big problem	Comments (place checkmark by any that are a major priority for you/client)	
Tracking date or time			
Staying focused			
Switching between tasks			
Holding information in memory			
Following conversations			
Following directions			
Remembering what I already did			
Getting and staying organized			
Initiating tasks			
Prioritizing tasks			
Finishing tasks			
Controlling impulses			
Interacting positively with people			
Getting thoughts out quickly			
Getting thoughts out accurately			
Understanding what I read			
Remembering what I read			
Organizing thoughts in writing			

III. Cognitive Profile

Check areas of concern:	For those that are checked, describe further and note any assessment results:
☐ **Attention** (e.g., sustained, divided, alternating)	
☐ **Working memory** (ability to hold information in memory long enough to act)	

(continued)

Check areas of concern:	For those that are checked, describe further and note any assessment results:
☐ **Episodic memory** (ability to remember daily events and personal experiences)	
☐ **Semantic memory** (ability to remember facts and knowledge-based information)	
☐ **Prospective memory** (ability to initiate a planned future action at a specific time)	
☐ **Procedural memory** (ability to learn procedures or steps, often without awareness)	
☐ **Retrograde amnesia** (loss of memory for events before injury)	
☐ **Declarative learning** (ability/rate of learning new information)	
☐ **Executive functions** (e.g., initiation, cognitive flexibility, inhibitory control)	
☐ **Awareness** (e.g., anosognosia, denial)	
☐ **Social communication** (e.g., social cognition, pragmatics)	
☐ **Language** (comprehension, expression, reading, writing)	

IV. Physical Profile

Check areas of concern:	For those that are checked, describe further, including current use of aids:
☐ **Visuoperceptual**	
☐ **Sensorimotor**	
☐ **Auditory**	

(continued)

234

V. Past and Current External Aid Use

Type of External Aid	Frequency of Use 0 = never, 3 = most days		How Helpful 0 = not helpful, 3 = very helpful	
	Before	**Now**	**Before**	**Now**
Paper Calendar *Describe:*				
• Enter scheduled events				
• Enter "things to do"				
• Refer to entries				
• Check off entries when done				
• Reschedule as needed				
• Other:				
Planner *Describe:*				
• Enter scheduled events				
• Enter "things to do"				
• Refer to entries				
• Check off entries when done				
• Reschedule as needed				
• Other:				
SMART Device *Describe:*				
• Enter scheduled events				
• Enter "things to do"				
• Assign tags				
• Refer to entries				
• Set alerts or reminders				
• Check off entries when done				
• Reschedule as needed				
• Take and save photos				
• Timer/stopwatch				
• Memo pad				
• Voice memos				
• Texting/messaging				

(continued)

Type of External Aid	Frequency of Use 0 = never, 3 = most days		How Helpful 0 = not helpful, 3 = very helpful	
	Before	Now	Before	Now
SMART Device *(continued)*				
• Voicemail				
• Other:				
• Apps:				
Other Aids				
• Voice recorder				
• Voicemail				
• Memo pad				
• Camera				
• Bulletin board				
• Whiteboard				
• Sticky notes				
• Filing cabinet				
• Pill box				
• Stopwatch				
• Calculator				
• Other:				
Other SMART Aids				
• Alexa/Apple/Google Home				
• SMART watch				
• SMART pen				
• Scanning pen				
• Screen reader (text-to-speech)				
• Speech-to-text				
• SMART glasses				
• Bluetooth tracker				
• Other:				

(continued)

VI. Client Preferences for External Aid

Appearance (e.g., color, style, size)	
Types of functions (e.g., calendar, to do list, budget, planner, reminders, tags, goals, logbook)	
Mode (e.g., electronic, written, auditory, graphic)	
Location/time of use (e.g., home, school, work, community; mornings, before bed, during class)	
Other	

VII. Other Tools, Strategies, Environmental Adaptations

Please describe (e.g., keep space neat, work in quiet, label items):

VIII. Supports and Resources

Family, friends, support workers:

Financial:

Baseline Probe for External Aid Use

Client:	Date:

Prompt:

Context where probe obtained:

Steps Recalled Independently:

Steps	Correct?	Comments

Other Comments/Observations:

Therapy Session Data Form—Target Acquisition, Mastery, Generalization (External Aid Use)

Client Name: **Date:**   **Location:**   **Others Present:**

Target: **Associated Aim:**   **Training Phase:**

Ingredients—Items: **Ingredients—Actions:**   **Ingredients—Motivators:**   **Measurement Plan:**

Check-in Info and Results of Homework:

Practice Data:	Retention Probe	Practice 1:	Practice 2:	Practice 3:	Practice 4:
External Aid Steps:					

(continued)

Therapy Session Data Form—Target Acquisition, Mastery, Generalization (Strategy Use) *(page 2 of 2)*

Practice Data:	Retention Probe	Practice 1:	Practice 2:	Practice 3:	Practice 4:
Comments:					

Session Summary/Analysis of Progress:

Feedback and Homework Provided (task, context, ingredients, tracking):

Plan for Next Session:

Progress Monitoring Form—
Target Acquisition, Mastery, Generalization (External Aid Use)

Client Name: **Target:**   **Training Phase:**

Select the summary measure being tracked (must use the same from each session):

☐ Retention probe result from start of each session

☐ Average of each session's practice trial results

☐ Other:

	Summary Measure			
	Date 1:	Date 2:	Date 3:	Date 4:
External Aid Steps:				
Ingredients:				
Prompts and Supports:				
Motivational:				
Other Measures:				

CHAPTER 9

Supporting Social Competence after Brain Injury

Changes in social functioning are among the most common and disabling consequences of acquired brain injury (ABI) and can have a major influence on family, school, work, and community outcomes. As a result, social skills are a common target of rehabilitation. Recent years have seen a shift from training discrete social skills to intervention aimed at improving social competence, consistent with the shift to a biopsychosocial model of disability described in Chapter 1. As many factors in addition to social skills can contribute to success in social interactions (Cavell, 1990), this shift in focus greatly increases our options for intervention. This chapter reflects that expanded focus and presents an overall framework for intervention aimed at meaningful improvement in social interactions.

The study of social functioning and the literature on social skills treatment for individuals with brain disorders use many different terms (Byom et al., 2020), which can make it confusing when seeking guidance on best methods. In this chapter, we will use the term *social behaviors*, which include behaviors that benefit the client and advance their social aims (*prosocial* behaviors, such as sharing speaking time in a conversation), and behaviors that are maladaptive, disadvantageous for the client, or have other social costs (*antisocial* behaviors, such as violating interpersonal space). Most social behaviors communicate something, so we include social communication in the category of social behaviors.

Typically in rehabilitation, the aim is to *increase social competence* rather than improve performance of specific social behaviors alone. The challenge is how to define social competence. The definition of social competence has been debated for more than 50 years (see the review in Rose-Krasnor, 1997), and social competence has been operationalized many different ways, such as by peer ratings of acceptance, counting number of friends, comparing performance of specific skills relative to "typical" behaviors, and measuring adherence to values of a social group. One possible reason there are so many definitions and measures of social competence is that it is subjective: social competence is defined by others in that person's life, and influenced not only by cognitive factors (e.g., our working memory constraints) but also by factors such as age, ethnicity and culture, workplace, and status (Prideaux, 1991). Judgments of social competence also can be influenced by in-the-moment variables, like the audience, mode of communication, and available time for an interaction. The subjective, context-dependent definition of social competence highlights the importance of focusing on each client's unique context and aims.

Consistent with a focus on the client in their social context, in this chapter social competence is defined according to Rose-Krasnor (1997). Rose-Krasnor proposed a "social competence prism" model, in which social competence emerges from social behaviors, is relative to that person's aims, and includes formation and maintenance of healthy relationships (Rose-Krasnor, 1997). She defined social competence as *effectiveness in interaction*, which is the *joint product of the individual and their environment*. In other words, social competence is not just one person's skill set, which means both partners can be treatment recipients. This view is expressed throughout the chapter and is reflected in our inclusion of everyday partners as recipients of training (see the example from the literature at the end of this chapter).

THE ROLE OF SOCIAL COGNITION

As defined in Chapter 2, social cognition refers to the ability to identify and interpret social signals (Schulkin, 2000). These signals can be spoken, written, gestured, signed (for speakers who use American Sign Language), or conveyed by body language, vocal intonation, or facial expression. The ability to identify and interpret social signals requires, at minimum, the ability to *recognize emotions* from others' affective and vocal displays, the ability to demonstrate *empathy*, and *theory of mind*, defined as the understanding that others have thoughts separate from one's own and these thoughts can influence behaviors (Premack & Woodruff, 1978). Some definitions of social cognition also include *social knowledge* (Ochsner & Lieberman, 2001), which is knowledge of the social norms of a particular social group, identified by age, race, culture, sex, gender, or other variables. Social cognition is required for social behaviors, including social communication as noted above.

Social cognition typically develops along with and is reflected in social behavior, but these two skill sets can be differentiated. A person can learn to execute a specific social behavior when cued, without understanding what that cue conveys [e.g., in the case of some children with Down syndrome (Cebula, Moore, & Wishart, 2010)]. Conversely, a person can "read" people well but be unable to perform target social behaviors [e.g., if they have severe aphasia (Siegal & Varley, 2006)]. Historically, social skills training models assumed that the core deficit in people with ABI was behavioral, that is, loss of the ability to execute social behaviors or even loss of knowledge about "appropriate" social behaviors. For that reason, traditional training often relied on didactic instruction (e.g., "A good listener sits upright, turns toward the speaker, and makes good eye contact"). Recent research has shown, however, that antisocial behaviors in many individuals with ABI have roots in impaired social cognition. Social cognition impairments have been shown in individuals with disorders such as medial temporal lobe epilepsy (Broicher et al., 2012); traumatic brain injury (TBI; Dennis et al., 2013; McDonald, 2013; Ryan et al., 2015; Spikman, Timmerman, Milders, Veenstra, & van der Naalt, 2012; Turkstra, Norman, Mutlu, & Duff, 2018); stroke (Nijsse, Spikman, Visser-Meily, de Kort, & van Heugten, 2019); primary central nervous system cancer (Pertz, Kowalski, Thoma, & Schlegel, 2021); and multiple sclerosis (Henry, Lannoy, Chaunu, Tourbah, & Montreuil, 2022).

When attempting to recognize others' emotions, individuals with impaired social cognition may make errors of *valence*, confusing positive and negative emotions (e.g., mistaking angry for enthusiastic), or errors of *magnitude* (e.g., mistaking angry for irritated). In general, recognition of basic emotions like *happy* is likely to be intact, with more errors on recognition of emotions with close visual neighbors (e.g., *fear* vs. *surprise*), subtle and complex emotions (e.g., *irritation* vs. *anger*); and emotions that require inferences about mental states or the social context (e.g., *embarrassment*) (Connolly, Lefevre, Young, & Lewis, 2019). In regard to theory of mind, individuals with ABI appear to have the most difficulty with complex theory of mind tasks, such as inferring meaning when someone's words do not match their behavior (e.g., as in sarcasm or deception) (McDonald, 2013). One question that remains outstanding in the literature is whether impairments on theory of mind tasks are true deficits or result because these are "second-person tasks" (Schilbach et al., 2013): at present, all theory of mind tasks ask the person to hypothesize about what one actor is thinking about another actor, rather than testing perception in first-person interaction (Beauchamp, 2017). Stimuli also tend to be relatively simple, with prolonged viewing times and a limited number of actors, so the extent to which findings capture theory of mind in everyday life is unknown.

In summary, emerging data on social cognition impairments in ABI suggest that assessment of social cognition should be the first step in intervention, as the client is unlikely to know which behavior to use if they don't recognize social cues. At the time of publication of this book, there was only one standardized test of emotion recognition or theory of mind that had been validated in individuals with ABI: the Test of Awareness of Social Inference (TASIT; (McDonald, Flanagan, Rollins, & Kinch, 2003) (see *www2. psy.unsw.edu.au/Users/Smcdonald/resources.html* for a description of available tests). Until more tests become available and, given the limits of existing assessment methods described above, informal assessment might be the primary option for clinicians.

THE ROLE OF OTHER COGNITIVE FUNCTIONS

Additional cognitive functions should be considered when assessing social functioning, particularly in populations like TBI, where links between cognitive impairments and social behaviors are well known (Rowley, Rogish, Alexander, & Riggs, 2017). In individuals with acquired brain disorders, the cognitive functions most likely to be affected are memory, particularly working and declarative memory; executive functions, including self-awareness; and attention, as described in Chapter 2. Reduced speed of information processing also may contribute to social cognition problems in some clinical groups, such as adults with schizophrenia (Lahera, Ruiz, Branas, Vicens, & Orozco, 2017) or multiple sclerosis (Pottgen, Dziobek, Reh, Heesen, & Gold, 2013) (though evidence for the latter is mixed; Cotter et al., 2016; Neuhaus et al., 2018), and also in older adults (German & Hehman, 2005; Rakoczy, Harder-Kasten, & Sturm, 2012). If a client with ABI asks the same question repeatedly, perhaps they are not missing their partner's cues that the repetitive questioning is aggravating, but rather that their declarative memory is impaired and they can't recall the answers. A client with poor executive function due to a stroke might make inappropriate comments because they're not able to inhibit the expression of their every thought. A client with multiple sclerosis and poor working memory might miss the point of a story because they can't keep the relevant details in mind long enough to put it all together. Impairments in divided attention might make a person seem tangential or egocentric because they are unable to focus on both a conversation and the work task they are performing. Another reason for poor social functioning is self-regulation fatigue: good social behavior takes self-regulation, and when we have mental fatigue, it is difficult to be on our best behavior (Kennedy & Coelho, 2005). People with ABI may be particularly vulnerable to self-regulation fatigue, as discussed in Chapter 2, so if social problems tend to occur after a task with high demands for self-control or near the end of the day, self-regulation or general cognitive fatigue should be considered as a possible explanation.

IDENTIFYING MEANINGFUL SOCIAL AIMS

Success in social interactions relies on many skills, including social cognition, declarative and procedural memory, working memory, and executive functions. The client needs to identify the appropriate time to use the skill, remember the correct skill to use, and be able to execute it in a timely and flexible manner, modifying target skills and behavior based on ongoing feedback from others. Many clients with ABI have impairments in all of these functions. Training discrete skills such as turn taking or eye contact also is unlikely to be effective unless those behaviors are directly relevant to the client's social aims, therapy is delivered with high dose in the target context, and targets are accurate. Thus, it is unsurprising that traditional didactic approaches in general have not generalized to everyday social interactions and improved quality of social life (Ylvisaker, Turkstra, & Coelho, 2005).

When a client presents with social aims, one useful tool for specifying targets is the International Classification of Functioning, Disability and Health (ICF), which was presented in Chapter 1 and has been a theme throughout this book. Consider Jade, a 25-year-old female who, 5 years after sustaining a TBI, sought therapy to help her "meet people." We return to Jade in the case example at the end of this chapter, but for now it is helpful to consider her strengths and limitations and the required elements for her intervention plan. Jade was highly motivated to seek therapy—to the point that she referred herself to the clinic—and had a clearly articulated aim and measurable deficits in social functions that could be the target of intervention. The likelihood of reaching her aim was greatly reduced, however, by her lack of access to social activities. She also lacked a regular social partner with whom to practice her new skills and who could provide support and cues to help Jade act in ways that fit her context and his own expectations. Compare this client to Deena, also 25 years old. Deena had more severe impairments in behavior regulation than Jade, and consistently made inappropriate comments in social interactions. She was equally motivated to improve her life in general but was quite happy with her social network. She was charismatic and engaging in first encounters, and although she was underemployed (only working part time), employees in her chosen line of work had a high tolerance for disinhibited language and the workplace was not open to the public. According to a traditional medical model, both of these individuals would be candidates for social skills training, as both have impairments in social behavior. For Jade, however, social skills training would be of limited benefit if she was not able to access social activities, and Deena did not need social skills intervention because she was happy with her quality of social life and accepted by her coworkers. The contrast between Jade and Deena shows how social skills training must occur in context and illustrates the factors to be considered in intervention planning.

ASSESSMENT OF SOCIAL FUNCTIONING

Social Cognition and Related Cognitive Functions

Intervention planning always begins with assessment. Historically, assessment of social competence in individuals with ABI focused on cataloging social behaviors. As literature on social problems after ABI began to identify cognitive mechanisms underlying these problems, however, assessment expanded to include evaluation of basic cognitive functions that were then linked to social behaviors (see Hartley, 1995, for examples). Current assessment also may include evaluation of social cognition, recognizing that, as noted above, a client is unlikely to employ prosocial behaviors if they do not recognize basic emotions or take the perspective of others. While standardized testing of nonsocial cognitive functions is a well-established practice, at the time of publication of this book, there were few standardized tests of social cognition other than TASIT, mentioned above. Thus, clinicians may be limited to informal assessment of clients' ability to recognize affect cues in others and appreciate that others have thoughts different from their own.

Social Behaviors

Social behaviors are judged by everyone who comes into contact with the person with ABI. They are so integral to human interaction that we all feel qualified to render an opinion, which makes sense given that social "appropriateness" is a subjective, context-specific judgment. Social behaviors also are incredibly diverse! If we tried to list all of the social behaviors that could be assessed as part of rehabilitation, that list would need to include greetings, farewells, and everything in between; in all social contexts; and with all communication methods. The complexity of measuring human social interaction is illustrated by the workplace communication matrix by Meulenbroek, Bowers, and Turkstra (2016). The matrix was only for the specific category of midlevel employment, a category that is made up of workers with specialized training, and nevertheless included five dimensions of communication with multiple different aspects in each (e.g., the "partner" dimension included both status and number of partners, with multiple options within those categories).

It is critical to remember that clinicians are likely to have different social standards than their clients, and expectations for social behavior change with age, culture, and context. Thus, determination of what constitutes a social problem will depend on the report of the client and people in their social life, rather than a standardized test score. An important consideration in social judgments is the effect of the rater's sex or gender versus that of the person being rated. Stafslien and Turkstra (2020) asked undergraduate students of both sexes to identify behaviors that were problematic if shown by a man or woman. While raters listed the same number of problem behaviors for men or women, female raters identified almost double the number of behaviors overall that would be a problem. Many studies of social behaviors, especially in TBI, are based on a mostly female group of close others rating a mostly male clinical group, raising questions about whether observer bias plays a role in our notions about social competence. If that close other is the person interacting with the person being rated, their opinion is critical, but it should not be the only source of rating information. Studies to date also have considered only sex (the biological construct) and not gender (the social construct), so results should be interpreted with caution.

While all members of the team participate in evaluating social behaviors, their role in everyday communication typically is assessed by speech-language pathologists when they evaluate *pragmatic communication ability*. A discussion of methods for evaluating pragmatic communication is beyond the scope of this book (see Byom et al., 2020; Sohlberg et al., 2019; Turkstra et al., 2017). In general, assessment of social behaviors uses a combination of questionnaires, such as the LaTrobe Communication Questionnaire (LCQ; Douglas, Bracy, & Snow, 2007) or the Profile of Functional Impairment in Communication (PFIC; Linscott, Knight, & Godfrey, 1996), and detailed examination of communication behaviors such as turn taking, topic maintenance, and other interpersonal behaviors in social interactions (Snow & Ponsford, 1995; Turkstra, McDonald, & Kaufmann, 1996). For children and adolescents with ABI, some standardized tests can be useful for evaluating language skills underlying pragmatic communication, such as linguistic inference (e.g., the Comprehensive Assessment of Spoken Language; Carrow-Woolfolk, 1999). For adults with ABI, however, as with the other aspects of social behavior and social cognition discussed earlier in this chapter, there is a critical shortage of well-validated standardized tests and measures (Beauchamp, 2017; Sohlberg et al., 2019). This may be inevitable given the context dependence of pragmatic communication and subjective nature of judgments of social appropriateness.

Assessment of social behaviors involves observation of the client as they engage in social interactions. This observation typically is done by either role-playing situations that are typical for the client in everyday life (e.g., pretending to greet a new person), or observing the client in daily social interactions with caregivers and others. Social behaviors often are assessed using informal measures, but there are also standardized tools. These include standardized caregiver checklists with questions about social performance in daily activities, such as the Pediatric Assessment of Disability Inventory (Haley, Coster, Ludlow, Haltiwanger, & Adrellos, 1992), the Functional Assessment of Communication Skills for adults (Frattali, Thompson, Holland, Wohl, & Ferketic, 1995), and the Behavior Rating Inventory of Executive Function (Roth, Isquith, & Gioia, 2005), which has child, adolescent, and adult versions, and also scales specific to social communication, such as the LCQ (Douglas et al., 2007).

When assessing behaviors using informal measures such as role playing or observing clients in clinical settings, it is important to keep in mind that clinical interactions differ from everyday social life in important ways. Clinicians tend to provide structure and support that are absent in everyday life. Our interactions with clients often are on a predetermined topic and have a question-and-answer format (Turkstra, 2001), which gives artificial structure to the conversation. We also typically evaluate clients in quiet settings with few distractions. As a result, assessment in clinic might overestimate the client's social ability. On the other hand, clinicians lack shared history that can support conversations with friends and family. We also have a status relationship with the client, a factor that is known to have a negative effect on aspects of social interaction (Togher, Hand, & Code, 1996). Thus, the best way to evaluate performance in social activities is to observe the client in everyday social interactions and ask caregivers and other communication partners to provide information about behaviors in these settings.

Social Competence

Early assessment of social functioning focused on discrete behaviors like those listed in the previous section and whether they were used in both clinical and everyday life settings (Walker, Irvin, Noell, & Singer, 1992). When overall social competence was measured, it often was via others' impressions, such as ratings of social acceptance by teachers or parents (Walker et al., 1992). In recent decades, however, individuals with disabilities have strongly advocated for rehabilitation that improves their everyday lives, which means using measures that capture outcomes important to the person (Hartley, 1995). This has led to the development of social competence assessment tools that include items specifically addressing an individual's participation in social life. Social participation can be assessed using either *objective* measures, which ask about outcomes that society in general would consider to be desirable (e.g., having friends, being involved in the community), or *subjective* measures, which ask about outcomes specific to the client (e.g., "Is your social life satisfactory to you?"). Most current scales are objective. These include the Pediatric Quality of Life Inventory (PEDsQL; Varni, Seid, & Rode, 1999) for children, the Craig Handicap and Reporting Assessment Technique (Whiteneck, Charlifue, Gerhart, Overholser, & Richardson, 1992), Community Integration Questionnaire–Revised (CIQ-R; Callaway et al., 2014), and Quality of Communication Life Scale (Paul et al., 2005) for adults. The clinician should keep in mind the objective nature of these instruments versus the subjective nature of social competence: each client has their own unique aims for social participation. When the client answers with a low number to a question like "Approximately how many times a month do you usually visit friends or relatives?" (a measure of community integration from the CIQ-R), the clinician should ask if this particular outcome is important to that client. People vary in the extent to which they seek social engagement, and there are marked differences across cultures (Larkins, Worrall, & Hickson, 2004), so not all items will apply to all clients.

Environmental Factors

The most important environmental factors in regard to social functioning are the everyday people with whom the client interacts. As clinicians, we rely on these individuals to provide cues and supports in everyday life and need to know their willingness and ability to do so. Thus, we often have discussions with partners about how they support the social competence of the person with brain injury, observe them informally in everyday interactions, and ask if they are willing to be part of the intervention process.

Unfortunately, there are few standardized methods for evaluating these social partners (the lack of validated, standardized measures is definitely a theme of this chapter!). One pair of validated tools is the Adapted Measure of Support in Conversation (MSC) and Measure of Participation in Conversation (MPC) (Togher, Power, Tate, McDonald, & Rietdijk, 2010), which capture the social competence of both parties in conversations between persons with TBI and their close others. Each person with TBI and their partner are given a conversational prompt (e.g., "We would like you to generate five ideas regarding what you have found useful during your recovery") and are video-recorded while discussing that topic for 5 minutes. Trained raters use the MSC and MPC scales to rate the recorded conversations on features such as naturalness of the conversation, the extent to which both participated, and whether the partner used behaviors that revealed competence of the person with TBI. The MSC and MPC have been effectively used to measure outcomes of partner training, discussed later in this chapter.

Environmental assessment also includes identification of social opportunities available to the client, including both the activities themselves and also practical factors like transportation and funds. Additional environment-related questions include whether the social context is private or public, the number of people and distractions, and the standards for social behavior (or costs of misbehavior) in that context. Research on intervention for social functioning in individuals with ABI (e.g., Finch, Copley, Cornwell, & Kelly, 2015) has revealed the importance of considering meaningful contexts for that person, so answers to questions about people and opportunities in the environment will be key factors in determining treatment targets.

Personal Factors

When a person has new cognitive impairments, it may take time before they are ready to be out in public or see premorbid friends. Readiness to be out in the social world, and readiness to use strategies and supports, might be the greatest predictors of response to therapy. Thus, attention to the factors discussed in Chapter 3 is critical for intervention planning. It is common for adolescents and adults with ABI to experience depression because of changes in their social abilities and social lives, particularly when some time has passed and premorbid friends have, as one man with TBI eloquently put it, "fallen away" (McWreath, 2005). As noted above, premorbid social style, skills, attitudes, and interests also must be considered when designing treatment so that targets are feasible and meaningful to that person.

In the next section, we use the PIE framework to review the key planning considerations specific to social functioning. We then return to the example of Jade as an illustration of the PIE process.

<u>PIE</u>: PLANNING INTERVENTION FOR SUPPORTING SOCIAL COMPETENCE

By now the reader will be familiar with the PIE framework. Chapter 5 provides a thorough description of the key elements involved in the treatment process. In this chapter, we review the elements that are specific to social competence targets and aims. For the sake of clarity, this chapter describes the PIE elements relevant to social competence targets under the distinct categories of *planning*, *implementation*, and *evaluation*, and the reader is referred to Chapter 5 for a reminder of how the PIE process is actually circular and iterative. In this chapter, we review assessment and target selection under planning, the application of treatment ingredients under implementation, and the selection and administration of treatment measures under evaluation. In practice, however, the clinician will have selected treatment ingredients and measurement tools as part of the planning process and will be conducting ongoing evaluation and treatment modification throughout therapy. We begin with a review of the two key components in the planning phase: assessment and selection of treatment targets and aims.

Assess and Hypothesize

The clinician will first consider the client's social behaviors and also cognitive, physical, and sensory abilities that can affect social behaviors, including social cognition. As discussed above, assessment may occur through standardized testing, observation in social activities, or interviews with the client and relevant support people. Some of this assessment can be done apart from social context, such as testing of cognitive functions. Assessment of social behaviors, however, is best done in context, as described above.

Clinical interviewing with the client and their social interaction partners is important in conducting a *needs assessment*. It begins with identifying the client's aims and relevant context factors, then uses task analysis to identify components that will be addressed in intervention. The following planning questions help to guide this process:

1. *What* is the specific need? This question is about the client's aims. Is the client a nursing-home resident who wants to increase engagement in social activities, or are they living at home with family members who are embarrassed by their behaviors out in the community? Is the client a child who laughs when another child gets hurt in school or an adolescent who wants to "fit in" socially with their preinjury peer group? Intervention for social functioning is always client-centered, as the client is unlikely to work on targets that are not personally meaningful and relevant, so collaboration with the client and everyday support people is essential in identifying intervention targets.

2. *What* is the target context? The answer to this question will help determine where training will take place, particularly if the client has poor executive function and declarative memory and thus is unlikely to generalize the behavior. This question also helps to identify available social supports, including people, as well as environmental modifications needed and standards for social behavior. It is cost-efficient for the clinician to see the target environment firsthand, as context factors will have a critical influence on the success of intervention. Money spent training social skills that require cues from nursing-home staff will be wasted if staff members are not available during social activities. The target environment may be something related to that person. We once identified a target of training a client to read a social script that he kept in his wallet, to reduce his long monologues about his accident (a complaint of his family when they were out in public with him), then discovered that he typically wore sweatpants with no pockets!

It is important to know if the client is expected to independently identify when they should use a target social behavior, as impairments in social understanding and metacognitive skills will influence the likelihood of success. Unlike other types of behavior, such as work routines, social behaviors tend to be unpredictable and variable, so it is very helpful to know if there are any environmental cues that will help the client identify when they need to execute a behavior. In general, low-frequency targets are more difficult to learn, as discussed in Chapter 6. If the client wishes to learn a joke to tell at parties, but only attends one party per year, there is not much opportunity to practice. This is not to say that low-frequency events are always poor treatment targets. A client may have an important upcoming event, such as the wedding of a child or an outing with a group, and learning a strategy or script for this type of event may be the most meaningful social intervention for that client. Hence, the assessment process should include identifying the target context for supporting the treatment aim.

In terms of candidacy for intervention, as with all cognitive rehabilitation, the client must have motivation and readiness to improve social functioning. The extent to which the client needs awareness and insight depends on the nature of the intervention. If intervention is mostly focused on training social scripts (Chapter 6) or use of external aids (Chapter 8), these could be learned as automatic behaviors without significant client insight. On the other hand, if the client will be using a metacognitive strategy (Chapter 7), such as "When I meet a new person, I will (1) smile at them, (2) share my name, and (3) not hug them," good awareness is a prerequisite. For interventions focused on partner training, the partner must have not only motivation and readiness to engage, but also the ability to modify their own behavior. As noted earlier, there are no standardized measures of partner willingness to engage or readiness to change, so assessment for these variables is typically informal.

Define Targets, Aims, and Measures

An important part of the planning process is to identify the desired target and aim. Because of the diversity, context dependence, and idiosyncratic and dynamic nature of social behaviors, intervention must clearly focus on targets that will help the client achieve their specific aim. Social behavior targets can include decreasing antisocial behaviors—that is, behaviors that have negative consequences for the client, such as the use of disinhibited language, sexually inappropriate behavior in public, repetitive questioning, talking off topic, or monopolizing a conversation. Targets also can include increasing prosocial targets, such as training social scripts and routines to increase positive participation in social activities, training close others in supportive strategies, modifying environmental demands, and educating others in that person's everyday life to increase tolerance and acceptance. Intervention for these targets can include ingredients to extinguish negative behaviors, as well as ingredients to substitute alternative behaviors that will have positive consequences for the client. At this juncture, the clinician will specify measurable targets and plan for multilevel evaluation. Examples of measurement are described in the later "PIE: Evaluation" section. One theme in the cognitive rehabilitation literature has particular relevance for clients with social aims: there is clear evidence across populations, aims, and targets that treatment must be individualized and meaningful to that person to be effective. Consistent with the definition of social competence as an emergent property of an interaction, as described earlier in this chapter, individualized and meaningful treatment includes considering the people and contexts in which the social behaviors will occur.

PIE: IMPLEMENTING INTERVENTION FOR SUPPORTING SOCIAL COMPETENCE

The planning process reviewed in the above section lays the groundwork for training that will be carried out in the implementation phase. The planning process will have generated: (1) the target client or stakeholder skills and knowledge, environmental modifications, or referrals that will meet the client's social participation aims; (2) measures to monitor performance; and (3) training stimuli to facilitate learning social skill components. The phases of intervention described in Chapter 5 (acquisition, mastery and generalization, maintenance) are equally applicable when training social function targets and the clinician should ensure that the selected ingredients match the phase of intervention (e.g., massed practice at the acquisition phase, distributed practice and fading of supports at the mastery/generalization phase).

Intervention for social functioning typically includes a combination of training social routines and strategies, making environmental modifications, identifying supports, and training caregivers or other communication partners. For example, Ted, who had sustained anoxic brain damage due to COVID-19, had problems in his community housing because he would yell at other residents when they changed the channel during his favorite television program. The clinician learned that Ted had moderate declarative learning impairments and performed best when he followed a routine. The clinician hypothesized that Ted's yelling was because the channel change altered his routine and that other residents might be changing the channel because they forgot it was Ted's viewing time. This hypothesis was supported by the clinician's observation that Ted did not yell when the channel was changed at other times and that other residents said they did not know that Ted had a favorite show he regularly watched. Thus, intervention included training Ted in a script to say when someone changed the channel, posting a television-watching schedule in a highly visible location so that other residents could easily remember Ted's and their viewing times, training care staff to stick to the viewing schedule and cue Ted's script, and planning to purchase video-recording capability for the television so that Ted could watch his favorite program whenever he wished.

The example of Ted clearly illustrates the inherent complexity of social behaviors. Due to this complexity, multiple targets likely will be required to address even just one antisocial behavior. The specific choice of targets also will depend on the client's declarative memory and executive function ability. For example, if procedural memory is the client's main route to new learning, then errorless learning and spaced retrieval (SR) are most appropriate and the client will need high-frequency practice of correct responses in target contexts (Chapter 6). By contrast, if the client has good insight and relatively good executive function, then metacognitive strategies can be trained (Chapter 7). Finally, some clients will benefit from using an external aid to support performance of prosocial behaviors (Chapter 8). Therefore, the forms shared throughout Chapters 5–8 may be used to document aims, targets, ingredients, and progress measures for improving social functioning. What is most important is conducting a thorough task analysis in order to identify the collection of targets that will lead to the desired change in social function.

In a review of social communication interventions for clients with TBI, Meulenbroek and colleagues (2019) identified effective treatment methods and ingredients that apply to all social targets. The one common ingredient across all studies was providing opportunities for practice, consistent with social behaviors typically being S (skill and habit) targets. Most studies used behavioral shaping and reinforcement ingredients, such as modeling social problem solving and self-monitoring of behavior; providing immediate corrective feedback and reinforcement, role-playing target behaviors, and eliciting peer feedback. Most studies involved some type of training in social strategies, such as strategies for self-monitoring or self-talk. Several studies in the Meulenbroek and colleagues review, as well as more recent research (e.g., Hoepner et al., 2021) used video feedback for either modeling of target behaviors or increasing self-awareness of problem behaviors, and education was a common ingredient across studies.

As social communication treatments reviewed by Meulenbroek and colleagues (2019) typically were "bundled" into a multifactored intervention, it was not possible to identify which ingredients were effective. Three themes emerged, however, and are worth noting for all ABI populations:

1. For individuals with acquired cognitive disorders, there is *little evidence that training discrete behaviors automatically generalizes to untreated contexts*. As with all targets in the S group, the skills required for learning discrete social behaviors (e.g., procedural learning) are not necessarily the same skills needed to generalize behaviors to novel contexts (e.g., executive functions, declarative recall). Social skills can be particularly challenging to generalize, given the complex, dynamic, and often unpredictable nature of social interactions in everyday life. Thus, as is true for all S targets, *change in performance in the desired context* should be specified as a target and treated with appropriate ingredients (e.g., variable cues, inclusion of partners in treatment).

2. Most social skills have developed over many millions of repetitions in that person's life and thus are highly proceduralized (i.e., automatic, routine). For those behaviors, *change requires many, many repetitions*.

3. There is growing evidence that *partner training* can effectively support social behavior in individuals with brain disorders. We provide an example at the end of this chapter using TBI Express (Togher et al., 2010), a multicomponent treatment program that yielded positive results in a single-blind randomized controlled trial (Togher, McDonald, Tate, Power, & Rietdijk, 2013). Communication partner training has its roots in aphasia (Kagan et al., 2001; Turner & Whitworth, 2006) and, among those with ABI, has mostly been used with adults with TBI (Behn et al., 2021; Hoepner et al., 2021) and dementia (O'Rourke, Power, O'Halloran, & Rietdijk, 2018; Swan et al., 2018; Williams, Perkhounkova, Herman, & Bossen, 2017). As noted in the case application below, it is not possible to identify effective ingredients in these multicomponent studies, but a theme across studies is the inclusion of education about brain injury and its effects on social interaction; training in supportive strategies; modeling and role-playing; immediate feedback on performance, particularly video feedback; and opportunities to practice.

All previous chapters have referenced the importance of involving everyday people in supporting the client in acquiring new knowledge, skills, and habits. However, the Meulenbroek and colleagues (2019) evidence above coupled with limitations often imposed on clinical practice (e.g., limited number of sessions, restrictions in conducting sessions outside of the clinic) suggest that partner training and environmental adaptations are especially critical for targets relating to improved social functioning.

One general recommendation for partner training is that stakeholders are formally involved in the process and that the burden on families and care providers is considered when asking them to provide supports. The literature suggests that lack of meaningful social interaction with the person with ABI is a significant source of long-term stress for families (Verhaeghe, Defloor, & Grypdonck, 2005), so families are likely to be motivated to participate in intervention that aims to improve social functioning. Families also can be stressed by having to change their own behaviors, however, and with the exceptions noted above, like TBI Express, studies of family training have not been methodologically strong (Boschen et al., 2007). Thus, when choosing an intervention approach, the clinician should carefully consider which method will fit for a particular family and lead to meaningful change.

When stakeholders are employers, they may need education about the potential benefits of providing social supports at work. Moving a person with ABI to a private workspace, so they are not engaged in distracting social conversations, may be an inconvenient and expensive undertaking for a business, and the clinician may need to provide concrete evidence of the potential for this arrangement to increase worker productivity. This is similar in school settings: some students with ABI need structure and advanced preparation to act appropriately when working in groups in class. This places an added burden on the teacher but might benefit all students in the class.

A benefit of considering the ICF in treatment planning is that the *why* of intervention is transparent from the outset, and the level at which outcome can be measured is easily observable. The specification of environmental and personal factors in this framework also helps identify factors that are beyond the clinician's control—if a person needs workplace social skills but is no longer employed, is unable to attend social events because of transportation, or is socially withdrawn because of depression, then the intervention plan may focus on referral to other specialists rather than direct intervention, and successful referral will be the criterion for successful outcome.

PIE: EVALUATING INTERVENTION FOR SUPPORTING SOCIAL COMPETENCE

Previous chapters described evaluation for targets and aims, and the same principles apply to evaluating gains in social behaviors and social competence. Table 5.3 in Chapter 5 includes examples of multilevel evaluation for social behavior targets. The measurement examples shared throughout Chapters 6–8 equally may be used for social behavior targets and aims. One addition for evaluating social competence is the use of ratings by others, such as the LCQ (Douglas et al., 2007) mentioned earlier in this chapter. When intervention includes partner training, evaluation also might include measures of the quality of the interaction, such as measures of support needed, participation in the conversation, or how the conversation burden is shared across partners (Barnes, 2020); see also the review in Behn and colleagues (2021).

PUTTING IT ALL TOGETHER: CASE APPLICATIONS

In the remainder of the chapter, we provide examples to show the integration of the PIE framework for social functioning intervention with actual clients. The first example is a group study conducted by Dahlberg and colleagues (2007); the second and third are individual studies (Hoepner et al., 2021; Rietdijk, Power, Brunner, & Togher, 2019). They are followed by a case example in which we revisit Jade, who was described in the introduction to this chapter.

Examples from the Literature

In what has become a classic study in the TBI rehabilitation literature, Braden and colleagues (Dahlberg et al., 2007) randomized 52 adults who were at least 1 year post-TBI to either treatment or deferred treatment social skills groups that met weekly for 12 weeks. According to the authors, the intervention had four key sets of ingredients: (1) It was delivered by a speech-language pathologist and social worker together, which provided different perspectives and models; (2) activities focused on self-awareness and self-identification of goals; (3) the group format was used "to foster interaction, feedback, problem solving, a social support system, and awareness that one is not alone" (p. 1564); and (4) the authors explicitly targeted generalization by assigning home practice, including family members in home practice and assessment, and providing opportunities to practice skills in the community. Additional ingredients included a consistent format for each meeting, with the opportunity for group sharing and feedback at the beginning of each meeting; use of goal attainment scaling (GAS; see Chapter 5) to individualize intervention targets; provision of a written treatment manual that participants and their families could use as a reference; and ingredients to support representation targets such as providing didactic information about consequences of injury.

Participants in the treatment group showed significantly more gains in social behaviors than those in the deferred treatment group, and gains were maintained over 9 months posttreatment and participants continued to improve in their social communication goals. Measures of social participation did not change, which the authors attributed to insensitivity of the social participation measures to changes in discrete behaviors, and perhaps to an "overly ambitious" aim of treating discrete behaviors and expecting global changes in social life. A key outcome of this study was that participants were up to 10 years postinjury and still continuing to improve, which supports the potential for intervention to benefit persons with ABI, even many years into the chronic stage.

Rietdijk and colleagues (2019) reported the results of a single-case ABA experimental study with two adults who had sustained moderate to severe TBI (msTBI), both of whom were rated by partners as having significant social communication deficits. Participants and their partners completed a telehealth version of TBI Express (Togher et al., 2010) that was a communication partner-training program, called TBIconneCT. Treatment dose was one 1.5-hour individual (participant plus partner) session per week for 10 weeks. Ingredients included didactic instruction, structured role-plays, video-recorded practice of conversations, use of a secure site for video uploading, review of recordings to identify communication difficulties and individualized strategies to address those difficulties, quotes from previous participants to explain the program, ingredients specifically to promote generalization, and email summaries of sessions and homework assignments. The primary outcome measure was frequency of occurrence of a conversation feature relevant to the aims of each participant.

One of the two participants in the study by Rietdijk and colleagues (2019) (P1) was a 33-year-old male with 14 years of education, who was 3 years post-TBI. P1 had a professional-level job preinjury and now worked part time as an administrative assistant. His partner (CP1) was a 33-year-old female with whom he had weekly contact, and together they aimed to have more enjoyable conversations that were less frustrating for the participants. P1's aims included being a more "responsive" listener, and CP1's aims included clarifying information for her partner less frequently. The primary outcome was frequency of target behaviors related to those aims in an extemporaneous conversation between P1 and CP1. The authors also asked participants to rate their own and the other person's social communication behaviors, collected process-related data such as frequency of home practice and technical problems, and asked participants to rate outcomes such as quality of life. Outcomes were measured at the conclusion of therapy and at 3 months posttreatment.

Results of the intervention illustrate the challenges of studying and interpreting the results of social skills intervention, and limitations of the treatment literature in general. First, it was not possible to obtain a stable baseline for either P1's or CP1's target behaviors because, as soon as they started the study, they changed their behavior so that it was in line with the targets (e.g., P1 doubled the number of his responsive behaviors from the first to the third baseline session). It is no surprise that intervention for social behavior is susceptible to the Hawthorne effect: social aims are easily understood by most people, and social errors are highly stigmatizing so individuals who are being observed are likely to be highly motivated not to make them. The Hawthorne effect is not problematic in and of itself; the challenge is whether those improvements can be maintained over time. Second, while the authors used an analysis method that considered each person's behavior in relation to the other's (e.g., if P1 was more responsive based on what CP1 said), the data are still summarized as one number that does not illustrate change over a conversation. Because social interactions are so dynamic, a single number does not capture behavior over time. Third, changes were not maintained over time, suggesting a need for ingredients such as reminders or "booster sessions" to provide opportunities for practice.

A last limitation, and one that is common in the ABI literature, is that TBIconneCT was a multicomponent, multi-ingredient intervention, and the authors did not specify treatment targets or ingredients, making it difficult to know which components or ingredients were effective. The study by Rietdijk and colleagues (2019) did show, however, that partner training in a virtual environment was feasible, could be delivered with fidelity, and had promise as a method to improve social behaviors in interactions with everyday communication partners.

Hoepner and colleagues (2021) described a 16-week intervention for two adults with TBI and their communication partners, which used joint video self-monitoring and coaching to increase both positive behaviors and awareness of social behaviors. Self- and proxy ratings on the LCQ improved for both dyads, and video review had the added benefit of increased accuracy of participants' ratings of their own behaviors. Although it was a small study, we include it here because it was, to our knowledge, the only study that (1) directly targeted awareness of both the person with TBI and their partner, operationalized as joint agreement on problem behavior ratings on the LCQ; (2) was based on an explicitly stated treatment theory (that motivational interviewing methods would improve awareness); (3) had a primary outcome of change in both partners in the dyad, via modified versions of the MPC and MSC described earlier in this chapter; and (4) included an outcome variable of success in identifying intervention targets with GAS, so video self-monitoring results were directly translated into intervention.

CASE APPLICATION—JADE

Methods for supporting social competence can include most of the interventions described in previous chapters, including training facts and simple routines, cognitive strategies, and external aids. In the following case application, the reader is encouraged to refer to the associated forms in other chapters and practice filling out the information provided in Jade's case.

Description of Client

Jade was a 25-year-old Latinx woman who referred herself for therapy 5 years after she sustained a TBI. Jade had received in- and outpatient rehabilitation for a few weeks after her injury but had not received any services for more than 4 years. As stated at the beginning of this chapter, Jade's aim was to meet people, and her opinion was that social skills training would help this happen. Jade was unemployed, although she very much wanted to work. She lived alone on the other side of town from her parents, a situation that appeared to suit them both.

Planning

Results of the interview with the client, as well as supplementary cognitive testing to evaluate memory, attention, and executive functions, revealed the following client profile:

Socio-cultural values. Jade reported that she enjoyed her independence (she had no assistance in the home) and did not seek social interaction with her parents, nor did they seek social interaction with her. She stated that friends had always complimented her on having a great sense of humor and that she had previously been known as outgoing and possessing a positive personality. Jade indicated that an older neighbor occasionally took her to community social events, but otherwise her activities were largely restricted to staying at home, attending a monthly ABI support group, and shopping. Jade stated that members of the ABI support group had been encouraging her for months to volunteer somewhere, but she really wasn't interested. Pre-accident she had greatly enjoyed socializing and meeting new people and had always had a boyfriend. She wasn't sure she wanted a long-term relationship, which her parents and support group members had all been encouraging, but she definitely wanted to meet men and enter into a relationship again. Jade was highly motivated to improve this aspect of her social life.

Cognitive findings. Jade's scores on the Repeatable Battery for Assessment of Neuropsychological Status (Randolph, 2001), a screening test of cognitive functions, were at the bottom of the normal range. In spontaneous conversation, Jade was observed to have mild word-finding difficulties. Somewhat reluctantly, Jade had asked her parents to complete a case history form, which she reviewed and made corrective notes on before providing it to the speech-language pathologist. From both her and her parents' descriptions, Jade had relatively good declarative memory in everyday life (Jade provided examples of remembering upcoming appointments, learning bus schedules, and remembering when sales were on at stores). By contrast, she showed poor executive function throughout the interview and assessment, at least in regard to control and flexibility: she perseverated on topics and comments and was often tangential and distractible. The clinic receptionist observed Jade to be "overly friendly" with men in the waiting room, seemingly with no awareness of the social cues from the women in the room. At the beginning of the assessment, Jade reported that "she felt better already" coming to the clinic, given the social opportunities it had afforded her while waiting for the appointment.

Physical and sensory functions. Jade reported that TBI-related sensory and motor limitations prohibited her from driving, but she was able to walk without assistance and had no difficulties with stairs, which supported her independence with using the transit system. She had no difficulty managing activities of daily living in her home.

Psychosocial functioning. Jade reported generally positive mental health, and this was corroborated by comments from her parents on the case history form. Boredom was a concern for Jade, and she indicated that she had to be careful to not spend hours online because her mood usually suffered when seeing everything that she was missing out on. She said that she was a night owl, preferring to stay up late and then sleep through the morning, which sometimes left her groggy or grumpy in the early afternoon. However, she was usually her positive and outgoing self by late afternoon.

Environmental variables. There was a bus stop right outside of Jade's apartment complex, and it connected with a number of other bus routes, allowing her easy access to many parts of the city. In addition, her neighbor was genuinely interested in helping her, as were the members and staff at the local brain injury association chapter. Negative environmental factors included reduced access to social events of interest to her due to bus schedules not matching event timing and location.

Jade's aim was to improve social functioning, particularly with regard to success in meeting men. A collaborative task analysis was completed to determine the potential contexts in which meeting new people might be possible and then the constellation of targets that would allow Jade to advance social behaviors in these contexts. Jade and the clinician collaborated to develop an acronym that described her target behavior in social situations, PRWD (pronounced "proud"), which stood for *Plain* language and tone, *Respect* other's space, *Wait* until you know the person better, and *Don't* mock. Together, they then decided on the following sequential targets:

1. Learn the acronym.
2. Implement a strategy in role-play contexts in the clinic to ensure she stays on track with the four requirements of the acronym.
3. Use a Reflection and Rating app on her smartphone to document performance and reflect on key success factors.
4. Train her neighbor to provide cueing support and encouragement at key times during a social interaction.

Learning the acronym was an R target and would be measured by the percent of accurate responses over increasing time intervals. Implementing the strategy was an S target and would be measured by independence in carrying out each step. Using the app was a volition target (R) to build and maintain her motivation and would be measured by ratings recorded in the app as well as a scale for Jade to rate her "commitment to stick with the program." Jade already knew how to use the app from an activity she had completed with the support group, so no S target was required to learn it. Training the neighbor was an S target and would be measured by his independence in providing cues prior to conversations getting too far off track.

Generalization to low-stakes social interactions outside of the clinic (when the neighbor could be present to cue and observe) was to be measured via Jade's and the neighbor's combined success ratings (following the format created for the Reflection and Rating app). The ultimate impact of the training would be measured by a Goal Attainment Scale describing Jade's level of satisfaction with her social life.

Implementation

To meet Jade's target of learning the acronym PRWD, the clinician implemented SR training with the added ingredient of high prompt variability, to promote generalization. Form 6.1 from Chapter 6 was used to plan and document the outcome of this training. In two sessions, Jade learned to cite the acronym and each component's meaning in response to a variety of social queries (e.g., "What would be appropriate in that situation?" "How could you have acted in that situation?").

Jade and the clinician then collaborated on determining each step of the PRWD strategy and decided on the following:

1. Say the acronym to herself.
2. Set the timer on her phone for 5 minutes × 2 occurrences.
3. When the timer goes off after the first 5 minutes, say the acronym to herself and self-affirm if her behaviors have met the criteria and redirect if not.
4. When the timer goes off after the second 5 minutes, say the acronym to herself and self-affirm if her behaviors have met the criteria and redirect if not.
5. Enter her Reflection (including key success factors) and Rating on the app.

While entering the Reflection and Rating in the app was part of the strategy, documenting and reviewing the ratings and success stories over time was a simultaneous ingredient for maintaining motivation.

The strategy was practiced during 10-minute role-plays with student volunteers in the clinic. Ingredients were modeling, opportunities for practice, error control via clinician cueing if Jade seemed to be veering too far from her plan before each 5-minute mark, and feedback on accuracy upon completion of the role-play. The clinician used Form 7.3 from Chapter 7 to plan and document the outcome of this training.

In the first strategy training session, Jade practiced the strategy 4 times, each time with the same volunteer partner and the same topics of conversation. In Session 2, the context was varied by alternating between different communication partners and introducing different conversation topics. Jade was able to independently implement all steps of the strategy by the end of Session 2. The neighbor joined the third strategy training session where Jade once again engaged in role-playing with the student volunteers, but this time the emphasis was on training the neighbor when and how to cue. The clinician used the ingredients of explanation followed by modeling, which was then faded to cueing. Jade collaborated in this training protocol by intentionally violating some of the target behaviors so that the neighbor had opportunities for practice. Jade also collaborated in the process by selecting the type of cueing she was comfortable with, something she would clearly recognize but that would be subtle and of no significance to anyone else around her (the neighbor would do an arm stretch out in front of him, as if relieving stiffness). The session plan and outcomes of the partner training were documented on Form 5.4 from Chapter 5. Jade reported that she greatly enjoyed instructing both the student volunteers and her neighbor.

For the generalization phase, Jade and her neighbor were asked to identify a low-stakes context outside of the clinic. "Low-stakes" was defined as low risk for negative consequences if Jade struggled to adhere to her target behaviors. They identified a park with unique sculptures where tourists often went and proposed some conversation topics that would fit in with meeting someone in that context. Jade agreed to use a logbook for her and the neighbor to collaboratively document observations and ratings to bring back to the clinic for discussion. They both agreed that areas of disagreement would only be addressed when meeting with the clinician. Jade said she would take responsibility for creating a graph to plot their combined ratings of each social interaction practice at the park, and the neighbor was in charge of documenting how frequently the arm-stretch cue was needed to keep Jade on track with her behaviors. Sessions with the clinician focused on reviewing the ratings and reflections/observations and discussing any changes that might be needed for the following session.

The generalization phase ended earlier than planned as Jade decided that she had enough social skills and did not see the need to develop new strategies or have further therapy. She reported feeling positive that she had made a contribution to student education, and mostly liked being in the waiting room and meeting new people. Therefore, she discharged herself from therapy, continued to pursue social opportunities via Brain Injury Association functions and outings with her neighbor, and expressed plans to find other ways to meet men at a range of local venues.

Evaluation

The evaluation plan described earlier was carried out as anticipated. Jade demonstrated accurate recall of the PRWD acronym for over 30 minutes in the second session. She additionally chose to text the acronym's meaning to the clinician several times prior to the next session, confirming effective recall over much longer intervals. Strategy implementation at the acquisition stage was evaluated by independence for each step, which she achieved for massed practice with the same partner and conversation topics in the first session and also for the initial foray into generalization (varying partners and topics but still in clinic) during the second session. For the partner training target, her neighbor was evaluated on (1) independence in using the arm-stretch cue and (2) doing so at the first clear sign that Jade's old behaviors were appearing. In a single training session, the neighbor achieved full independence in using the correct cue and was rated as using it at the right moment 80% of the time.

Generalization data from the park included the combination of Jade's 1–10 rating of her overall implementation of the PRWD behaviors and the neighbor's 1–10 rating. For the three sessions completed before Jade discharged herself from therapy, ratings increased from 9/20 (Jade 6/10 plus neighbor 3/10) to 12/20 (Jade 7/10 plus neighbor 5/10) to 13/20 (Jade 8/10 plus neighbor 5/10). Jade had also documented her "commitment to stick with the program" as 5/5 in each of the three sessions, even though she decided to discontinue therapy after the third session. Jade elected not to review the success parameters she had prepared for the Goal Attainment Scale describing satisfaction with her social life and instead reported that her social skills were "much better" and that she had enjoyed the opportunity to be an instructor for the students in the clinic. Jade retained a positive relationship with her neighbor, and he expressed a commitment to continue supporting her as much as possible.

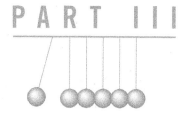

PART III

SPECIAL CONSIDERATIONS

CHAPTER 10

Cognitive Rehabilitation in the Inpatient Setting

Tessa Hart, Mary K. Ferraro,
and Amanda R. Rabinowitz

In this chapter, we consider how best to achieve the goals of cognitive rehabilitation in the inpatient rehabilitation setting. As we will see, both the constraints of the setting and the cognitive characteristics of many inpatients with brain injury pose obstacles to achieving the foundational goals expressed earlier in this volume: to promote positive change in *functional outcomes* and to improve the *sense of well-being* of clients—in this case, hospitalized patients. We contend that in most inpatient settings, there is little opportunity to help patients *directly* to improve their cognitive function. Rather, the inpatient team must use knowledge of each patient's cognitive status to implement methods for the *optimal teaching and training* of functional tasks, and to *minimize patient and family distress.*

We begin with a brief discussion of the challenges to cognitive rehabilitation in the inpatient setting. Using the extant literature and our experience with inpatient rehabilitation, we then propose some practical approaches for this difficult phase of recovery. Our focus is mainly on traumatic brain injury (TBI), particularly moderate to severe TBI (msTBI), given that few persons with mild brain injuries require inpatient treatment. However, much of the discussion below will also apply to patients with other types of brain injury causing severe and often diffuse cognitive impairment, such as cerebral anoxia/hypoxia and encephalitis.

THE CHALLENGES OF INPATIENT REHABILITATION

Time and Team Constraints on Treatment

There are significant constraints affecting the time allotted to inpatient rehabilitation. We are clinical researchers working in the United States, but many other developed nations face similar limitations. The skyrocketing cost of health care in recent decades has led to draconian cutbacks in inpatient lengths of stay, both in acute/emergency care and on the rehabilitation unit. In the last 25 to 30 years, TBI rehabilitation stays have dropped from an average of about 6 weeks to just over 2 weeks (Kreutzer et al., 2001; Lamm et al., 2019). At the same time, average acute care hospitalizations for TBI have declined from almost a month to just over 2 weeks (Kreutzer et al., 2001; Traumatic Brain Injury Model Systems Center, 2020). This means that compared to years past, patients with msTBI are admitted to rehabilitation "sicker, quicker"—with more acute injuries, and typically in less stable condition both medically and cognitively. Truncated hospitalization also means that the families of inpatients are often in acute distress when they arrive at the rehabilitation unit. Far from being ready to absorb information and guidance, they are frequently distracted and sleep-deprived as they struggle to process the injury and its consequences, both logistically and emotionally.

With less time to work with patients, the overall aims addressed by the inpatient rehabilitation team have also been constrained. Discharge planning begins on Day 1, and the team must focus closely on basic skills for safety and maximal independence in the home or the next level of care. While these are certainly worthy aims, some experienced therapists may find it disappointing not to be able to address more complex goals related to societal participation, such as parenting or return to school or work. Less treatment time also means less opportunity to develop relationships with the patient and family, to enjoy their successes, and to learn firsthand about the evolution of cognitive and behavioral recovery.

Time limitations and stricter documentation and reimbursement requirements have also constrained the team's ability to solve problems collectively, educate one another, and coordinate care. While clinicians know that ideal treatment means using effective strategies consistently across the team, the increasing demands on nurses and therapists mean less opportunity to communicate with one another to identify those strategies and ensure that everyone puts them in place.

Cognitive and Behavioral Status of Inpatients

The typical inpatient with msTBI is unlikely to be able to engage in many of the cognitive rehabilitation procedures described in this volume. Sleep–wake disturbance with daytime fatigue, pain from musculoskeletal injuries, sensory disturbances, and side effects of various medications are only a few of the factors affecting participation in rehabilitation. Moreover, as a consequence of shorter stays in acute care, many patients arrive to inpatient rehabilitation units with impaired consciousness and/or in post-traumatic amnesia (PTA; also called posttraumatic confusion). One study of inpatients with msTBI revealed that over half were still in PTA 1 month after injury (Nakase-Richardson, Yablon, & Sherer, 2007). In concert with the data on the duration of hospital care, this suggests that many inpatients with msTBI remain in PTA for their entire hospital stays.

PTA becomes evident as a patient emerges from coma, but can also occur without any loss of consciousness. The manifestations of PTA are variable across patients but can include frank delirium, extreme distractibility, emotional lability, and disordered behavior such as restlessness, agitation, and aggression. There is rapid and unpredictable fluctuation in cognition and behavior within and across days, although often (thankfully) with an improving trend. This instability makes even the first step of the PIE process described in Chapter 5—assessment—quite challenging, as treatment plans based on cognitive status may become obsolete literally overnight.

Regardless of other symptoms, the hallmark of PTA is disorientation to time, place, and circumstances, and dense anterograde amnesia, that is, the inability to recall ongoing events. PTA is considered to end at the point where a patient is at least grossly oriented and able to recall salient events from day to day, although anterograde memory usually remains inconsistent. The duration of PTA (which includes the length of coma, if any) is generally considered to be the most sensitive index of the severity of diffuse injury in TBI (Povlishock & Katz, 2005), with prognosis for favorable recovery of functional independence diminishing as PTA extends beyond a few weeks (Nakase-Richardson et al., 2011). Although it is tempting to think that one could shorten PTA duration using procedures such as frequent reorientation, the available evidence suggests that PTA reflects pathophysiological changes in the brain that in most cases resolve over time but cannot be reversed with medications or behavioral interventions. For example, while serial assessment of orientation is important for tracking purposes, more frequent assessment does not expedite clearance from PTA (Alderson & Novack, 2002). Nor is there evidence that "orientation groups" or use of external aids such as calendars serve to improve day-to-day recall (Langhorn, Holdgaard, Worning, Sørensen, & Pedersen, 2015; Watanabe, Black, Zafonte, Millis, & Mann, 1998). Thus, rehabilitation teams have little recourse but to administer the most effective treatments and help patients and families cope with PTA for the duration. In this context, the memory deficits exhibited by patients in PTA deserve special attention, as understanding them helps to pinpoint the approaches to cognitive rehabilitation that will succeed in the inpatient setting—and the ones that will not.

Deficits in Declarative Memory

Recall that Chapter 2 described two major brain systems supporting human learning and memory: the declarative (or *explicit*) system and the nondeclarative (or *implicit*) system. The declarative system is highly localized in medial temporal regions and is more vulnerable to injury or insult than the nondeclarative system, which is phylogenetically older and more diffusely represented; that is, it contains more redundancy in brain tissue (Camina & Güell, 2017). Patients in PTA, and those with anterograde amnesia due to anoxic brain injury or encephalitis, have virtually no ability to store new declarative memories. This means that they are unable to use semantic memory to acquire new facts ("My name is Jane and I am your speech therapist"), nor can they retain episodic memories such as what they had for breakfast, whether they even *had* breakfast, or what they worked on in therapy a few hours beforehand.

Unfortunately, declarative memory deficits appear not to affect only *new* information. Retrograde amnesia of variable duration affects memory for events immediately preceding the injury (Levin, 1990), but there is also evidence that more remote memories may be unstable during PTA. Inpatients with TBI are routinely asked about preinjury interests, hobbies, and relationships, or to supply details of medical history, on the assumption that autobiographical memory is intact, even if the patient is confused as to current or recent events. However, this assumption was called into question by a study that examined personal semantic memory—that is, recall of items such as schools attended, hobbies, and activities—across three periods of life (childhood, early adulthood, and recent life) in 20 patients in PTA and 20 healthy controls (Roberts, Spitz, Mundy, & Ponsford, 2018). Patients were significantly less accurate than controls, and there was no temporal gradient, meaning that early memories were as vulnerable as more recent ones. Thus, autobiographical questions run the risk of providing inaccurate information to the treatment planning process (Ponsford, Sloan, & Snow, 2012). In an observational study conducted on an inpatient TBI unit by Valitchka and Turkstra (2013), some patients in PTA were asked questions about their medical histories that were used to develop care plans (e.g., for diabetes) without verification from another informant.

In contrast, the nondeclarative memory system is relatively spared, although it may not be functioning normally. Amnestic patients are able to learn new procedures, for example, context-specific action sequences such as a dressing routine adapted for hemiparesis, and they can form emotional associations, including fear and anxiety, to specific stimuli. A classic example of these two systems at work (or not) is found in the patient whose declarative memory system draws a complete blank when, at the end of one therapy, is asked, "Where do you go next?" only to turn spontaneously in the correct direction for the next therapy because the patient's nondeclarative system has learned the navigation sequence. Unfortunately, the patient may also have established an anxiety response to the therapist who keeps asking questions the patient cannot answer. Negative emotional responses to treatment staff may be inadvertently conditioned by such communications, even though patients lack any memory of the anxiety-provoking events. When repeated over the hours, days, and weeks of a hospital stay, "unanswerable" questions may cast a negative emotional pall over a patient's experience of rehabilitation and provoke behaviors that function to escape or avoid contact with staff. Patients may also (implicitly) learn to terminate the interaction by saying, "I don't know" (Turkstra, 2013). The observational study cited above confirmed that disoriented patients are routinely asked numerous questions that depend on declarative recall, and that "I don't know" was a frequent response (Valitchka & Turkstra, 2013).

APPROACHES TO COGNITIVE REHABILITATION FOR INPATIENTS

Given the many and daunting challenges discussed above, what might be feasible and evidence-informed approaches to the goals of cognitive rehabilitation—improving functional outcomes and sense of well-being—at this early and often turbulent stage of recovery? The answer is easy to express, but very difficult to accomplish in practice. The entire treatment team must share a common understanding of patients' cognitive abilities and limitations and what these mean for optimal treatment approaches; and all must work in concert to adapt the social, physical, and teaching environments to maximize patients' functional gains while minimizing their distress. Later in this chapter, we describe an example of how one facet of this rather ambitious vision was implemented on a dedicated TBI unit.

In the discussion below, we use the framework of the Rehabilitation Treatment Specification System (RTSS; Hart et al., 2019), introduced in Chapter 4, to propose some considerations and recommendations for meeting the cognitive rehabilitation needs of inpatients with TBI.

Targets of Treatment

According to the RTSS, treatment targets are the proximal and measurable functional changes intended to be brought about by a treatment. Targets fall into three broad groups: those intended to improve organ function; those addressing skills and habits; and those concerned with changing the cognitive or affective representations underlying knowledge, beliefs, attitudes, and intentions. In the context of cognitive rehabilitation, *organ function targets* refer to treatments that act directly on brain tissue, such as medications and neuromodulation techniques. Rehabilitation therapists also use "low-tech" methods for the target of improved arousal, such as positioning a somnolent patient in a more upright position, which stimulates the reticular activating system via vestibular connections.

While a detailed review is beyond the scope of this chapter, psychotropic medications have a definite place in inpatient cognitive rehabilitation. Drugs that improve attention and arousal, in particular, may help the patient to benefit from training and teaching. For example, Willmott and Ponsford (2009) showed that methylphenidate had robust effects on information-processing speed in inpatients at an average of 46 days post-TBI. The interested reader is referred to Bhatnagar and colleagues' review of psychotropic medications applicable to TBI rehabilitation (Bhatnagar, Iaccarino, & Zafonte, 2016).

Targets focused on improving *skills* and *habits* are arguably the *sine qua non* of inpatient rehabilitation. Shorthand terms such as ambulation/wheelchair/gait/dressing/bathing/grooming/swallowing *training* refer to structured opportunities to practice specific routines to improve their accuracy, speed, or automaticity. These practice opportunities, along with various cues and types of feedback, enable the broad mechanism of action: "learning by doing" (Hart et al., 2014). As noted above, even patients in PTA or with other sources of declarative memory deficits should be able to learn procedural skills by virtue of a more intact nondeclarative memory system. This has been empirically supported: a clinical trial comparing active to deferred rehabilitation of activities of daily living (ADL) for patients in PTA showed superior gains on FIM scores for those receiving active ADL training (Trevena-Peters et al., 2018). An economic analysis of the trial data showed that structured training of ADL during PTA resulted in significant cost savings from fewer hospital days and less use of medication compared to deferred care (Mortimer, Trevena-Peters, McKay, & Ponsford, 2019). Another secondary analysis revealed that agitation did not limit therapy participation, nor was agitation exacerbated by such treatment (Trevena-Peters, Ponsford, & McKay, 2018).

The trial noted above used a specific systematic instruction technique for ADL training that was introduced in Chapter 4: errorless learning (EL). As the name implies, EL is learning in which errors are deliberately prevented or minimized during the learning process. Why is this so important for inpatients with TBI? The reason is that errors are helpful for learning *only* if the declarative memory system is working well (Ponsford et al., 2014). Consider a tennis lesson; if at the end of the session your coach says,

"You would do better if you held the racquet further down," you will remember that correction and apply it to future lessons using your declarative memory system. If you have a poorly functioning or absent declarative memory system, the correction may be forgotten and the wrong racquet placement "stamped in" by your intact nondeclarative memory system as you engage in repeated, but incorrect, practice sessions. By the same token, a therapist who wraps up a session by reviewing "how to do better next time" with a memory-impaired patient is more likely than not to see the same errors, or perhaps new ones, in the next session. Instead, the therapist should prevent errors to the extent possible by using cue saturation, modeling, or even hand-over-hand guidance until the patient has mastered the sequence.

EL can be used to promote optimal functioning in daily living tasks that are familiar (e.g., dressing, grooming, mobility), as well as tasks with new procedures or equipment that are incorporated to ensure safety, for example, donning a helmet to protect a skull defect or completing tub or toilet transfers with safety rails. One limitation of nondeclarative learning is that it tends to be context- and task-dependent, so therapists should train skills in environments resembling each patient's home setup to the extent possible. At the very least, an attempt should be made to keep the training environment, and definitely the task sequence, invariant.

Although several factors influence the effectiveness of EL, including the type of task and the stage of learning, the best rule of thumb is *always* to use EL for skill-related targets with patients in PTA or those who have impaired declarative recall for other reasons. Inpatients who have cleared PTA and are oriented, with adequate day-to-day recall, may be able to benefit from discovery learning, in which they are permitted to experiment with the best ways of completing tasks and encouraged to notice and correct errors. The most effective discovery learning is likely to include therapist prompts to help the patient consider what went wrong with an attempted approach and to generate a plan for subsequent attempts (Skidmore, 2015). Table 10.1 contrasts the clinical features and ingredients of EL and discovery learning.

We have mentioned skills related to mobility, self-care, and safety. But what about skills involved in compensating for the memory deficits that are so prevalent? On many inpatient units, it is common practice to supply memory-impaired patients with notebooks, schedules, and calendars, and to devote therapy time to teaching them how to use these memory aids. Except in unusual circumstances, such as the case of a high-functioning patient who is completing work or school tasks while in the hospital, we recommend that this practice be minimized. Even if EL were to be used to prompt the use of a "memory book," that book is unlikely to resemble a tool that the patient will use to enhance functioning outside the hospital, meaning that the therapy time devoted to such training may not contribute to meeting the overall aims of the inpatient team. Of course, patients who are able to use them should be given schedules and written materials to help navigate their days, and therapists might experiment with aids that the family could use to structure time at home, such as a calendar of appointments or a list of tasks to accomplish during the day. But a detailed exploration of evolving patient needs and preferences with regard to memory aids, including preinjury strategies, is best accomplished in outpatient treatment.

Many *representation targets*, such as the learning of new facts and information, rely on the declarative memory system. Inpatient rehabilitation units for patients with

TABLE 10.1. Errorless Learning and Discovery Learning Contrasted

	Errorless learning	Discovery learning
Primary memory system	Nondeclarative (implicit, procedural)	Declarative (explicit)
Suggested use	Training representation and skill/habit targets for clients with moderate to severe impairments in declarative learning and memory; and skill/habit targets for clients with mild impairments in declarative learning and memory	Representation targets for clients with mild impairments in declarative learning and memory
Contextual factors	Keep context as invariant as possible (e.g., environment, materials, task sequences).	Vary contextual factors to promote generalization.
Role of error	• Errors should be minimized (prevented or corrected immediately). • Errors are easy to spot, as the desired response is specified in detail. • Guessing is discouraged.	• Errors may be discussed or processed to enhance future performance. • Self-evaluation may be encouraged. • Form of desired response may vary. • Guessing or brainstorming is permitted.
Speed of learning	Depends on dose of repetition (practice) of correct response Typically requires multiple trials	Depends on factors such as target complexity, aspect, and desired outcome; variability; meaning to client; and consequences May be learned in a single trial
Generalization of learning	Learning is hyperspecific to task and context and not amenable to verbal description, so generalization must be carefully programmed using variable stimuli.	Client can consciously generalize target to novel stimuli and contexts, providing the client is aware of potential application of target and recognizes when and where target can be applied.
Main ingredients	• Instructions focus on mastery of one step at a time. • Forward/backward chaining may be used to reinforce correct sequence of actions. • Cues are provided to constrain performance to minimize errors (saturation cueing, hand-over-hand guidance). • Feedback, if any, is provided within task.	• Instructions may invite patient to figure out how to complete a task or meet a goal. • Cues may be open-ended or Socratic-type questions. • Feedback may be terminal and include self-evaluation.

intact cognition are ideal places to provide patient education—information about the causes and consequences of the disability, ways to continue progress at home, and recommendations for ongoing care. For many inpatients with TBI, however, the information delivered via traditional patient education will not be retained. Those who have cleared PTA may well benefit from a structured approach to learning about their injuries as well as their current status and rationale for treatment, and such information may even improve engagement with therapies (Pegg et al., 2005).

For patients with impaired declarative memory, representation targets should include providing factual information not with the goal of long-term retention, but for reassuring the person in the moment—that is, addressing *affective* representations for the aim of improving the sense of well-being. Confusion is often accompanied by anxiety, and answering patients' questions, simply and truthfully, can help to relieve it. At each encounter with a memory-impaired patient, clinicians should reintroduce themselves, provide basic information about what will happen in the session and why, and avoid "quizzing" questions that, as noted above, can exacerbate anxiety and frustration. Each member of the team should also have access to the same basic narrative about the injury circumstances and other salient facts so that any such information provided to the patient is consistent.

Recipients of Treatment

The vast majority of inpatients with TBI are discharged with ongoing needs—for supervision and guidance if not direct care at home, and for additional medical and therapeutic treatment. Successful transition from the inpatient setting to a more permanent living situation requires a great deal of new learning, as well as planning and organization of tasks, schedules, and unfamiliar systems, such as equipment suppliers and benefits and entitlements programs. Since most people with TBI cannot manage these cognitive demands at this stage of recovery and may not be fully aware of their limitations and associated needs, other *treatment recipients* must be involved: family members or other persons identified to serve as caregivers after discharge. Both skill-related and representation targets are appropriate for caregiver training. Accurate, understandable information about the injury, its consequences, and prognosis has been repeatedly cited by caregivers as a paramount need (Bond, Draeger, Mandleco, & Donnelly, 2003; Dams-O'Connor, Landau, Hoffman, & St. De Lore, 2018; Kreutzer, Serio, & Bergquist, 1994). Caregivers may also need to learn skills such as wound care, medication management, implementation of safety measures, and how to assist the patient with personal hygiene, grooming, and ambulation. Given that patients' needs and abilities, as well as their cognitive and behavioral status, will continue to fluctuate in unpredictable ways following discharge, preparing caregivers for all eventualities is a very tall order. Ideally, the inpatient team should focus on the skills and information needed for the first few weeks or months, correct misinformation to which the family may have been exposed, and effect a transition to a next level of care that will meet patients' and caregivers' evolving concerns.

The literature offers few guidelines for preparing caregivers for discharge. A recent scoping review produced mostly qualitative studies and descriptive examples of caregiver education for msTBI at the inpatient level (Hart et al., 2018). Qualitative findings have reinforced the commonsense notions that caregivers need simple explanations in lay terms, that written information is helpful as a memory aid, and that education and training are more effective when spread throughout the inpatient stay rather than squeezed in right before discharge (Smith & Testani-Dufour, 2002). Clinical experience also suggests that information and skill training should be coordinated among team members to avoid contradictory messages and tailored to the cultural concerns and emotional status of caregivers. Some units offer a prepackaged education series for family members covering the main sequelae of TBI and common treatment issues. In our experience, these programs tend to be less valuable than information targeted to the patient's status and the specific questions raised by potential caregivers. In fact, hearing about problems such as agitation or seizures may be frightening unless they apply to one's family member.

For patients who are agitated and confused, it is vital to provide family members and other visitors with education and training on this phase of recovery. Training should address representation targets such as increased knowledge and skill targets such as how to maintain a calming environment. This is important not only because relatives may be discomfited by the behaviors, but also because familiar people who are able to remain calm and reassuring may be very helpful in reducing the agitation. Family members should also be counseled to refrain from quizzing memory-impaired patients or asking them questions that depend on declarative recall. On some units, therapists record patients' progress in a simple log that travels with the patient so that family members may consult it for information when they come to visit.

With truncated lengths of stay and the pressures on staff and family alike, it is increasingly difficult to offer comprehensive education and training to caregivers. One wishes for an enhanced case management approach, similar to the process used in the U.S. Veterans Health Administration (Cross, 2009; Perla, Jackson, Hopkins, Daggert, & VanHorn, 2013), in which patients and families are followed after discharge to facilitate referrals and to solve emerging problems and meet evolving needs. Such an approach, offering resource facilitation and troubleshooting by phone or video for 6 months after discharge from inpatient TBI rehabilitation, is currently being tested in a pragmatic randomized trial among six Traumatic Brain Injury Model System centers (Fann et al., 2021).

Other recipients of treatment may include people who play important roles in the patient's life, such as employers or teachers, who may need to be educated about the patient's status and trained to adapt work or school responsibilities to accommodate injury-related limitations. As with the development of memory compensations, however, the outpatient setting more often confers the appropriate time and place for detailed recommendations to work or school personnel.

Ingredients of Treatment

In the RTSS, *ingredients* are defined very broadly as "anything said, done, or applied by a treatment provider to address a treatment target" (Hart & Ehde, 2015, p. 129). Although we cannot list every ingredient used in inpatient TBI rehabilitation, several types of ingredients deserve special mention for this population at this level of care. We have already specified some ingredients for effecting different types of training and teaching approaches in Table 10.1. Two other categories with special importance for inpatients with TBI are *environmental* ingredients and *volition* ingredients.

The environment serves as an ingredient when it is modified to address a treatment target. Perhaps the most common example in inpatient TBI rehabilitation is reducing noise and clutter in the environment to allow a distractible patient to focus on a task. For agitated and/or confused patients, published recommendations for the physical environment include minimizing restraint, avoiding overstimulation, and maintaining a quiet and consistent milieu. With regard to the social environment, recommendations include maintaining consistent treatment staff, providing frequent reassurance, and evaluating/managing the effects of visitors (Ponsford et al., 2014). For patients who become more agitated in the presence of unfamiliar people (e.g., one-to-one "sitters"), video monitoring may be helpful. Lights should be dimmed at night to promote rest and to serve as a reminder to staff to maintain a quiet atmosphere. Careful observation sometimes reveals times of day when a patient seems less distracted and more engaged so that therapy schedules may be adjusted to maximize performance. The same principle can be applied to identifying activities that seem to calm or motivate a specific patient.

Volition, which is roughly equivalent to effort expended by a recipient on a treatment activity, is a central concept in the RTSS (see Chapter 4). By definition, all skill-related targets and all representation targets require volition: one must engage in practice in order to improve a skill, and one must (at least) attend to information in order to process it. *Volition ingredients* are clinician actions that are designed to maximize patient effort. There are two situations in which attention to volition ingredients is particularly important. One is when the treatment involves activity that occurs without the clinician's supervision, for example, a home exercise program. The other is when the treatment is "known to be painful, difficult, or disliked . . . [or when recipients have] organic impairments in motivation and drive, or deficits in learning" (Hart et al., 2019, p. 176). It is the latter circumstance that is most relevant for inpatient TBI rehabilitation.

Volition ingredients overlap with those used to facilitate task performance. For example, the cueing methods listed in Table 10.1 may be considered volition ingredients to the extent that they help patients to engage and expend effort in tasks. However, different volition ingredients may be needed to counteract active resistance to treatments that patients perceive as aversive or unnecessary. Depending on the cognitive status of the patient, these may include switching to a more preferred task that addresses the same target; redirection to promote engagement through indirect means; various forms of persuasion and provision of rationales for tasks; and offering rewards and reinforcements for task engagement. Some patients enjoy competing with themselves (or others) and will engage in order to try to surpass a goal, and some will respond to graphic representations of their progress from one session to the next. Team members should let each other know when they find successful volition ingredients for a given patient to promote better performance across different therapies.

A TEAM APPROACH TO COGNITIVE REHABILITATION ON AN INPATIENT TBI UNIT

We now turn from a general discussion of principles to a specific example of how one inpatient TBI unit created a plan to put some of those principles in practice. Within a multidisciplinary quality improvement group, we developed and implemented an evidence-informed staff training series and patient care protocol to better meet the cognitive needs of inpatients with msTBI. Below we describe the steps undertaken and the interim results of the program, which is ongoing as of this writing.

A basic requirement for any initiative of this kind is protected time for staff to meet, discuss, and plan programmatic improvements. In the case of our program, one of us (Ferraro) is an education coordinator for TBI, with responsibilities for staff training and quality improvement across the continuum of care. On the inpatient TBI unit, supervisors in physical, occupational, and speech therapies, nursing, and neuropsychology also have time allotted for staff training and program development. In a meeting to discuss ideas for quality improvement on the inpatient unit, the needs of patients with severe memory impairment (e.g., patients in PTA) came to the fore. It was felt that frontline staff did not always know the memory capabilities of each patient, and for patients in PTA, staff did not fully understand the nature of the memory impairment and were using well-intended but inappropriate practices. For example, patients in PTA were quizzed with orientation questions multiple times per day and were asked to provide other kinds of information dependent on declarative recall. Thus, *step 1* was the decision to focus on developing a protocol that would help staff to identify patients in PTA, to understand the nature of their memory impairments, and to change clinical interactions with such patients to better meet their needs.

We decided to focus solely on identification of PTA and communication with patients for two main reasons. First, we had begun to receive grant-supported consultation from Lyn Turkstra, who had reminded us of the negative aspects of repeated quizzing and questioning and had pointed us to the observational study confirming its frequency on inpatient units (Valitchka & Turkstra, 2013). Second, we believed that full-scale training in multiple evidence-based methods at once, such as incorporating instruction in EL techniques as well as communication, would exceed our resources. Since quality improvement is a never-ending process, we reasoned that staff training in systematic instruction methods could be accomplished in a later phase.

Once we had selected the area of focus, *step 2* entailed deciding on specific, measurable changes to be achieved by the staff training protocol to be developed. Guided by the literature on best practices (e.g., Ponsford et al., 2014) and the experience of our consultant, we determined that tracking orientation on a routine basis was important to monitor the presence/absence of PTA, but that orientation questions should be asked only once per day at most. We decided that each patient's treating speech therapist would track PTA using the Orientation Log (O-Log; Jackson et al., 1998) and keep the team apprised of PTA/declarative memory status. Patients deemed to be in PTA would be placed on the "PTA protocol" (described below) until the speech therapist determined that they had cleared. Aside from the O-Log questions administered in speech therapy, a patient on the PTA protocol was not to be quizzed on orientation questions or asked any other questions dependent on declarative memory. Only questions based in the here-and-now, such as "How many plants can you see on that windowsill?" or "Are you hungry/cold/tired/in pain?" were permitted. Other communications should focus on providing patients with information and reassurance, in addition to specific therapy instructions.

Having decided to banish questions that clinicians typically use for gathering history and establishing rapport, we identified different sources of information for the former, and alternative means for the latter. We established that personal and medical history should be obtained only from the medical record and/or reliable friends or family members. We assumed that rapport could best be maintained by reintroducing oneself to the patient at each encounter, and by reexplaining the purpose of treatment as often as needed to allay anxiety about what was taking place.

For implementation of this plan, in *step 3*, we developed the PTA protocol itself. This involved creating a variety of materials, including a staff training series about the different types of memory disorders and their implications for clinical practice; color-coded door signs, folders, and other items to alert staff to patients on the protocol; and a plan for a training rollout. A "dos and don'ts" list was developed for staff with daily treatment responsibilities; it is illustrated in Figure 10.1. A less detailed list was supplied to personnel with regular but not daily patient contact (e.g., nutrition, housekeeping, and chaplaincy staff). A colored folder that traveled with each patient included a page of basic personal and injury-related information (called a "ME page"), which the treatment team could consult instead of asking the patient questions.

Step 4 was the all-important rollout of training to clinical staff. This entailed PowerPoint presentations, handouts, and videotaped role-play illustrations of the dos and don'ts. A recorded version of the training was made available for staff with weekend and evening shifts, which was particularly important for reaching all nursing staff. Attending physiatrists were given responsibility for the training of new medical residents. Therapy and nursing supervisors, who had participated in the design of the protocol, were tasked with providing direct feedback to frontline therapists responsible for implementing the new procedures.

An important question is how to evaluate the success of quality improvement initiatives. Early in the process, we realized that we could conduct a "natural experiment" to assess the effects of the protocol rollout. Inspired by the study of Valitchka and Turkstra (2013), we conducted a similar observational study on the inpatient TBI unit before and after the implementation of the PTA protocol, with frontline staff unaware of the purpose of the observations. We found ample evidence of the desired decrease in questions demanding declarative recall, with a corresponding decrease in memory-impaired

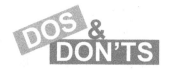

Do introduce yourself; state your name and purpose	Don't assume they remember you
Do provide information	Don't ask the individual to recall information
Do focus questions on the here and now	Don't quiz them for explicit information
Do establish habits and routines Same sequence, same way each time	Don't use lengthy verbal explanations
Do help them avoid making errors by modeling, step by step prompting	Don't expect them to remember what they've been told
Do evaluate their learning by what they do, not by what they say	Don't encourage them to "guess" or "try" after a failed verbal or physical attempt

FIGURE 10.1. Reference sheet for therapists and RNs.

patients saying, "I don't know" or giving answers that were unrelated to the question. Other details of our findings, including qualitative data from treatment staff regarding the perceived impact of the protocol, are found in our published report (Hart et al., 2020). In addition, interested readers may download all of the materials created for this protocol at *https://mrri.org/innovations/mossrehab-post-traumatic-amnesia-pta-protocol/.*

Our efforts are far from complete. We continue to provide training in the PTA protocol when new staff arrive, and we are aware that keeping our unit aligned with evidence-informed practice requires constant attention to the other needs of inpatients with TBI. However, we do believe that the PTA protocol initiative has succeeded in helping our inpatient staff to provide more consistent and streamlined team rehabilitation to a particular group of memory-impaired patients with specific needs.

CONCLUSIONS

The treatment of inpatients with msTBI is quite challenging, due to not only resource limitations affecting the duration and scope of treatment, but also the cognitive and behavioral difficulties that can interfere with conventional therapies and medical care. These challenges are best met with a teamwide effort to adapt all teaching, training, and communication practices to the needs of patients and families in this highly dynamic phase of recovery. Functional outcomes and patient well-being can be optimized by using systematic instruction and communication techniques geared toward patients' residual cognitive abilities. Concerted attention to family education and training, the effects of the physical and social environment, and strategies to maximize patient volition will also help to enable the best transition to the community and the next level of care.

CHAPTER 11

Computer-Based Cognitive Rehabilitation

In this chapter, we discuss computer-based cognitive rehabilitation (CBCR), sometimes described as "brain training." Before discussing specific CBCR approaches, we first describe the roots of this approach and how it relates to the principles of rehabilitation discussed in Chapter 4. We then present studies illustrating the main methods and themes of CBCR research and, based on that research, suggest guidelines for using CBCR in clinical practice. To illustrate those guidelines, we provide a case example in which CBCR could be part of a treatment plan to achieve functional change.

As described in Chapter 1, cognitive rehabilitation encompasses a broad range of interventions. Historically, these interventions were divided into two theoretically distinct categories: therapies aimed at *restoration* and therapies aimed at *compensation*. Restorative techniques, also called *process-specific interventions*, focused on improving a particular cognitive skill such as attention, language, or memory. Restorative approaches are the focus of most CBCR activities. In contrast, compensation techniques focused on training skills and strategies that would circumvent cognitive challenges, so clients could complete cognitive tasks in everyday life (Institute of Medicine, 2011; Sohlberg & Mateer, 2001).

The concepts of *target* and *mechanism of action* from the Rehabilitation Treatment Specification System (RTSS; see Chapter 4) help clarify the assumptions that led clinicians to dichotomize treatments as restorative or compensatory. As clinicians and researchers, we initially assumed that targets for restorative therapies were *cognitive processes* (e.g., improving memory), whereas targets of compensatory approaches were *behavior* (e.g., increasing likelihood of arriving on time for appointments). Furthermore, it was assumed that the mechanism of action for restorative approaches was *neuroplasticity*, whereas the mechanism for compensatory approaches was *skill acquisition*. While this dichotomy can be useful in describing aspects of certain interventions, most of our cognitive rehabilitation treatments cannot be neatly categorized. For example, studies of interventions described as restorative often measure outcomes using standardized neuropsychological tests, but test scores also can improve with "compensatory"-type approaches. For example, Goal Management Training, a strategy-based intervention, has been associated with improved scores on standardized executive function tests in adults with frontal-lobe damage (Stamenova & Levine, 2019); metacognitive attention strategy training was shown to improve scores of children with traumatic brain injury (TBI) on a test of nonverbal intelligence (Chan & Fong, 2011); and a self-generation learning strategy resulted in improved standardized memory test scores in adults with multiple sclerosis (Goverover, Chiaravalloti, Genova, & DeLuca, 2017). We also know that neuroplasticity underlies any sustained behavioral change and can be mediated by psychological and contextual factors (see the discussion of neuroplasticity in Chapter 4). As illustrated throughout this text, the practice of cognitive rehabilitation has evolved, with an emphasis on the interdisciplinary, integrative, and functional aspects of therapies that are designed to help clients with cognitive impairments fully participate in meaningful life activities.

In the early years of cognitive rehabilitation practice, clinicians aiming to "restore" or remediate cognitive function often used workbooks and paper-and-pencil-based drills. Since the advent of personal computers in the 1980s, these strategies have been largely replaced by CBCR (Lynch, 2002). Like the analogue methods of old, CBCR focuses on hierarchical, high-dose, drill-type activities, but with one critical addition: according to CBCR advocates, the computer platform allows delivery of therapy in a way that "maximizes brain plasticity" by including features such as adaptive delivery (tasks get more difficult as users improve), instant feedback and reinforcement, and the opportunity for easily accessible, high-dose independent practice. Activities are often gamified, with points systems and competitions, which increases their appeal to consumers. The practicality and accessibility of CBCR, along with its intense commercialization, have popularized this approach, and it is understandable that clients would want to avail themselves of its advantages. Another appeal was that, at least initially, some vendors claimed that CBCR could restore cognition after acquired injury or reverse cognitive decline in dementia. These claims were tempered in the United States after the 2016 Federal Trade Commission fined one company for false advertising ("Lumosity to Pay $2 Million," 2016), but the same claims still exist on websites in other countries and the term *neuroplasticity-based* is ubiquitous in CBCR advertising.

Broadly defined, neuroplasticity is the ability of the nervous system to respond to intrinsic and extrinsic stimuli by reorganizing its structure, function, and connections (definition from the American Congress of Rehabilitative Medicine at *https://acrm.org/ acrm-communities/neuroplasticity/*). Neuroplasticity is complex, as adaptation can occur at multiple levels, from molecules to synapses, networks, and behavior, making it difficult to extrapolate research findings examining changes at one level (e.g., neuronal firing) to another level (e.g., behavior). In their review of neuroplasticity in rehabilitation, Cramer and colleagues (2011) identified common themes that emerge across diverse central nervous system conditions, including the dependence on experience and the role of motivation and attention. The fact that plasticity after injury can be moderated by external experience is good news for clinicians and clients who engage in treatment, as external experience is the crux of all of our therapies. What we have learned is that interventions that aim to promote plasticity can be expected to have maximum impact when coupled with optimal training and experience (Cramer et al., 2011).

Chapter 4 reviewed the key principles of neuroplasticity with relevance to rehabilitation following brain damage, based on the work by Kleim and Jones (2008). Research over the past three decades has shown that the ideal approach for exploiting neuroplasticity and achieving functional change is to provide the opportunity for high-intensity, high-frequency repetition of meaningful and functional skills, in a context that is as similar as possible to the one in which those skills will be used. The brain changes in response to both internal input [e.g., medications that change neuronal responses, level of motivation (Crocker et al., 2013)] and external input (e.g., training and instruction), as well as contextual factors (e.g., people and location involved in training). The Plan, Implement, and Evaluate (PIE) framework is designed to provide optimal conditions for neuroplasticity that leads to functional change.

Because CBCR is of interest to many clients, clinicians should be knowledgeable about CBCR approaches and understand the science. Thus, in this section, we summarize the main themes of research on CBCR for clients with acquired cognitive impairments, and use the PIE framework to describe a case study that incorporated CBCR as part of a client's cognitive rehabilitation program. As a systematic review of the CBCR literature is beyond the scope of the chapter, we refer interested readers to recent reviews in a variety of client populations (e.g., Dardiotis et al., 2018; Fernandes, Richard, & Edelstein, 2019; Fernandez Lopez & Antoli, 2020; Fetta, Starkweather, & Gill, 2017; Niemeijer, Svaerke, & Christensen, 2020; Sigmundsdottir, Longley, & Tate, 2016).

WHAT DOES THE RESEARCH SAY?

There are two general types of CBCR studies. The first is studies linking CBCR to changes in brain activity either during or after performance of computerized cognitive tasks, typically measured via neuroimaging methods. The aim of these studies is generally to identify CBCR *mechanisms of action* (see Chapter 4). Most studies of this type have had small sample sizes and combined CBCR with other behavioral interventions, making it challenging to draw conclusions about CBCR specifically. For example, Yuan and colleagues (Yuan, Treble-Barna, Sohlberg, Harn, & Wade, 2017) measured cortical network connectivity in 10 children with TBI and 11 comparison peers, before and after CBCR. Brain network connectivity showed small but significant changes in the TBI group posttreatment, with the balance of local and long-tract connections changing toward typical values. Participants also received metacognitive coaching, however, so the brain changes could not be clearly linked to CBCR. Two studies compared neuroimaging findings before and after CBCR for attention in clients with multiple sclerosis (e.g., Cerasa et al., 2013; Filippi et al., 2012) and showed brain changes and improvements on the Stroop Test but not on other neuropsychological measures. By contrast, a study of CBCR in adults with mild cognitive impairment (Vermeij et al., 2017) showed changes in task performance but not imaging measures. Given mixed findings like these, and recent critiques of neuroimaging research in general (e.g., Botvinik-Nezer et al., 2020; Elliott et al., 2020), further work in this area is needed.

The second, and more common, type of CBCR studies are studies measuring behavioral outcomes, typically performance on neuropsychological tests. These are of most interest to clinicians. There have been several large studies of CBCR in typical adults (e.g., Stojanoski, Wild, Battista, Nichols, & Owen, 2021) as well as studies in adults with acquired brain disorders (e.g., Chen, Thomas, Glueckauf, & Bracy, 1997; Cooper et al., 2017; Mahncke et al., 2021; Zickefoose, Hux, Brown, & Wulf, 2013). The greatest number of studies are in adults with TBI or multiple sclerosis, and the following paragraphs review exemplar studies to illustrate the research landscape.

Zickefoose and colleagues (2013) compared the use of computer-delivered drills (without the recommended associated strategy training) from the Attention Process Training-3 (APT-3; Sohlberg & Mateer, 2011) to drills from Lumosity (The Lumosity Team, 2010) in a study of four adults with a history of severe TBI. The study used a single-subject A-B-A-C-A design, where A was assessment, B was either APT-3 or Lumosity, and C was whichever program the participant hadn't completed in B. Treatment was delivered over 20 sessions within 1 month. Generalization was operationalized as accuracy on a series of probes constructed to test attention on novel stimuli. All four participants improved on the trained tasks, and most rated the tasks as enjoyable. One participant showed near-transfer—that is, improved on the probe stimuli—although that participant was at ceiling when the treatment started; the three others did not show evidence of generalization.

Dymowski, Ponsford, and Willmott (2016) compared strategy training to computer-based drills to determine the effects of individualized strategy training on attention, beyond the effects of attention drills. The authors reported improvements on speed of processing tests following both interventions with more improvements observed following strategy training but noted limited generalization to questionnaire and interview data. They concluded that the variability in attention deficits and everyday attentional requirements between clients required individualized goals and approaches to rehabilitation. Their conclusion supports the findings by Serino and colleagues (2006), who compared the efficacy of working memory drills to a general stimulation approach using nonspecific drills. Participants were nine clients with severe deficits in working memory following brain injury. Unlike what occurred in most studies, the results were positive in showing improvements on tests of working memory that generalized to everyday functioning. What was different about this study was that participants were selected based on their attention profiles such that working memory drills matched their working memory deficits. The previously reviewed studies, and most of those in the literature, tend to use the same computer drills, regardless of the participant's cognitive profile and do not personalize the drills.

In a randomized controlled clinical trial (RCT) of 126 U.S. service members with mild TBI, Cooper and colleagues (2017) compared psychoeducation and medical management of symptoms alone to one of three cognitive rehabilitation approaches: CBCR alone; traditional cognitive rehabilitation, which included clinician-guided CBCR, education about cognitive strategies, and strategy training; and integrated rehabilitation, which included traditional cognitive rehabilitation plus mindfulness, anxiety reduction, and counseling ingredients. Intervention was delivered over 6 weeks. There was no differential effect of treatment arm on neuropsychological test scores (all improved); participants in the two therapist-directed arms made significantly more self-reported gains in functional cognition than those in the CBCR alone or psychoeducation arms; and in general, participants in the integrated arm reported the greatest psychological benefits. Gains were mostly maintained at 12 and 18 weeks after treatment. The authors attributed the benefits of clinician-directed intervention to benefits of the therapeutic alliance, team-based milieu, and focus on function. The study had several limitations, including heterogeneity in mental health across participants and underspecification of ingredients and targets in all treatment arms. The results, however, are consistent with those of other studies: CBCR showed near-transfer to similar neuropsychological tasks but not far-transfer to functional activities.

Hildebrandt and colleagues (2007) randomized 42 adults with multiple sclerosis to receive either CBCR completed at home (n = 17) or no treatment (n = 25). Participants in the CBCR group were asked to use CBCR software to train for 30 minutes per day, 5 days per week, for 6 weeks. At baseline, about half of the participants in each group had cognitive test scores in the impaired range, although the domains of impairment differed between groups. Participants in the CBCR group showed significant improvements on neuropsychological tests matched to CBCR activities, and at posttest only 25% still had impairments on one of the baseline tests. Test performance in the control group remained unchanged. The authors attributed their positive findings versus negative findings in previous studies to increased intensity of treatment, a focus on specific cognitive domains (e.g., working memory) rather than a broad range of cognitive functions, and tailoring outcome measures to match study tasks. A strength of this study was that there was no therapist involvement, so it was possible to isolate the effects of CBCR alone. In addition to measuring only near-transfer, the main limitation was that there was no active control, so it was not possible to determine if gains were attributable to CBCR per se versus general cognitive engagement.

Mahncke and colleagues (2021) addressed the limitation of studies like the one just reviewed, comparing an off-the-shelf CBCR suite of activities to off-the-shelf computer games in an RCT of 83 U.S. active-duty Service Members and Veterans. Outcomes were scores on neuropsychological tests and self-reported measures of everyday function, symptoms, and mood. Participants were offered 1 hour of training per day, 5 days per week, for 13 weeks. CBCR consisted of 23 exercises selected to target speed and accuracy of cognitive processing, and computer games were selected to target aspects of cognition such as executive functions. Participants self-administered both treatments, with weekly telephone calls from a coach who "focused on motivating participants, rewarding progress with praise, aligning participant real-world goals with specific features of the exercises/games they were using, [and] helping participants define and adhere to a training schedule" (Mahncke et al., 2021, p. 1997). Results showed that participants in the CBCR group exhibited 3.9 times more improvement on the neuropsychological tests than controls, with no significant between-groups difference in self-reported everyday function, symptoms, or mood. Results were largely consistent at follow-up, with one unexpected finding: participants in the control group had significantly more improvement in posttraumatic stress. The authors concluded that there was a need for more specificity in designing and implementing these types of interventions.

Strengths of the study by Mahncke and colleagues (2021) were the inclusion of an active control, use of accessible activities in both groups, and careful consideration of potential confounds such as engagement, time on task, and regression to the mean. Limitations included a mismatch between CBCR group treatment tasks, which focused on speed, and outcome measures, which were untimed, raising questions about the mechanism of action for improvements. Also problematic was the underspecification of treatment ingredients for both groups, particularly the control group (e.g., the authors stated that "reaction time" was a target in some tasks, which seems similar to the "speed" requirement in CBCR) (Whyte & Turkstra, 2021).

What is clear from the CBCR literature is that generalization or far-transfer does not occur with repeated administration of computer drills alone. Like the study by Cooper and colleagues (2017) in adults, a number of pediatric studies have shown positive findings from hybrid approaches of computerized drills integrated with strategy training. For example, a pilot study evaluated an integrated intervention approach with the active ingredients being attention drills and cognitive strategies personalized to match individual participant profiles in 11 adolescents (Sohlberg et al., 2014). Results showed variable changes on attention measures, with different participants improving on different neuropsychological measures. The most consistent and positive change was found in participants' individualized Goal Attainment Scales. This small pilot study suggested that key treatment ingredients include individualized training that personalizes drills and cognitive strategies, active encouragement of engagement and motivation, and promotion of generalization through homework.

In their introduction to a 2016 special issue of *Neuropsychological Rehabilitation* that was dedicated to brain training, van Heugten, Ponds, and Kessels (2016) suggested that computerized cognitive training may offer the most benefit when incorporated into a therapeutic milieu rather than administered alone. In other words, CBCR is a collection of ingredients that can be applied to achieve a target, and these ingredients are most effective if they are tightly linked to the target outcome measure (e.g., training and outcome tasks have similar cognitive characteristics). Van Heugten and colleagues also suggested that individualized training is likely optimal and that we need to learn more about participant characteristics that predict treatment response. Results of the studies described here are consistent with that view. We would add that there also is a need to specify targets and ingredients more fully in CBCR research, so clinicians can replicate results in their own practice.

TRANSFER OF LEARNING

A theme throughout this book is *generalization* or *transfer of training*, the importance of which is highlighted by the above CBCR study results. Transfer of training refers to the degree to which a learned behavior or skill will be executed in a new situation. *Near-transfer* refers to application of a learned task or behavior to a task that is very similar to the original learned task, and *far-transfer* occurs when there is application of the learned task to another task that is conceptually related to the original trained task but very different in task parameters (Engelmann, 1980). For CBCR, near-transfer would be, for example, transfer of attention training task gains to an attention test, and far-transfer would be the client perceiving that attention in everyday life has improved. Between these outcomes might be intermediate transfer to an everyday task that requires attention (e.g., sorting pills in a medication organizer; Li, Alonso, Chadha, & Pulido, 2015). As that example shows, measures of far-transfer often are aims rather than targets, which means a change in outcome requires achieving more than just one target. A mismatch between targets and outcome measures likely contributes to the lack of change in far-transfer measures in CBCR and other studies.

Near- and far-transfer of gains from practice in the clinic to performance in everyday settings are more likely to occur when there is overlap and similarity between the skills practiced and the real-life tasks (Ehlhardt, Sohlberg, Glang, & Albin, 2005;

Toglia, Johnston, Goverover, & Dain, 2010). This is particularly true for individuals with poor declarative memory or executive functions, who need support in making the connection between clinic tasks and everyday life. For CBCR, practicing cognitive skills on a computer alone is most likely to lead to changes in everyday tasks if the computer tasks are related to those everyday tasks, limit context variance, and directly promote transfer (e.g., include elements of the target task, have variable stimuli) (Li et al., 2015).

Below we suggest a set of principles for implementing CBCR based on the current intervention and neuroplasticity literature. We then use the PIE framework to describe a clinical case in which CBCR activities were used as ingredients to achieve targets and aims related to everyday life.

Principles for Implementing CBCR

I. Carefully consider candidacy.

- The client's primary cognitive challenge should be in attention or working memory. Unlike declarative learning and memory, the literature suggests that these cognitive domains might be improved by high-dose practice. Accordingly, the client's responses to the clinical interview should match the results of standardized neuropsychological testing. For example, if the client describes frustration with sustaining their attention, this should be evidenced by low scores on a standardized test of sustained attention.
- Prerequisites for CBCR should be fluency with and high motivation to engage in computer exercises without an overlay of psychosocial or somatic concerns that could be primary drivers of cognitive complaints. For example, clients who are not comfortable with computers or for whom screens elicit headaches would not be good candidates.
- Clients should have *sufficient* residual cognitive resources to complete exercises, including attention sufficient for task completion and enough insight to motivate participation.

II. Ensure that the treatment includes targets and active ingredients that embody the Kleim and Jones (2008) principles. These include:

- Exercises individualized to the client's neuropsychological profile and delivered with high intensity. Clinicians will choose those drills that match the impairment profile shown on standardized tests.
- Ingredients for cognitive strategy training integrated with the cognitive exercises (i.e., combine "bottom-up" and "top-down" methods). For example, a mindfulness breathing strategy might be integrated with drills working on distractibility or selective attention.
- Strategies individualized to address functional needs in the client's everyday life, and systematic training in strategy use.
- Ingredients designed to engage and motivate clients. Self-reflection on performance and explicitly linking drills and strategies to functional aims are examples of ingredients that can increase engagement.
- Active targeting of generalization or far-transfer, with ongoing monitoring of changes on meaningful functional tasks affected by the attention or memory impairment being addressed. For example, repeated measurement and discus-

sion of progress toward a functional aim should be incorporated into treatment sessions.

III. Ensure that treatment targets and aims are related to the cognitive impairment being addressed and that the treatment aims are meaningful to the client. Treatment aims should be functional and relate to the underlying cognitive impairment being targeted by the drills and strategies.

Below we describe a therapy program, completed with a client from our clinic, that illustrates the application of these principles.

CASE APPLICATION—KAI

Description of Client

Kai was a 19-year-old male in his second year of college, where he was majoring in music with a focus on the violin. He and several friends were playing catch with a frisbee in a spiral stairwell when Kai slipped and fell several flights. He experienced a brief loss of consciousness. His friends took him to the student health center, where he was diagnosed with a concussion and a sprained ankle. Initial cognitive symptoms included disorientation and memory and attention challenges that manifested as not being able to remember conversations. Somatic symptoms included headache, nausea, and sleep disturbance. Kai was given accommodations in his classes to lighten his workload and be able to avoid screen viewing. He took frequent rest breaks. After 8 weeks, all of his symptoms had resolved with the exception of ongoing difficulty sustaining his attention and experiencing severe headaches about once a day. He was referred to a concussion and brain injury clinic on campus that was part of a Communication Disorders and Sciences program, where he received cognitive rehabilitation.

Planning

A *clinical interview* revealed that Kai was a well-adjusted college student with no previous psychosocial or educational concerns outside of the presenting problems that arose with the onset of his concussion. He had a solid group of friends, was active in several campus groups, and had received A's and B's in all his general education and major courses. His parents lived 2 hours from his college and had been down several times to check on his recovery and provide support. Kai's primary focus in college was music. He was a dedicated violinist and played in a symphony that was a collaboration between the community and the college. Kai's main concern was an inability to "focus" when playing his violin. Prior to the concussion, he practiced several hours a day in a campus studio, and now was only able to play in 20-minute increments before his mind wandered or he became frustrated with not being able to play well. These "attention and concentration" issues were not as disruptive in his nonmusic courses, as he reported that they were easy classes and not demanding. Kai also was challenged by headaches that had improved in frequency and intensity but still were bothersome.

The clinician administered several *formal cognitive assessments* to test her hypothesis that Kai had diminished working memory, which made it difficult for him to focus on his music as he played. She administered the Test of Everyday Attention (TEA; Robertson, Ward, Ridgeway, & Nimmo-Smith, 1994), the Behavior Rating Inventory of Executive Function (BRIEF; Roth et al., 2005), and a memory screen that looked at declarative memory. Results on the tests confirmed her hypothesis that Kai had a mild decline in working memory and no other memory concerns. He had lower than expected scores in the TEA subtests on sustained attention and working memory and on the working memory, suppression, and inhibition scores on the BRIEF. The memory screen revealed no impairments. The testing supported his clinical report.

The clinician and Kai collaboratively identified a *treatment aim* to increase the duration and quality of his violin practice. They developed two Goal Attainment Scales as listed below to make a scale for levels of progress that would be anticipated after 8 weeks of treatment. After a review of treatment options, they decided to do a trial of *computer-based cognitive exercises* integrated with *cognitive strategy training*. Additionally, Kai was interested in receiving information on *headache management strategies*. He was able and willing to engage in a home program between sessions that included completing the computer exercises, practicing his strategies, and recording what headache strategies he used and their effect.

The clinician selected initial computer exercises that matched Kai's profile on the attention tests and developed a reminder sheet with the initial cognitive and headache management strategies that had been selected by Kai.

Implementation

Kai attended eight weekly 50-minute sessions. Each session was structured as follows:

- 5-minute check-in on homework/generalization data in order to plan session accordingly
- 35 minutes on attention computer drills with integration of cognitive strategy practice
- 10 minutes for planning and updating home program and adjusting datasheets, computer exercises and loading the computer exercises on the thumb drive

Computer exercises. The clinician selected computer exercises that tapped into sustained attention and working memory and matched Kai's profile of clinical complaints and test results. Based on the findings in the literature, the clinician informed Kai that he would need to be able to complete a minimum of three computer sessions each week, including the clinic session, and Kai believed that was doable. He had a laptop, and the computer training program came with thumb drives that could be loaded with the client's exercises. Completion of each exercise generated (1) accuracy or timing data as well as error profiles (e.g., distribution of errors) and (2) ratings for both effort and motivation and whether the strategy was used and if it helped. The clinician and Kai reviewed these data at their session and made adjustments. For example, if Kai consistently rated an exercise as highly effortful and thus had low motivation, the clinician would decrease difficulty level even if accuracy was acceptable. Conversely, if he rated exercises as easy or average and achieved 80% accuracy or better after several trials, she increased the difficulty level. The clinician encouraged Kai to engage in self-reflection on his performance and participate in the adjustments.

Cognitive strategy training. Kai was shown a number of examples of different types of strategies designed to improve attention. He elected to use self-talk or verbal mediation. He developed a key phrase "reset" to use when he noticed his mind wandering during the computer exercises or during his violin practice. After a few sessions, he developed a second key phrase "keep going" to encourage him to not stop when he grew frustrated.

Psychoeducation for headache management. The clinician gave Kai a link to a headache management website that she had learned about from a concussion course that was developed by a neurologist. Kai was asked to review assignments, select management strategies that resonated with him, and to chart when he used strategies and any perceived benefit.

Evaluation and Outcome Measurement

Measurement data included:

Session data. Session targets were set for each of the three treatment domains. Targets for the computer-based attention training were based around completion and advancement in the computer program. Targets for the cognitive strategy training were for accuracy in using Kai's self-talk strategy.

Generalization data. Generalization measures focused on completing aspects of the home program and using Kai's cognitive strategies during his violin practice.

Impact measures. There were three types of treatment impact measures, including GAS, pre- and post-comparison on the TEA and the BRIEF to evaluate changes in attention, and a pre- and post-comparison of scores on a headache impact questionnaire. The two Goal Attainment Scales were the treatment aims and are depicted below. Kai achieved Level 2 for the number of minutes able to practice without losing focus and Level 0 for the quality of practice. Performance on the subtests of the TEA and indices on the BRIEF improved on the attention areas targeted and remained stable in the other areas. There was a slight improvement on his reported headache impact score.

Goal Attainment Scale	Number of minutes able to rehearse before losing focus	Self-rating on quality of rehearsal for past 3 days (1 = poor; 5 = excellent)
Level 2 (much more than expected)	41–50 minutes	5
Level 1 (more than expected)	31–40 minutes	4
Level 0 (expected)	21–30 minutes	3
Level –1 (baseline)	11–20 minutes	2
Level –2 (below expected)	Less than 11 minutes	1

SUMMARY

Kai is an example of one clinical case. There were no controls or experimental manipulation; thus, it is not possible to discern the relative contribution of the three types of intervention. For example, it is not known whether strategies or attention drills alone would have resulted in therapeutic change. The improvement on the specific areas of attention observed to be impaired and activated by the attention drills suggests that the targeted drills may have been helpful. Unlike many of the experimental studies that deliver decontextualized, generic attention drills and do not personalize drills and integrate strategy training, this case followed the candidacy recommendations and used the treatment ingredients currently supported in the literature and relevant guidelines.

CHAPTER 12

Cognitive Rehabilitation
for Functional Cognitive Symptoms

Rose Dunn, Pauline Mashima, Katharine Seagly, Brigid Waldron-Perrine, Diane Paul, McKay Moore Sohlberg, and Kelly Ann Peña[1]

When considering the practice of cognitive rehabilitation, we thought it important to devote a chapter to discussing treatment of individuals with *functional symptoms*. Functional symptoms are genuine, distressing, often disabling to the person, and are accompanied by distinctive clinical features that cannot be fully explained by another recognized neurological or medical condition (Schmidtke, Pohlmann, & Metternich, 2008; Stone et al., 2015). The lack of consensus on nomenclature for individuals with functional symptoms continues to be problematic, with varying labels used in clinical practice and scientific literature, including "psychogenic," "psychosomatic," "conversion disorder," "nonorganic," "cogniform disorder," or "medically unexplained." This chapter will use the term *functional* in accordance with recent trends for diagnostic terminology (Ball et al., 2020; Edwards, Stone, & Lang, 2014; Stone et al., 2015), and because of preliminary evidence that the word "functional" is preferred by clients (Ding & Kanaan, 2016). Functional neurological disorder (FND) is often used as an umbrella term for these conditions.

Functional symptoms can include cognitive symptoms (e.g., memory loss, inability to focus), motor dysfunction (e.g., paralysis, tremor), speech changes (e.g., stuttering, dysphonia), sensory dysfunction (e.g., vision changes, pain), and episodes of altered awareness (e.g., dissociative or functional seizures). Clients with functional symptoms are seen in a variety of medical settings, and symptoms vary widely among clients,

---

[1] On behalf of the Joint Committee on Interprofessional Relations Between the American Psychological Association and the American Speech–Language–Hearing Association.

with many presenting as polysymptomatic. Many individuals with functional symptoms have a comorbid neurological disorder and/or experienced a precipitating physical event or trauma before developing functional symptoms (Kutlubaev, Xu, Hackett, & Stone, 2018; Stone et al., 2009). In other words, a notable percentage of clients present for treatment with both functional symptoms *and also* symptoms related to identifiable pathology [e.g., traumatic brain injury (TBI), epilepsy]. This chapter focuses on functional cognitive symptoms (FCS), which constitute a large proportion of clients with functional symptoms. For example, clients with FCS comprise an estimated 12–56% of new referrals in cognitive or memory disorders clinics (Bharambe & Larner, 2018; Bhome, McWilliams, Huntley, Fleming, & Howard, 2019; Elsey et al., 2015; Pennington, Ball, & Swirski, 2019; Pennington, Hayre, Newson, & Coulthard, 2015; Wakefield et al., 2018). Given these high base rates, it is likely that clinicians have worked with or will work with clients with FCS during their careers, perhaps often.

Despite the high prevalence of FCS, development of evidence-based guidelines and training in treatment approaches have historically been neglected, making it challenging for clinicians working with this population. Clients with functional symptoms report higher levels of disability and distress than clients with other identified neurological diagnoses, which underscores the immense need for targeted interventions for FCS (Carson et al., 2011). These clients are also at high risk for iatrogenic effects secondary to misdiagnosis and delays in appropriate intervention (Stone et al., 2015). Fortunately, there has been increasing awareness and acceptance of functional symptoms as an important clinical issue in recent years. Although more randomized controlled trials are needed, emerging evidence has elucidated general principles and approaches that can be effective when working with clients with functional symptoms (Nicholson et al., 2020; Nielsen et al., 2015). Most of the existing literature and research has focused on noncognitive functional symptoms (e.g., functional motor disorders, functional speech disorders, functional seizures), however, and there is currently no evidence-based consensus on how to treat FCS. More research is needed to develop gold-standard treatments for functional cognitive conditions. In the interim, cognitive rehabilitation clinicians need resources to inform their work with these clients, who frequently present for evaluation and treatment. Thus, using the existing scientific literature on functional symptoms, this chapter provides an overview of what is currently known about FCS and proposes a client-centered, practical approach for cognitive rehabilitation treatment of clients with FCS.

ETIOLOGIES

Historically, functional symptoms were thought to result from emotional trauma and other psychological causes. Although psychological factors can increase the risk for developing functional symptoms, many individuals with functional symptoms do not endorse any history of traumatic events or psychological diagnoses (Kranick, Gorrindo, & Hallett, 2011). Current etiological models have moved away from erroneous mind-versus-body dichotomies and instead propose that development and maintenance of functional symptoms can best be understood via a biopsychosocial framework. Psychological factors to consider include history of adverse childhood events, comorbid psychological conditions, and illness beliefs. Social factors may include social benefits (e.g., increased support from family) or avoidance of undesired activities (e.g., a stressful work environment) due to symptoms. Biological factors, as noted above, often include a precipitating physical injury (e.g., a concussion) or medical illness (e.g., epilepsy, COVID-19) that precedes the onset of functional symptoms. The combination of these three factors underscores the utility of an integrated biopsychosocial approach to treatment, as opposed to the historical approach of solely referring to a psychiatrist or psychologist for treatment.

ASSESSMENT

Given that functional symptoms can be highly varied and may present differently depending on the time point, setting, and treating provider, interprofessional assessment and collaboration are crucial for diagnosis and treatment planning. The need for diagnostic criteria is supported by evidence that clients with longer symptom duration have poorer outcomes, whereas early diagnosis predicts good outcomes (Gelauff & Stone, 2016). One common misconception is that functional conditions are a diagnosis of exclusion (i.e., a diagnosis made by ruling out all other conditions), as opposed to diagnosing based on clinical features (Lidstone, Araújo, Stone, & Bloem, 2020). However, recent research efforts have focused on identifying "positive" clinical signs that can be used to make an affirmative diagnosis of functional symptoms (Espay et al., 2018; McWhirter, Ritchie, Stone, & Carson, 2020).

As with any diagnosis, the potential for misdiagnosis of FND must be acknowledged and carefully considered, as this has significant implications for prognosis and treatment. FND is often diagnosed by a neurologist, and referral to a specialist with expertise in neurological diagnosis is recommended (Bennett et al., 2021). It is, however, important for all clinicians engaged in cognitive rehabilitation to be knowledgeable about positive clinical signs of FND. As Lidstone and colleagues (2020) highlighted, missing another medical or neurological condition can cause profound harm to the client, but misdiagnosing FND as another neurological condition can be just as harmful. While more longitudinal studies are needed, existing data suggest that when a specialist makes an FND diagnosis, FND can be diagnosed as accurately as other neurologic and psychiatric conditions (Gelauff & Stone, 2016).

Unfortunately, although there are emerging diagnostic criteria for FND, at present there are no validated diagnostic criteria specifically for FCS. As with all clients with FND, clients with FCS are at high risk for iatrogenic effects if symptoms are not accurately diagnosed and appropriately treated in a timely manner (McWhirter et al., 2020). Many individuals with FCS undergo unnecessary, duplicative, and costly tests and evaluations, as well as inappropriate treatment, without receiving an accurate explanation for their symptoms. Without a clear understanding of their diagnosis, clients are denied the opportunity to make informed treatment decisions (Barnett, Davis, Mitchell, & Tyson, 2020).

Although there is no consensus on diagnostic criteria for functional cognitive conditions, experts in the field have described the utility of "internal" and "external" inconsistencies as markers for FCS (Bennett et al., 2021; Duffy, 2016; McWhirter et al., 2020). Internal inconsistency has been described as the ability to perform a task well at certain times but with significantly impaired ability at other times, particularly when the client's performance on the task is the focus of attention (Ball et al., 2020). For example, a client may demonstrate excellent working memory and detailed recall of recent events during casual conversation but severely impaired performance on simple tasks of attention and recall during formal testing. Another example of internal inconsistency is a client who successfully maintains a cognitively challenging job but demonstrates significant difficulty on much simpler cognitive tasks during treatment sessions. It is important to highlight that these inconsistencies must be distinguished from the fluctuations over time that can be observed in other conditions, such as delirium, Lewy body dementia, or cognitive fatigue after acquired brain injury, or from medication effects.

Evidence of external inconsistencies can also suggest functional symptoms (Stone et al., 2015). External inconsistencies are incongruencies between the client's presentation and what typically occurs in neurological conditions affecting cognition. For example, after a concussion, a client with FCS may report a marked increase in cognitive symptoms 6 months after the event with no other precipitating cause. This is incongruent with expected concussion recovery, in which cognitive symptoms improve rather than worsen over time. Another example is a client concerned about dementia who is able to easily recall detailed information about their recent medical experiences (e.g., appointment dates, clinicians' names, test results) but reports an inability to recall the names of family members and close friends with whom they regularly interact. This presentation is incongruent with neurological conditions affecting memory, in which we would typically expect overlearned, remote information to be more intact than new information. Although further empirical validation of positive clinical signs of FCS is needed to improve diagnostic accuracy, these clinical signs should trigger further investigation by the client's physician and treatment team. Rather than jumping to conclusions based on one observation, the treatment team should collaborate to determine if there are converging patterns of positive clinical signs. Neuropsychological testing, which emphasizes performance and symptom validity measurement, can provide objective evidence for internal and external inconsistencies, and assist with diagnosis and treatment recommendations.

When assessing clients with possible functional symptoms, clinicians may encounter behaviors that feel "exaggerated," which can raise questions about the presence of consciously feigned symptoms for secondary gain, such as attention from others (as seen in factitious disorder) or financial gain (as seen in malingering). Clinicians may find themselves attempting to disentangle whether symptoms are consciously or unconsciously produced, which is difficult, if not impossible in many cases (Stone, Carson, & Sharpe, 2005). While it is important for treating clinicians to thoroughly consider external factors that may be reinforcing symptoms (e.g., avoiding a stressful work setting, receiving increased care from spouse), a brief trial of client-centered treatment can be provided to improve functioning without making a determination regarding volition. Clinicians are encouraged to be aware of natural biases they may have to ensure that these biases do not impede a nonjudgmental and collaborative approach. If clients feel that their clinician is doubting the veracity or validity of their symptoms, they may (consciously or unconsciously) exhibit increased severity of symptoms (Ahern, Stone, & Sharpe, 2009; Bennett et al., 2021; O'Connell, Jones, Chalder, & David, 2020). In turn, clinicians can become frustrated by this increase in symptoms and resulting lack of progress, creating a vicious cycle (Barnett et al., 2020).

COMMON PRESENTATIONS OF FCS

Presentations of FCS can be very heterogeneous. The following are examples that may be encountered within the context of cognitive rehabilitation (Stone et al., 2015).

FCS as the Primary Concern

> Miguel was a 44-year-old attorney who presented to outpatient cognitive rehabilitation with complaints of memory problems for the previous year after a concussion. A neurological exam and neuroimaging were normal, and neuropsychological testing indicated above-average cognitive abilities. During the initial evaluation with his speech-language pathologist, Miguel provided a detailed description of his recent errors and memory lapses, recalling exactly when and where they occurred. The accuracy of his report was verified by his husband. He had disengaged from household responsibilities he once took pride in doing, such as grocery shopping and cooking, due to fear of memory lapses. Despite these cognitive symptoms, he had been recently promoted at work, and he consistently receives positive feedback about his performance from his partners at his law firm.

Individuals may present with FCS as the sole concern or chief complaint. Although they may also have other comorbid functional symptoms, such as dizziness or vision changes, the cognitive symptoms are causing the most distress and/or having the most impact on functioning.

FCS as a Component of Another Functional Neurological Disorder

> Nia, a 53-year-old financial manager, participated in physical therapy after being diagnosed with a functional movement disorder after hospitalization 2 years previously. Her primary symptoms at that time were functional weakness and tremor in her legs. Although she was receptive to the diagnosis and treatment approach, progress had been somewhat slow. When discussing perceived barriers, she reported difficulty attending to information during therapy sessions due to extreme distractibility, as well as difficulty implementing treatment strategies at home due to forgetfulness. Although not reported during her initial evaluation, it became evident as sessions progressed that cognitive symptoms were limiting treatment progress and daily functioning. On neuropsychological testing, Nia performed better on more challenging tasks than easier tasks (e.g., better performance on free recall than recognition memory tasks).

Research suggests that clients with other functional neurological disorders, such as functional movement disorders, also may report cognitive complaints (Matin et al., 2017). Although cognitive complaints may be a "background" symptom to primary complaints, cognitive rehabilitation may be warranted if symptoms impact daily functioning or engagement with other therapies (e.g., physical therapy, cognitive-behavioral therapy). Because individuals with functional neurological conditions are often polysymptomatic, interdisciplinary treatment and collaboration (e.g., collaborative goal setting) are often needed to optimize functioning across symptom domains.

Functional Cognitive Symptoms with Comorbid Medical or Neurological Conditions

> William was a 26-year-old nurse who sustained a moderate TBI with a loss of consciousness of 4 hours. While in acute care, his treatment team was impressed with his rapid cognitive recovery. He was quickly transferred to an inpatient rehabilitation facility, and initial evaluations suggested an excellent prognosis. Within a few days, he was able to accurately recall detailed and complex information from the previous days. At the same time, his family was expressing concerns to the team that he was unable to recall basic autobiographical information, such as how many children he had and the state where he was raised. A few days later, these memory problems began to present during therapy sessions, and his carryover between sessions deteriorated from excellent to poor. Medical workup did not reveal an explanation for the recent rapid decline. After collecting information across sessions, his treatment team noted his memory difficulties seemed more pronounced when he was being directly asked or "tested," as opposed to when he was engaging in casual conversation about the day's events. He was becoming increasingly anxious about whether these memory issues would become permanent.

As previously mentioned, physical injury, medical illness, and neurological conditions are risk factors for developing functional symptoms. For example, a systematic review and meta-analysis found that 22% of clients with functional seizures had a history of epileptic seizures (Kutlubaev et al., 2018). The term *functional overlay* is often used when core symptoms caused by another recognized medical or neurological condition are complicated by additional functional features (Stone, Reuber, & Carson, 2013). Clinicians are encouraged to be mindful that a client's presentation cannot always be clearly delineated as functional versus another medical/neurological condition and instead may include features of both. Although this comorbidity can pose clinical challenges, many of the treatment principles described below are still applicable.

TREATMENT PRINCIPLES AND STRATEGIES

With increased research and clinical efforts in recent years, clinics specializing in the treatment of functional symptoms have been developed. However, given the limited number of specialized clinics and the prevalence rates of clients with functional symptoms, rehabilitation clinicians working outside of these specialty clinics need to be informed of how to meet the treatment needs of this client population. This section will outline general principles and techniques that have been suggested from extant research and experts in the field (Bennett et al., 2021; Duffy, 2016; Nicholson et al., 2020; Nielsen et al., 2015). Given the heterogeneity of functional presentations, treatment interventions will need to be personalized based on the client's particular symptom presentation, beliefs, goals, and response to treatment; and factors maintaining symptoms.

Interprofessional Approach

As many clients with functional symptoms present as polysymptomatic, interprofessional collaborative treatment is recommended. It is imperative that all clinicians use similar language and consistent messaging when working with the client and their family. A team meeting at the onset of treatment and regular team huddles are beneficial to ensure that all clinicians are working toward common targets and remaining current on progress across disciplines. Performance advancement can quickly become stalled if one clinician is working on a high-level cognitive aim (e.g., the client independently taking notes), while another clinician from a different profession is not aware of that aim and may be unintentionally reinforcing a lower level of functioning (e.g., writing out notes for the client). Clinicians should frequently model and reinforce the team's collaborative approach with the client (e.g., "You did fantastic with your note taking today. I'm going to let your physical therapist know so you can use this during your sessions with them as well."). Co-treatment sessions are another helpful means to ensure skills and independence are generalizing to other areas of functioning.

Client Education

Personalized education is essential to ensure the clients' understanding of their symptoms throughout the course of treatment. Information should be presented in a validating, collaborative manner. Published consensus recommendations (Nicholson et al., 2020; Nielsen et al., 2015; Stone, Carson, & Hallett, 2016) suggest that the following client education ingredients can be useful:

1. Assure the client that you believe them and are taking their concerns seriously. It is important to say this explicitly (e.g., "The symptoms you are experiencing are very real, and they are impacting your quality of life. Is it OK if we work together to help you address these symptoms?"). This is particularly important when clients report prior negative experiences with other health care providers.

2. Highlight that functional symptoms are common (e.g., "Functional cognitive symptoms are actually very common even though many people have not heard of them. I have worked with many other individuals with concerns similar to yours.").

3. Emphasize that symptoms can get better (e.g., "We aren't always sure what causes functional symptoms, but fortunately we do know these symptoms can get better.").

4. Emphasize that self-help will be a key component of treatment and progress (e.g., "We are going to work together as a team to help you get back to doing the things you care about. I am also going to ask you to take the strategies you learn in our sessions and apply them throughout your daily routine at home, work, etc. Our goal is for you to become independent in using these strategies.").

5. Provide printed or online peer-reviewed information specific for functional symptoms, or links to peer-reviewed resources from organizations specializing in functional neurological disorders. These online resources not only reinforce important education and a sense of hope for clients but can also facilitate a sense of community with other individuals with functional symptoms. An example of a website with support and information for both providers and clients with FND is *https://fndhope.org.*

6. Avoid emphasis on finding a psychological origin unless the client is making this link on their own. If the client has identified specific "triggers" for functional symptoms, such as increased stress, then this can be helpful when developing self-help strategies.

7. With the client's consent, it can be helpful to involve members of the client's support network when providing education.

Additional educational ingredients are provided below within each of the treatment approaches. Anecdotally, we have observed that for a subset of clients with FCS, education and reassurance are sufficient to improve functioning, but many clients require further intervention. Additional research is needed to determine which clients will benefit from education alone.

Stepwise Goal Approach

At the beginning of treatment, it is recommended that time be spent identifying the client's personal and cultural values and goals, which can be translated into a structured, stepwise goal approach. These values-driven goals should be referenced regularly throughout the course of treatment. It can be particularly helpful to keep these goals and associated targets in a written format (e.g., visual chart), so that checking off target achievements can be used as a source of positive reinforcement for progress. The focus should be on high-level, personalized, activity-based (i.e., functional) targets, with clear timelines for accomplishment (e.g., "Now that you've successfully gotten back to managing meal-planning for your family, I feel confident you'll be able to prepare a simple dish following a recipe by the end of the week."). Involving members of the client's support network in goal-setting discussions is also crucial so that they can reinforce the same goals outside of sessions with an appropriate level of support.

The following questions can be helpful starting points in assessing a client's values and goals:

- "If your symptoms were not getting in the way, what kinds of things would you want to be doing? Walk me through what you would like a typical day to look like."
- "I want you to think about times in which you've felt most fulfilled. What would I find you doing during those times?"
- "If you felt really confident that your symptoms could get better, what kinds of big goals would you set for yourself?"

Chapter 3 on psychological mindedness offers additional information and tools for exploring personal values to guide interactions with clients, identify areas for desired changes, inform approaches to care, and maximize engagement in rehabilitation by linking treatment targets to values-based, person-centered life goals.

Operant Conditioning Approach

An operant conditioning approach has been proposed as a potentially useful treatment approach for functional symptoms (Hardin & Carson, 2019; Jimenez, Aboussouan, & Johnson, 2019; Speed & Mooney, 1997). This type of approach involves the clinician providing positive reinforcement via verbal praise and attention when the client demonstrates progress or independently engages in self-help strategies to improve functioning. When the client shows behaviors or patterns that the clinician is working to reduce, the clinician avoids giving excessive attention to these behaviors. For example, if a client is making frequent errors on a bill-paying task, the clinician might say, "Hmm. This seems to be one of those moments when your mind's signal is glitchy. That's OK; it happens. We've talked about some ways to help your brain get unstuck and back on track. Shall we try one of those now?" With this approach, there is minimal to no discussion about the specific errors, and the conversation quickly turns to selecting self-help techniques. The clinician should give ample attention and praise when the client effectively uses a self-help technique, such as initiating the use of a calculator or a task checklist. This may look very different than interventions used with other client groups, in which error feedback may be used to increase the client's insight into deficits and self-monitoring of errors.

Members of the client's support network also need education on how to respond when the client is exhibiting difficulty. Well-meaning members of the client's support network may frequently step in to assist the client with tasks, which can maintain symptoms and reduce self-efficacy. Thus, it can be helpful to provide close others with concrete examples of how they can respond in a supportive manner that also promotes optimal client functioning. Inviting close others to practice these approaches with the client during treatment sessions can be beneficial.

Promoting Realistic Expectations for Cognition

During the initial phase of treatment, it is important to understand how the client conceptualizes and responds to their symptoms. Unhelpful illness beliefs, for example that symptoms will be permanent, can be poor predictors of successful outcomes (Sharpe et al., 2010). Some individuals with FCS become hyper-focused on normal, everyday cognitive errors (Stone et al., 2015). "Memory perfectionism" has been used in the literature to describe clients who have unrealistically high standards for their memory (Pennington et al., 2015). For these clients, psychoeducation about the frequency of cognitive errors in healthy individuals can be beneficial.

It is important to note that while there is emerging evidence to support the efficacy of cognitive-behavioral therapy (CBT) in treating functional conditions, some individuals with functional symptoms may be resistant, at least initially, to engaging in treatment with a mental health provider. Thus, cognitive rehabilitation clinicians would benefit from being familiar with basic CBT-informed strategies to promote realistic expectations and optimize progress. Specifically, when clients engage in avoidance behaviors (e.g., deferring all tasks to a family member, avoiding social interactions due to fear of memory lapses), it can be beneficial to provide education on how avoidance may provide short-term relief from unwanted thoughts and feelings but will actually maintain symptoms in the long run.

Clinicians should discuss with clients and their families how gradual exposure to challenging activities will allow the client's brain to "challenge" unhelpful beliefs and relearn that they can be successful with implementation of self-help tools, whereas avoidance does not provide this opportunity for change. For example, clients with FCS may believe, "If I go to the grocery store by myself, I'll forget an item and feel like a failure." Instead, the clinician can encourage the client to consider and test out alternative potential outcomes, such as, "If I go to the grocery store, I will need to bring a list of items and double check the list before I leave. Needing to rely on a list in the past has made me feel embarrassed, but I know that it might help me be successful, which would build my confidence." Readers may refer to Chapter 3 on psychological mindedness for additional information and tools about CBT-informed strategies.

Addressing "Overfocus"

Research suggests that excessive effort or self-attention can interfere with performance in individuals with functional symptoms. For example, clients with functional motor disorders who are unable to walk may be able to walk backward or run when engaged in tasks that divert attention away from deliberate, effortful processes (McWhirter et al., 2020). It is thought that diverting attention allows automatic movement-control processes to take over, which, in turn, improves performance (Nielsen et al., 2015). Similarly, it has been hypothesized that clients with FCS may demonstrate more difficulty when striving to perform on cognitive tests but then exhibit intact cognitive abilities when less effort is being exerted, such as during casual conversation or when multitasking (McWhirter et al., 2020). If this pattern is present for clients, it can be helpful to make them aware of how such "overfocus" can negatively impact functioning. Showing the client specific, in-the-moment examples of overfocus can be illustrative and promote mindfulness of internal patterns. The clinician can then guide the development of self-awareness and self-help strategies for the client to "reset" when they notice excessive effort or focus. For example, it may be beneficial for a client to step away from a task for a few minutes and distract themselves with a more automatic or relaxing activity (e.g., doing the dishes, stretching) before resuming the more cognitively demanding task.

Again, this approach frequently looks different than traditional cognitive rehabilitation approaches in which we often encourage clients to concentrate fully on a task and minimize distractions. Chapter 3 reviews acceptance and commitment therapy (ACT; Hayes et al., 2016) as a method that does not focus directly on symptom alleviation and instead emphasizes the benefits of acknowledging internal experiences/symptoms in a nonjudgmental manner and mindfully shifting one's attention to pursue valued activities in the present moment.

Self-Management Strategies

The focus of cognitive rehabilitation for FCS is to teach client-specific management strategies to restore function, promote self-efficacy, and support successful reengagement in meaningful activities. Chapter 7 provides instruction on cognitive strategy training. Direct teaching and guided practice seek to empower clients to achieve treatment targets, followed by gradual weaning from therapeutic support to effective self-management in daily situations. Reinforcing healthy behaviors that can impact cognition (e.g., sleep hygiene, education about medication effects, management of cerebrovascular risk factors, exercise, relaxation) can foster a proactive attitude of prevention and maintaining wellness.

MONITORING PROGRESS AND CONCLUDING TREATMENT

Clinicians should discuss outcome monitoring and a set discharge process from the onset of treatment to reinforce expectations for progress and highlight that treatment is time-limited and has the end goal of self-management. Monitoring of progress is particularly important when working with clients with FCS given the aforementioned risks for iatrogenic effects. Clinicians must be mindful of the fact that certain treatment approaches and/or settings can reinforce or exacerbate functional symptoms in some clients, and a prolonged course of treatment in the absence of improvement is strongly discouraged. It is important to be transparent with clients that progress toward goals will be collaboratively monitored and routinely discussed, and if the client is not advancing toward their identified goals, then services may need to be discontinued. In these situations, clinicians can emphasize that discontinuing therapy that is not advancing the client toward their goals may allow the client to spend more time on meaningful activities (Gilmour et al., 2020). Some clients with chronic, severe symptoms may require higher levels of care, such as a specialized functional disorders clinic or inpatient rehabilitation, before they can benefit from outpatient services. It is still unclear which treatment setting is best for clients with functional symptoms and is likely highly variable depending on the client. Outcome monitoring can assist with making these decisions.

The heterogeneity and variability of symptoms, as well as the discrepancy between objective measures/clinician ratings and the clients' subjective experiences of symptoms, can complicate outcome measurement in functional symptoms (Nicholson et al., 2020). Pick and colleagues (2020) conducted a systematic review of outcome measurement in FND to identify existing measures, develop recommendations, and guide future research. They concluded that there is a dearth of functional disorder-specific outcome measures and much more research is needed. In the interim, the authors recommended measures assessing quality of life and general functioning, such as the Short Form Health Survey (SF) scales (Ware, Kosinski, & Keller, 1996), which can help identify clinically meaningful change during treatment. Assessing change in illness beliefs and symptom attributions across treatment, with tools such as the Illness Perception Questionnaire (Weinman, Petrie, Moss-Morris, & Horne, 1996), may provide helpful information as important mediators of treatment response. Given the heterogeneity of symptoms, use of personalized assessments such as Goal Attainment Scales (see Chapter 5) may also be beneficial for tracking progress.

When concluding treatment, it is recommended that the clinician and client collaboratively develop a written self-management plan that includes self-help strategies proven to be beneficial in therapy, future goals with realistic time frames, and plans for

how to address potential setbacks/relapses. Symptom relapse is common in this population, and clients ought to be prepared with a personalized plan to get back on track
should this occur. It can also be helpful to engage in role-playing exercises with clients
before discharge, so they know how to educate future health care providers about both
their diagnosis and also the treatment approaches that work best for them. If the client will be discharged to a different setting, a summary letter or phone consultation is
recommended to ensure that the next clinician is informed of treatment approaches that
were effective.

Glossary of Key Memory and Learning Terms

Term	Description
Anterograde amnesia	Impairment in the ability to encode, store, or retrieve information encountered after the amnesia-causing event.
Consolidation	The time-dependent processes that stabilize a memory representation after initial acquisition.
Declarative learning	The process of consciously acquiring new long-term declarative memories.
Declarative memory	The conscious, intentional recollection of experiences (episodic memory) and information (semantic memory). Synonymous with *explicit memory.*
Distributed practice	Practice that occurs over a series of sessions spaced over time. Practice is often conducted in an expanded rehearsal format, where there is a gradual increase in the time interval between the practice trials.
Elaboration	A process that encourages a deeper level of processing than simply rehearsing. Examples are creating a visual image or trying to remember a special feature of target information.
Episodic memory	A subtype of declarative memory that is memory for temporally related events and comprises our autobiographical memory.
Errorless learning	An approach that minimizes opportunities for error responses during training.
Explicit memory	Synonymous with *declarative memory.*

Term	Description
Implicit memory	Synonymous with *nondeclarative memory.*
Long-term memory	A theoretically unlimited-capacity system for durable storage of learned information and behaviors. Comprised of declarative and nondeclarative memory systems.
Maintenance	Preservation of memories or skills over time.
Metacognition	Knowledge about one's own thinking, typically described as including two linked processes: the ability to monitor one's thoughts and the ability to regulate thinking. The ability to use strategies to help remember information is an example of metacognitive ability.
Nondeclarative learning	The process of acquiring new long-term memories without conscious awareness.
Nondeclarative memory	A subtype of long-term memory that is inaccessible to conscious awareness but evidenced in behavior. Examples are priming, emotional associations, and performance of procedures. Synonymous with *implicit memory.*
Posttraumatic amnesia (PTA)	The state of confusion and inability to form new memories after a traumatic brain injury. In addition to the memory disorder, PTA can include delirium, extreme distractibility, emotional lability, restlessness, agitation, and aggression.
Priming	The nondeclarative process whereby exposure to an item influences the performance on a subsequent item.
Procedural memory	The subtype of nondeclarative memory that underlies performance of motor and cognitive tasks without conscious recall. Use of correct grammar without declarative knowledge of grammatical rules is an example of procedural memories.
Prospective memory	The initiation of intended actions at a future time.
Retrieval	The process of recovering a declarative memory, either automatically or strategically, and either independently or when provided with cues.
Retrograde amnesia	Impairment in memory for information and events experienced prior to the event that caused the amnesia.
Semantic memory	The subtype of declarative memory comprised of facts and concepts.
Working memory	A limited-capacity system for both short-term storage of information and also active manipulation of that information for either storage or retrieval.

Mindfulness Resources

MINDFULNESS BOOKS

- *Mindfulness for Beginners* by Jon Kabat-Zinn. Boulder, CO: Sounds True.
- *Wherever You Go, There You Are* by Jon Kabat-Zinn (practical guide to mindfulness meditation). New York: Hachette Books.

MINDFULNESS APPS AND WEBSITES

- Headspace (meditation app geared toward beginners with some free content, including a basics course of the foundation and common techniques of mindfulness and meditation).
- Insight Timer (free meditation app with up to 100,000 guided meditations).
- Mindful.org (website and magazine about mindfulness).

MINDFULNESS RESEARCH RESOURCES

- American Mindfulness Research Association (Altadena, CA), which has a monthly newsletter.
- Center for Healthy Minds (University of Wisconsin–Madison).

References

Adams, G. L., & Engelmann, S. (1996). *Research on direct instruction: 25 years beyond DISTAR.* Seattle: Educational Achievement Systems.

Ahern, L., Stone, J., & Sharpe, M. C. (2009). Attitudes of neuroscience nurses toward patients with conversion symptoms. *Psychosomatics, 50*(4), 336–339.

Alderson, A. L., & Novack, T. A. (2002). Measuring recovery of orientation during acute rehabilitation for traumatic brain injury: Value and expectations of recovery. *Journal of Head Trauma Rehabilitation, 17*(3), 210–219.

American Speech–Language–Hearing Association. (2021). *Interprofessional Education/Interprofessional Practice (IPE/IPP).* Retrieved from *www.asha.org/practice/ipe-ipp.*

Anderson, N. D., & Craik, F. I. (2006). The mnemonic mechanisms of errorless learning. *Neuropsychologia, 44*(14), 2806–2813.

Armistead-Jehle, P. (2010). Symptom validity test performance in U.S. veterans referred for evaluation of mild TBI. *Applied Neuropsychology, 17*(1), 52–59.

Asnaani, A., & Hofmann, S. G. (2012). Collaboration in multicultural therapy: Establishing a strong therapeutic alliance across cultural lines. *Journal of Clinical Psychology, 68*(2), 187–197.

Baddeley, A. D. (1995). The psychology of memory. In *Handbook of memory disorders* (pp. 3–25). Oxford: John Wiley & Sons.

Baddeley, A., Eysenck, M. W., & Anderson, M. C. (2009). *Memory.* New York: Psychology Press.

Baddeley, A., & Hitch, G. (1974). Working memory. In G. Bower (Ed.), *The psychology of learning and motivation: Advances in research and theory* (Vol. 8, pp. 47–89). New York: Academic Press.

Baddeley, A., & Wilson, B. A. (1994). When implicit learning fails: Amnesia and the problem of error elimination. *Neuropsychologia, 32*(1), 53–68.

Baker, S. K., Gersten, R., & Scanlon, D. (2002). Procedural facilitators and cognitive strategies: Tools for unraveling the mysteries of comprehension and the writing process, and for providing meaningful access to the general curriculum. *Learning Disabilities Research & Practice, 17*(1), 65–77.

Ball, H. A., McWhirter, L., Ballard, C., Bhome, R., Blackburn, D. J., Edwards, M. J., . . . Carson, A. J. (2020). Functional cognitive disorder: Dementia's blind spot. *Brain, 143*(10), 2895–2903.

Barnes, S. (2020). Right hemisphere damage and other-initiated repair in everyday conversation. *Clinical Linguistics & Phonetics, 34*(10–11), 910–932.

Barnett, C., Davis, R., Mitchell, C., & Tyson, S. (2020). The vicious cycle of functional neurological disorders: A synthesis of healthcare professionals' views on working with patients with functional neurological disorder. *Disability and Rehabilitation, 40*(10), 1–10.

Baron, L. S., & Arbel, Y. (2022). An implicit-explicit framework for intervention methods in developmental language disorder. *American Journal of Speech–Language Pathology, 31*(4), 1557–1573.

Baumeister, R. F., Tice, D. M., & Vohs, K. D. (2018). The strength model of self-regulation: Conclusions from the second decade of willpower research. *Perspectives on Psychological Science, 13*(2), 141–145.

Beauchamp, M. H. (2017). Neuropsychology's social landscape: Common ground with social neuroscience. *Neuropsychology, 31*(8), 981–1002.

Beck, A. T., & Weishaar, M. (2005). Cognitive therapy. In *Current psychotherapies* (7th intr. ed., pp. 238–268). Belmont, CA: Thomson Brooks/Cole.

Beck, J. S. (2011). *Cognitive behavior therapy.* New York: Guilford Press.

Beer, J. S., & Ochsner, K. N. (2006). Social cognition: A multi level analysis. *Brain Research, 1079*(1), 98–105.

Behn, N., Francis, J., Togher, L., Hatch, E., Moss, B., & Hilari, K. (2021). Description and effectiveness of communication partner training in TBI: A systematic review. *Journal of Head Trauma Rehabilitation, 36*(1), 56–71.

Benigas, J., Brush, J., & Elliot, G. (2016). *Spaced retrieval step by step: An evidence-based memory intervention.* Baltimore: Health Professions Press.

Bennett, K., Diamond, C., Hoeritzauer, I., Gardiner, P., McWhirter, L., Carson, A., & Stone, J. (2021). A practical review of functional neurological disorder (FND) for the general physician. *Clinical Medicine (London), 21*(1), 28–36.

Bharambe, V., & Larner, A. (2018). Functional cognitive disorders: Memory clinic study. *Progress in Neurology and Psychiatry, 22*, 19–22.

Bhatnagar, S., Iaccarino, M. A., & Zafonte, R. (2016). Pharmacotherapy in rehabilitation of post-acute traumatic brain injury. *Brain Research, 1640*, 164–179.

Bhome, R., McWilliams, A., Huntley, J. D., Fleming, S. M., & Howard, R. J. (2019). Metacognition in functional cognitive disorder—A potential mechanism and treatment target. *Cognitive Neuropsychiatry, 24*(5), 311–321.

Blair, C., & Raver, C. C. (2014). Closing the achievement gap through modification of neurocognitive and neuroendocrine function: Results from a cluster randomized controlled trial of an innovative approach to the education of children in kindergarten. *PLoS One, 9*(11), e112393.

Blakemore, S. J., & Choudhury, S. (2006). Development of the adolescent brain: Implications for executive function and social cognition. *Journal of Child Psychology and Psychiatry, 47*(3–4), 296–312.

Bond, A. E., Draeger, C. R. L., Mandleco, B., & Donnelly, M. (2003). Needs of family members of patients with severe traumatic brain injury: Implications for evidence-based practice. *Critical Care Nurse, 23*(4), 63–72.

Boschen, K., Gargaro, J., Gan, C., Gerber, G., & Brandys, C. (2007). Family interventions after acquired brain injury and other chronic conditions: A critical appraisal of the quality of the evidence. *NeuroRehabilitation, 22*(1), 19–41.

Botvinik-Nezer, R., Holzmeister, F., Camerer, C. F., Dreber, A., Huber, J., Johannesson, M., . . . Schonberg, T. (2020). Variability in the analysis of a single neuroimaging dataset by many teams. *Nature, 582*(7810), 84–88.

Bourgeois, M., Lenius, K., Turkstra, L. S., & Camp, C. (2007). The effects of cognitive teletherapy on reported everyday memory behaviours of persons with chronic traumatic brain injury. *Brain Injury, 21*(12), 1245–1257.

Boutron, I., Altman, D. G., Moher, D., Schulz, K. F., Ravaud, P., & Group, C. N. (2017). CONSORT statement for randomized trials of nonpharmacologic treatments: A 2017 update and a CONSORT extension for nonpharmacologic trial abstracts. *Annals of Internal Medicine, 167*(1), 40–47.

Bouwens, S. F., van Heugten, C. M., & Verhey, F. R. (2009). The practical use of goal attainment scaling for people with acquired brain injury who receive cognitive rehabilitation. *Clinical Rehabilitation, 23*(4), 310–320.

Bovend'Eerdt, T. J., Botell, R. E., & Wade, D. T. (2009). Writing SMART rehabilitation goals and achieving goal attainment scaling: A practical guide. *Clinical Rehabilitation, 23*(4), 352–361.

Bracy, O. L. (1983). Computer based cognitive rehabilitation. *Cognitive Rehabilitation, 1*(1), 7–8, 18.

Broadbent, D. E., Cooper, P. F., FitzGerald, P., & Parkes, K. R. (1982). The cognitive failures questionnaire (CFQ) and its correlates. *British Journal of Clinical Psychology, 21*(1), 1–16.

Broicher, S. D., Kuchukhidze, G., Grunwald, T., Kramer, G., Kurthen, M., & Jokeit, H. (2012). "Tell me how do I feel"—emotion recognition and theory of mind in symptomatic mesial temporal lobe epilepsy. *Neuropsychologia, 50*(1), 118–128.

Brune, M., & Brune-Cohrs, U. (2006). Theory of mind—evolution, ontogeny, brain mechanisms and psychopathology. *Neuroscience & Biobehavioral Reviews, 30*(4), 437–455.

Butler, R. W., Copeland, D. R., Fairclough, D. L., Mulhern, R. K., Katz, E. R., Kazak, A. E., . . . Sahler, O. J. Z. (2008). A multicenter, randomized clinical trial of a cognitive remediation program for childhood survivors of a pediatric malignancy. *Journal of Consulting and Clinical Psychology, 76*(3), 367.

Byom, L., O'Neil-Pirozzi, T. M., Lemoncello, R., MacDonald, S., Meulenbroek, P., Ness, B., . . . On behalf of the Academy of Neurologic Communication Disorders Traumatic Brain Injury Writing, C. (2020). Social communication following adult traumatic brain injury: A scoping review of theoretical models. *American Journal of Speech-Language Pathology, 29*(3), 1735–1748.

Callaway, L., Winkler, D., Tippett, A., Migliorini, C., Herd, N., & Willer, B. (2014). *The Community Integration Questionnaire-Revised (CIQ-R)*. Melbourne, Australia: Summer Foundation.

Camina, E., & Güell, F. (2017). The neuroanatomical, neurophysiological and psychological basis of memory: Current models and their origins. *Frontiers in Pharmacology, 8*, 438.

Carroll, E., & Coetzer, R. (2011). Identity, grief and self-awareness after traumatic brain injury. *Neuropsychological Rehabilitation, 21*(3), 289–305.

Carrow-Woolfolk, E. (1999). *Comprehensive Assessment of Spoken Language*. Circle Pines, MN: American Guidance Service.

Carson, A., Stone, J., Hibberd, C., Murray, G., Duncan, R., Coleman, R., . . . Sharpe, M. (2011). Disability, distress and unemployment in neurology outpatients with symptoms "unexplained by organic disease." *Journal of Neurology, Neurosurgery, and Psychiatry, 82*(7), 810–813.

Cavell, T. A. (1990). Social adjustment, social performance, and social skills: A tri-component model of social competence. *Journal of Clinical Child Psychology, 19*(2), 111–122.

Cebula, K. R., Moore, D. G., & Wishart, J. G. (2010). Social cognition in children with Down's syndrome: Challenges to research and theory building. *Journal of Intellectual Disability Research, 54*(2), 113–134.

Centers for Disease Control and Prevention. (2015). *Report to Congress on traumatic brain injury in the United States: Epidemiology and rehabilitation*. www.cdc.gov/traumaticbraininjury/pdf/TBI_Report_to_Congress_Epi_and_Rehab-a.pdf.

Cepeda, N. J., Pashler, H., Vul, E., Wixted, J. T., & Rohrer, D. (2006). Distributed practice in verbal recall tasks: A review and quantitative synthesis. *Psychological Bulletin, 132*(3), 354–380.

Cerasa, A., Gioia, M. C., Valentino, P., Nisticò, R., Chiriaco, C., Pirritano, D., . . . Quattrone, A. (2013). Computer-assisted cognitive rehabilitation of attention deficits for multiple sclerosis: A randomized trial with fMRI correlates. *Neurorehabilitation and Neural Repair, 27*(4), 284–295.

Chan, D. Y. K., & Fong, K. N. K. (2011). The effects of problem-solving skills training based on metacognitive principles for children with acquired brain injury attending mainstream schools: A controlled clinical trial. *Disability and Rehabilitation, 33*(21–22), 2023–2032.

Charters, E., Gillett, L., & Simpson, G. (2015). Efficacy of electronic portable assistive devices for people with acquired brain injury: A systematic review. *Neuropsychological Rehabilitation, 25*(1), 82–121.

Chaytor, N., & Schmitter-Edgecombe, M. (2003). The ecological validity of neuropsychological tests: A review of the literature on everyday cognitive skills. *Neuropsychology Review, 13*(4), 181–197.

Chen, S. H., Thomas, J. D., Glueckauf, R. L., & Bracy, O. L. (1997). The effectiveness of computer-assisted cognitive rehabilitation for persons with traumatic brain injury. *Brain Injury, 11*(3), 197–209.

Cherry, K. E., Hawley, K. S., Jackson, E. M., & Boudreaux, E. O. (2009). Booster sessions enhance the long-term effectiveness of spaced retrieval in older adults with probable Alzheimer's disease. *Behavior Modification, 33*(3), 295–313.

Chesnutt, J. C. (2021). Evolving science to inform emerging concussion practices. *American Journal of Speech-Language Pathology, 30*(4), 1592–1597.

Chu, Y., Brown, P., Harniss, M., Kautz, H., & Johnson, K. (2014). Cognitive support technologies for people with TBI: Current usage and challenges experienced. *Disability and Rehabilitation: Assistive Technology, 9*(4), 279–285.

Ciaramelli, E., Neri, F., Marini, L., & Braghittoni, D. (2015). Improving memory following prefrontal cortex damage with the PQRST method. *Frontiers in Behavioral Neuroscience, 9*, 211.

Cicerone, K. D., Dahlberg, C., Malec, J. F., Langenbahn, D. M., Felicetti, T., Kneipp, S., . . . Catanese, J. (2005). Evidence-based cognitive rehabilitation: Updated review of the literature from 1998 through 2002. *Archives of Physical Medicine and Rehabilitation, 86*(8), 1681–1692.

Cicerone, K. D., & Giacino, J. T. (1992). Remediation of executive function deficits after traumatic brain injury. *NeuroRehabilitation, 2*(3), 12–22.

Cicerone, K. D., & Wood, J. C. (1987). Planning disorder after closed head injury: A case study. *Archives of Physical Medicine and Rehabilitation, 68*(2), 111–115.

Cole, E. (1999). Cognitive prosthetics: An overview to a method of treatment. *NeuroRehabilitation, 12*(1), 39–51.

Connolly, H. L., Lefevre, C. E., Young, A. W., & Lewis, G. J. (2019). Sex differences in emotion recognition: Evidence for a small overall female superiority on facial disgust. *Emotion, 19*(3), 455–464.

Cooper, D. B., Bowles, A. O., Kennedy, J. E., Curtiss, G., French, L. M., Tate, D. F., & Vanderploeg, R. D. (2017). Cognitive rehabilitation for military service members with mild traumatic brain injury: A randomized clinical trial. *Journal of Head Trauma Rehabilitation, 32*(3), E1–E15.

Cooper, D. B., Bunner, A. E., Kennedy, J. E., Balldin, V., Tate, D. F., Eapen, B. C., & Jaramillo, C. A. (2015). Treatment of persistent post-concussive symptoms after mild traumatic brain injury: A systematic review of cognitive rehabilitation and behavioral health interventions in military service members and veterans. *Brain Imaging and Behavior, 9*(3), 403–420.

Cooper, D. B., Curtiss, G., Armistead-Jehle, P., Belanger, H. G., Tate, D. F., Reid, M., . . . Vanderploeg, R. D. (2018). Neuropsychological performance and subjective symptom reporting in military service members with a history of multiple concussions: Comparison with a single concussion, posttraumatic stress disorder, and orthopedic trauma. *Journal of Head Trauma Rehabilitation, 33*(2), 81–90.

Cotter, J., Firth, J., Enzinger, C., Kontopantelis, E., Yung, A. R., Elliott, R., & Drake, R. J. (2016). Social cognition in multiple sclerosis: A systematic review and meta-analysis. *Neurology, 87*(16), 1727–1736.

Cramer, S. C., Sur, M., Dobkin, B. H., O'Brien, C., Sanger, T. D., Trojanowski, J. Q., . . . Vinogradov, S. (2011). Harnessing neuroplasticity for clinical applications. *Brain, 134*(6), 1591–1609.

Crocker, L., Heller, W., Warren, S., O'Hare, A., Infantolino, Z., & Miller, G. (2013). Relationships among cognition, emotion, and motivation: Implications for intervention and neuroplasticity in psychopathology. *Frontiers in Human Neuroscience, 7*(261).

Cross, G. (2009). *Care management of Operation Enduring Freedom (OEF) and Operation Iraqi Freedom (OIF) veterans.* Department of Veterans Affairs. www.va.gov/vhapublications/publications.cfm?pub=2.

Crosson, B., Barco, P. P., Velozo, C. A., Bolesta, M. M., Cooper, P. V., Werts, D., & Brobeck, T. C. (1989). Awareness and compensation in postacute head injury rehabilitation. *Journal of Head Trauma Rehabilitation, 30*(5).

Cunningham, R., & Ward, C. (2003). Evaluation of a training programme to facilitate conversation between people with aphasia and their partners. *Aphasiology, 17*(8), 687–707.

Dahlberg, C. A., Cusick, C. P., Hawley, L. A., Newman, J. K., Morey, C. E., Harrison-Felix, C. L., & Whiteneck, G. G. (2007). Treatment efficacy of social communication skills training after traumatic brain injury: A randomized treatment and deferred treatment controlled trial. *Archives of Physical Medicine and Rehabilitation, 88*(12), 1561–1573.

Dams-O'Connor, K., Landau, A., Hoffman, J., & St. De Lore, J. (2018). Patient perspectives on quality and access to healthcare after brain injury. *Brain Injury, 32*(4), 431–441.

Dardiotis, E., Nousia, A., Siokas, V., Tsouris, Z., Andravizou, A., Mentis, A.-F. A., . . . Nasios, G. (2018). Efficacy of computer-based cognitive training in neuropsychological performance of patients with multiple sclerosis: A systematic review and meta-analysis. *Multiple Sclerosis and Related Disorders, 20*, 58–66.

Davis, A. M., Cockburn, J. M., Wade, D. T., & Smith, P. T. (1995). A subjective memory assessment questionnaire for use with elderly people after stroke. *Clinical Rehabilitation, 9*(3), 238–244.

de Joode, E., van Heugten, C., Verhey, F., & van Boxtel, M. (2010). Efficacy and usability of assistive technology for patients with cognitive deficits: A systematic review. *Clinical Rehabilitation, 24*(8), 701–714.

Dennis, M., Simic, N., Bigler, E. D., Abildskov, T., Agostino, A., Taylor, H. G., . . . Yeates, K. O. (2013). Cognitive, affective, and conative theory of mind (ToM) in children with traumatic brain injury. *Developmental Cognitive Neuroscience, 5*, 25–39.

Dewar, B. K., Patterson, K., Wilson, B. A., & Graham, K. S. (2009). Re-acquisition of person knowledge in semantic memory disorders. *Neuropsychological Rehabilitation, 19*(3), 383–421.

Diamond, A. (2013). Executive functions. *Annual Review of Psychology, 64*, 135–168.

DiLollo, A., & Favreau, C. (2010). Person-centered care and speech and language therapy. *Seminars in Speech and Language, 31*(2), 90–97.

Ding, J. M., & Kanaan, R. A. (2016). What should we say to patients with unexplained neurological symptoms?: How explanation affects offence. *Journal of Psychosomatic Research, 91*, 55–60.

Dobson, D., & Dobson, K. S. (2018). *Evidence-based practice of cognitive-behavioral therapy.* New York: Guilford Press.

Dollaghan, C. A. (2007). *The handbook for evidence-based practice in communication disorders.* Baltimore: Paul H. Brookes.

Donovan, J. J., & Radosevich, D. J. (1999). A meta-analytic review of the distribution of practice effect: Now you see it, now you don't. *Journal of Applied Psychology, 84*(5), 795–805.

Dörfler, E., & Kulnik, S. T. (2020). Despite communication and cognitive impairment—person-centred goal-setting after stroke: A qualitative study. *Disability and Rehabilitation, 42*(25), 3628–3637.

Douglas, J. M., Bracy, C. A., & Snow, P. C. (2007). Exploring the factor structure of the La Trobe Communication Questionnaire: Insights into the nature of communication deficits following traumatic brain injury. *Aphasiology, 21*(12), 1181–1194.

Douglas, N. F., Campbell, W. N., & Hinckley, J. J. (2015). Implementation science: Buzzword or game changer? *Journal of Speech, Language, and Hearing Research, 58*(6), S1827–S1836.

Duffy, J. R. (2016). Functional speech disorders: Clinical manifestations, diagnosis, and management. *Handbook of Clinical Neurology, 139*, 379–388.

Duncan, J., Emslie, H., Williams, P., Johnson, R., & Freer, C. (1996). Intelligence and the frontal lobe: The organization of goal-directed behavior. *Cognitive Psychology, 30*(3), 257–303.

Dunlosky, J., Hertzog, C., Kennedy, M., & Thiede, K. (2005). The self-monitoring approach for effective learning. *Cognitive Technology, 10*, 4–11.

Dunlosky, J., Rawson, K. A., Marsh, E. J., Nathan, M. J., & Willingham, D. T. (2013). Improving students' learning with effective learning techniques: Promising directions from cognitive and educational psychology. *Psychological Science in the Public Interest, 14*(1), 4–58.

Dymowski, A. R., Ponsford, J. L., & Willmott, C. (2016). Cognitive training approaches to remediate attention and executive dysfunction after traumatic brain injury: A single-case series. *Neuropsychological Rehabilitation, 26*(5–6), 866–894.

Edwards, M. J., Stone, J., & Lang, A. E. (2014). From psychogenic movement disorder to functional movement disorder: It's time to change the name. *Movement Disorders, 29*(7), 849–852.

Ehlhardt, L. A., Sohlberg, M. M., Glang, A., & Albin, R. (2005). TEACH-M: A pilot study evaluating an instructional sequence for persons with impaired memory and executive functions. *Brain Injury, 19*(8), 569–583.

Ehlhardt, L. A., Sohlberg, M. M., Kennedy, M., Coelho, C., Ylvisaker, M., Turkstra, L., & Yorkston, K. (2008). Evidence-based practice guidelines for instructing individuals with neurogenic memory impairments: What have we learned in the past 20 years? *Neuropsychological Rehabilitation, 18*(3), 300–342.

Elliott, M. L., Knodt, A. R., Ireland, D., Morris, M. L., Poulton, R., Ramrakha, S., . . . Hariri, A. R. (2020). What is the test-retest reliability of common task-functional MRI measures?: New empirical evidence and a meta-analysis. *Psychological Science, 31*(7), 792–806.

Elsey, C., Drew, P., Jones, D., Blackburn, D., Wakefield, S., Harkness, K., . . . Reuber, M. (2015). Towards diagnostic conversational profiles of patients presenting with dementia or functional memory disorders to memory clinics. *Patient Education and Counseling, 98*(9), 1071–1077.

Engel, G. L. (1977). The need for a new medical model: A challenge for biomedicine. *Science, 196*(4286), 129–136.

Engelmann, S. (1980). *Direct instruction* (Vol. 22). Englewood Cliffs, NJ: Educational Technology.

Engelmann, S., & Carnine, D. (1991). *Theory of instruction: Principles and applications* (rev. ed.). Eugene, OR: ADI Press.

Englert, C. S., Raphael, T. M., Anderson, L. M., Anthony, H. M., & Stevens, D. D. (1991). Making strategies and self-talk visible: Writing instruction in regular and special education classrooms. *American Educational Research Journal, 28*(2), 337–372.

Espay, A. J., Aybek, S., Carson, A., Edwards, M. J., Goldstein, L. H., Hallett, M., . . . Morgante, F. (2018). Current concepts in diagnosis and treatment of functional neurological disorders. *JAMA Neurology, 75*(9), 1132–1141.

Evald, L. (2015). Prospective memory rehabilitation using smartphones in patients with TBI: What do participants report? *Neuropsychological Rehabilitation, 25*(2), 283–297.

Fann, J. R., Hart, T., Ciol, M. A., Moore, M., Bogner, J., Corrigan, J. D., . . . Hammond, F. M. (2021). Improving transition from inpatient rehabilitation following traumatic brain injury: Protocol for the BRITE pragmatic comparative effectiveness trial. *Contemporary Clinical Trials, 104*, 106332.

Fasotti, L., Kovacs, F., Eling, P. A., & Brouwer, W. H. (2000). Time pressure management as a compensatory strategy training after closed head injury. *Neuropsychological Rehabilitation,* 10(1), 47–65.

Ferguson, J. E., MacLennan, D. L., Cates, L. P., Rich, T. L., & Hughes, A. M. (2021). *Just One Thing (JOT): Custom care plans.* http://z.umn.edu/justonething.

Ferguson, S., Friedland, D., & Woodberry, E. (2015). Smartphone technology: Gentle reminders of everyday tasks for those with prospective memory difficulties post-brain injury. *Brain Injury,* 29(5), 583–591.

Fernandes, H. A., Richard, N. M., & Edelstein, K. (2019). Cognitive rehabilitation for cancer-related cognitive dysfunction: A systematic review. *Support Care Cancer,* 27(9), 3253–3279.

Fernandez Lopez, R., & Antoli, A. (2020). Computer-based cognitive interventions in acquired brain injury: A systematic review and meta-analysis of randomized controlled trials. *PLoS One,* 15(7), e0235510.

Fetta, J., Starkweather, A., & Gill, J. M. (2017). Computer-based cognitive rehabilitation interventions for traumatic brain injury: A critical review of the literature. *Journal of Neuroscience Nursing,* 49(4), 235–240.

Filippi, M., Riccitelli, G., Mattioli, F., Capra, R., Stampatori, C., Pagani, E., . . . Rocca, M. A. (2012). Multiple sclerosis: Effects of cognitive rehabilitation on structural and functional MR imaging measures—An explorative study. *Radiology,* 262(3), 932–940.

Finch, E., Copley, A., Cornwell, P., & Kelly, C. (2015). A systematic review of behavioural interventions targeting social communication difficulties following traumatic brain injury. *Archives of Physical Medicine and Rehabilitation,* 97(8), 1352–1365.

Fisher, A., Bellon, M., Lawn, S., Lennon, S., & Sohlberg, M. (2019). Family-directed approach to brain injury (FAB) model: A preliminary framework to guide family-directed intervention for individuals with brain injury. *Disability and Rehabilitation,* 41(7), 854–860.

Fisher, A., Lennon, S., Bellon, M., & Lawn, S. (2015). Family involvement in behaviour management following acquired brain injury (ABI) in community settings: A systematic review. *Brain Injury,* 29(6), 661–675.

Fleming, J. M., Strong, J., & Ashton, R. (1996). Self-awareness of deficits in adults with traumatic brain injury: How best to measure? *Brain Injury,* 10(1), 1–16.

Fleming, J. M., Strong, J., & Ashton, R. (1998). Cluster analysis of self-awareness levels in adults with traumatic brain injury and relationship to outcome. *Journal of Head Trauma Rehabilitation,* 13(5), 39–51.

Frampton, S. B., Guastello, S., Hoy, L., Naylor, M., Sheridan, S., & Johnston-Fleece, M. (2017). *Harnessing evidence and experience to change culture: A guiding framework for patient and family engaged care.* National Academy of Medicine. https://nam.edu/harnessing-evidence-and-experience-to-change-culture-a-guiding-framework-for-patient-and-family-engaged-care.

Frattali, C., Thompson, C., Holland, A., Wohl, C., & Ferketic, M. (1995). *American Speech–Language–Hearing Association Functional Assessment of Communication Skills for Adults.* Rockville, MD: American Speech–Language–Hearing Association.

Gallistel, C. R., & Balsam, P. D. (2014). Time to rethink the neural mechanisms of learning and memory. *Neurobiology of Learning and Memory,* 108, 136–144.

Gambrill, E. (2012). *Critical thinking in clinical practice: Improving the quality of judgments and decisions* (3rd ed.). Hoboken, NJ: John Wiley & Sons.

Gasquoine, P. G. (2016). Blissfully unaware: Anosognosia and anosodiaphoria after acquired brain injury. *Neuropsychological Rehabilitation,* 26(2), 261–285.

Gelauff, J., & Stone, J. (2016). Prognosis of functional neurologic disorders. *Handbook of Clinical Neurology,* 139, 523–541.

German, T. P., & Hehman, J. A. (2005). Representational and executive selection resources in "theory of mind": Evidence from compromised belief-desire reasoning in old age. *Cognition,* 101(1), 129–152.

Gilmour, G. S., Nielsen, G., Teodoro, T., Yogarajah, M., Coebergh, J. A., Dilley, M. D., . . . & Edwards, M. J. (2020). Management of functional neurological disorder. *Journal of Neurology, 267*(7), 2164–2172.

Glang, A., Singer, G., Cooley, E., & Tish, N. (1992). Tailoring direct instruction techniques for use with elementary students with brain injury. *Journal of Head Trauma Rehabilitation, 7*(4), 93–108.

Gloster, A. T., Walder, N., Levin, M., Twohig, M., & Karekla, M. (2020). The empirical status of acceptance and commitment therapy: A review of meta-analyses. *Journal of Contextual Behavioral Science, 18*, 181–192.

Goia, G., Isquith, P., Guy, S., & Kenworthy, I. (2000). *Behavior Rating Scale of Executive Function BRIEF Professional Manual*. Lutz, FL: PAR.

Goverover, Y., Chiaravalloti, N., Genova, H., & DeLuca, J. (2017). A randomized controlled trial to treat impaired learning and memory in multiple sclerosis: The self-GEN trial. *Multiple Sclerosis Journal, 24*(8), 1096–1104.

Graham, S., & Harris, K. R. (2003). Students with learning disabilities and the process of writing: A meta-analysis of SRSD studies. In H. L. Swanson, K. R. Harris, & S. Graham (Eds.), *Handbook of learning disabilities* (pp. 323–344). New York: Guilford Press.

Grant, M., & Ponsford, J. (2014). Goal attainment scaling in brain injury rehabilitation: Strengths, limitations and recommendations for future applications. *Neuropsychological Rehabilitation, 24*(5), 661–677.

Greenberg, D. L., & Verfaellie, M. (2010). Interdependence of episodic and semantic memory: evidence from neuropsychology. *Journal of the International Neuropsychological Society, 16*(5), 748–753.

Griffiths, G. G., Sohlberg, M. M., Kirk, C., Fickas, S., & Biancarosa, G. (2016). Evaluation of use of reading comprehension strategies to improve reading comprehension of adult college students with acquired brain injury. *Neuropsychological Rehabilitation, 26*(2), 161–190.

Haley, S. M., Coster, W. J., Ludlow, L. H., Haltiwanger, J. T., & Adrellos, P. J. (1992). *Pediatric Evaluation of Disability Inventory: Development, standardization, and administration manual*. Boston: New England Medical Center Hospital/Trustees of Boston University.

Hammer, D. (1997). Discovery learning and discovery teaching. *Cognition and Instruction, 15*(4), 485–529.

Han, K., Chapman, S. B., & Krawczyk, D. C. (2020). Cognitive training reorganizes network modularity in traumatic brain injury. *Neurorehabilitation and Neural Repair, 34*(1), 26–38.

Hardin, A. S., & Carson, C. (2019). Interdisciplinary treatment of functional neurological symptom disorder in an inpatient rehabilitation setting: A case report. *PM & R: Journal of Injury, Function, and Rehabilitation, 11*(6), 661–664.

Harris, K. R., & Pressley, M. (1991). The nature of cognitive strategy instruction: Interactive strategy construction. *Exceptional Children, 57*(5), 392–404.

Harris, R. (2009). *ACT with love: Stop struggling, reconcile differences, and strengthen your relationship with acceptance and commitm*. Oakland, CA: New Harbinger.

Hart, T., Buchhofer, R., & Vaccaro, M. (2004). Portable electronic devices as memory and organizational aids after traumatic brain injury: A consumer survey study. *Journal of Head Trauma Rehabilitation, 19*(5), 351–365.

Hart, T., Dijkers, M. P., Whyte, J., Turkstra, L. S., Zanca, J. M., Packel, A., . . . Chen, C. (2019). A theory-driven system for the specification of rehabilitation treatments. *Archives of Physical Medicine and Rehabilitation, 100*(1), 172–180.

Hart, T., Driver, S., Sander, A., Pappadis, M., Dams-O'Connor, K., Bocage, C., . . . Cai, X. (2018). Traumatic brain injury education for adult patients and families: A scoping review. *Brain Injury, 32*(11), 1295–1306.

Hart, T., & Ehde, D. M. (2015). Defining the treatment targets and active ingredients of rehabilitation: Implications for rehabilitation psychology. *Rehabilitation Psychology, 60*(2), 126.

Hart, T., Ferraro, M., Rabinowitz, A., Fitzpatrick DeSalme, E., Nelson, L., Marcy, E., . . . Turkstra, L. (2020). Improving communication with patients in post-traumatic amnesia: development and impact of a clinical protocol. *Brain Injury, 34*(11), 1518–1524.

Hart, T., Tsaousides, T., Zanca, J. M., Whyte, J., Packel, A., Ferraro, M., & Dijkers, M. P. (2014). Toward a theory-driven classification of rehabilitation treatments. *Archives of Physical Medicine and Rehabilitation, 95*(1, Suppl.), S33–S44.

Hartley, L. L. (1995). *Cognitive-communicative abilities following brain injury: A functional approach.* San Diego, CA: Singular Publishing Group.

Haslam, C. (2018). The tyranny of choice: Deciding between principles of errorless learning, spaced retrieval and vanishing cues. In C. Haslam & R. P. C. Kessels (Eds.), *Errorless learning in neuropsychological rehabilitation: Mechanisms, efficacy and application* (pp. 180–192). London: Routledge.

Haslam, C., & Kessels, R. P. C. (Eds.) (2018). *Errorless learning in neuropsychological rehabilitation: Mechanisms, efficacy and application.* Current Issues in Neuropsychology. London: Routledge.

Hawley, K. S., Cherry, K. E., Boudreaux, E. O., & Jackson, E. M. (2008). A comparison of adjusted spaced retrieval versus a uniform expanded retrieval schedule for learning a name-face association in older adults with probable Alzheimer's disease. *Journal of Clinical and Experimental Neuropsychology, 30*(6), 639–649.

Hayes, S. C., Strosahl, K. D., & Wilson, K. G. (2009). *Acceptance and commitment therapy.* Washington, DC: American Psychological Association.

Hayes, S. C., Strosahl, K. D., & Wilson, K. G. (2016). *Acceptance and commitment therapy: The process and practice of mindful change.* New York: Guilford Press.

Henry, A., Lannoy, S., Chaunu, M.-P., Tourbah, A., & Montreuil, M. (2022). Social cognition and executive functioning in multiple sclerosis: A cluster-analytic approach. *Journal of Neuropsychology, 16*(1), 97–115.

Herbert, M. S., Afari, N., Robinson, J., Listvinsky, A., Bondi, M. W., & Wetherell, J. L. (2018). Neuropsychological functioning and treatment outcomes in acceptance and commitment therapy for chronic pain. *Journal of Pain, 19*(8), 852–861.

Hettema, J., Steele, J., & Miller, W. R. (2005). Motivational interviewing. *Annual Review of Clinical Psychology, 1*, 91–111.

Higginbotham, J., & Moulton, B. (2017). *Appraising change: Making evidence-informed decisions in speech-language pathology.* Ultra-Blue Capital, LLC. www.therapy-science.com.

Hildebrandt, H., Lanz, M., Hahn, H. K., Hoffmann, E., Schwarze, B., Schwendemann, G., & Kraus, J. A. (2007). Cognitive training in MS: Effects and relation to brain atrophy. *Restorative Neurology and Neuroscience, 25*(1), 33–43.

Hilderbrand, E. (2017). *The identicals.* New York: Little, Brown and Company.

Hillary, F. G., Schultheis, M. T., Challis, B. H., Millis, S. R., Carnevale, G. J., Galshi, T., & DeLuca, J. (2003). Spacing of repetitions improves learning and memory after moderate and severe TBI. *Journal of Clinical and Experimental Neuropsychology, 25*(1), 49–58.

Hoepner, J. K., Sievert, A., & Guenther, K. (2021). Joint video self-modeling for persons with traumatic brain injury and their partners: A case series. *American Journal of Speech-Language Pathology, 30*(2S), 863–882.

Hoepner, J. K., & Turkstra, L. S. (2013). Video-based administration of the La Trobe Communication Questionnaire for adults with traumatic brain injury and their communication partners. *Brain Injury, 27*(4), 464–472.

Hofmann, S. G., Asnaani, A., Vonk, I. J., Sawyer, A. T., & Fang, A. (2012). The efficacy of cognitive behavioral therapy: A review of meta-analyses. *Cognitive Therapy and Research, 36*(5), 427–440.

Holland, A. L., & Ryan, R. L. (2020). *Counseling in communication disorders: A wellness perspective* (3rd ed.). San Diego, CA: Plural.

Hopper, T., Drefs, S. J., Bayles, K. A., Tomoeda, C. K., & Dinu, I. (2010). The effects of modified spaced-retrieval training on learning and retention of face-name associations by individuals with dementia. *Neuropsychological Rehabilitation, 20*(1), 81–102.

Hopper, T., Mahendra, N., Kim, E., Azuma, T., Bayles, K. A., Cleary, S., & Tomoeda, C. K. (2005). Evidence-based practice recommendations for individuals working with dementia: Spaced-retrieval training. *Journal of Medical Speech-Language Pathology, 13*(4), xxvii–xxxiv.

Horn, S. D., DeJong, G., & Deutscher, D. (2012). Practice-based evidence research in rehabilitation: An alternative to randomized controlled trials and traditional observational studies. *Archives of Physical Medicine and Rehabilitation, 93*(8, Suppl.), S127–S137.

Horn, S. D., & Gassaway, J. (2010). Practice based evidence: Incorporating clinical heterogeneity and patient-reported outcomes for comparative effectiveness research. *Medical Care, 48*(6, Suppl.), S17–S22.

Horvath, A. O., & Luborsky, L. (1993). The role of the therapeutic alliance in psychotherapy. *Journal of Consulting and Clinical Psychology, 61*(4), 561–573.

Huckans, M., Pavawalla, S., Demadura, T., Kolessar, M., Seelye, A., Roost, N., . . . Storzbach, D. (2010). A pilot study examining effects of group-based cognitive strategy training treatment on self-reported cognitive problems, psychiatric symptoms, functioning, and compensatory strategy use in OIF/OEF combat veterans with persistent mild cognitive disorder and history of traumatic brain injury. *Journal of Rehabilitation Research and Development, 47*(1), 43–60.

Institute of Medicine. (2011). *Cognitive rehabilitation therapy for traumatic brain injury: Evaluating the evidence.* Washington, DC: National Academies Press.

International Classification of Functioning, Disability and Health. (2001). World Health Organization. www.who.int/standards/classifications/international-classification-of-functioning-disability-and-health.

Irish, M., & Vatansever, D. (2020). Rethinking the episodic-semantic distinction from a gradient perspective. *Current Opinion in Behavioral Sciences, 32*, 43–49.

Jackson, W. T., Novack, T. A., & Dowler, R. N. (1998). Effective serial measurement of cognitive orientation in rehabilitation: The Orientation Log. *Archives of Physical Medicine and Rehabilitation, 79*(6), 718–720.

Jacobs, K., Leopold, A., Hendricks, D., Sampson, E., Nardone, A., Lopez, K., . . . Scherer, M. (2017). Project Career: Perceived benefits of iPad apps among college students with traumatic brain injury (TBI). *Work, 58*(1), 45–50.

James, W. (1890). *Principles of psychology.* New York: Henry Holt.

Jamieson, M., Cullen, B., McGee-Lennon, M., Brewster, S., & Evans, J. J. (2014). The efficacy of cognitive prosthetic technology for people with memory impairments: A systematic review and meta-analysis. *Neuropsychological Rehabilitation, 24*(3–4), 419–444.

Jiménez, F. J. R. (2012). Acceptance and commitment therapy versus traditional cognitive behavioral therapy: A systematic review and meta-analysis of current empirical evidence. *International Journal of Psychology and Psychological Therapy, 12*(3), 333–358.

Jimenez, X. F., Aboussouan, A., & Johnson, J. (2019). Functional neurological disorder responds favorably to interdisciplinary rehabilitation models. *Psychosomatics, 60*(6), 556–562.

Jones, F., & Riazi, A. (2011). Self-efficacy and self-management after stroke: A systematic review. *Disability and Rehabilitation, 33*(10), 797–810.

Judge, K. S., Yarry, S. J., & Orsulic-Jeras, S. (2009). Acceptability and feasibility results of a strength-based skills training program for dementia caregiving dyads. *Gerontologist, 50*(3), 408–417.

Kagan, A., Black, S. E., Felson Duchan, J., Simmons-Mackie, N., & Square, P. (2001). Training volunteers as conversation partners using "supported conversation for adults with aphasia" (SCA): A controlled trial. *Journal of Speech, Language, and Hearing Research, 44*, 624–638.

Kangas, M., & McDonald, S. (2011). Is it time to act?: The potential of acceptance and commitment therapy for psychological problems following acquired brain injury. *Neuropsychological Rehabilitation, 21*(2), 250–276.

Kaschel, R., Sala, S. D., Cantagallo, A., Fahlböck, A., Laaksonen, R., & Kazen, M. (2002). Imagery mnemonics for the rehabilitation of memory: A randomised group controlled trial. *Neuropsychological Rehabilitation, 12*(2), 127–153.

Kavale, K. A., & Forness, S. R. (2000). What definitions of learning disability say and don't say: A critical analysis. *Journal of Learning Disabilities, 33*(3), 239–256.

Kay, T., Cavallo, M. M., Ezrachi, O., & Vavagiakis, P. (1995). Head injury family interview: A clinical and research tool. *Journal of Head Trauma Rehabilitation, 10*(2), 12–31.

Keith, R. A., & Lipsey, M. W. (1993). The role of theory in rehabilitation assessment, treatment, and outcomes. In R. L. Glueckauf, L. B. Sechrest, G. R. Bond, & E. C. McDonel (Eds.), *Improving assessment in rehabilitation and health* (pp. 33–58). Thousand Oaks, CA: SAGE.

Kennedy, M. R. T., & Coehlo, C. (2005). Self-regulation after traumatic brain injury: A framework for intervention of memory and problem solving. *Seminars in Speech and Language, 26*, 242–255.

Kennedy, M. R. T., Coelho, C., Turkstra, L., Ylvisaker, M., Moore Sohlberg, M., Yorkston, K., . . . Kan, P.-F. (2008). Intervention for executive functions after traumatic brain injury: A systematic review, meta-analysis and clinical recommendations. *Neuropsychological Rehabilitation, 18*(3), 257–299.

Kennedy, M. R. T., Linhart, S., & Brady, B. (2006). *Metamemory for narratives after traumatic brain injury: Does timing matter?* Unpublished manuscript.

Kessels, R. P. C. (2017). Application of errorless learning in dementia. In C. Haslam & R. P. C. Kessels (Eds.), *Errorless learning in neuropsychological rehabilitation* [ebook]. London: Routledge.

Kim, A. H., Vaughn, S., Wanzek, J., & Wei, S. (2004). Graphic organizers and their effects on the reading comprehension of students with LD: A synthesis of research. *Journal of Learning Disabilities, 37*(2), 105–118.

Kim, A. S. N., Wong-Kee-You, A. M. B., Wiseheart, M., & Rosenbaum, R. S. (2019). The spacing effect stands up to big data. *Behavior Research Methods, 51*(4), 1485–1497.

Kim, H., & Xu, H. (2019). Exploring the effects of social media features on the public's responses to decreased usage CSR messages. *Corporate Communications, 24*(2), 287–302.

Kim, H. J., Burke, D. T., Dowds, M. M., Boone, K. A., & Park, G. J. (2000). Electronic memory aids for outpatient brain injury: Follow-up findings. *Brain Injury, 14*(2), 187–196.

Kiresuk, T. J., & Sherman, R. E. (1968). Goal attainment scaling: A general method for evaluating comprehensive community mental health programs. *Community Mental Health Journal, 4*(6), 443–453.

Kirsch, N. L., Levine, S. P., Fallon-Krueger, M., & Jaros, L. A. (1987). Focus on clinical research: The microcomputer as an "orthotic" device for patients with cognitive deficits. *Journal of Head Trauma Rehabilitation, 2*(4), 77–86.

Kleim, J. A., & Jones, T. A. (2008). Principles of experience-dependent neural plasticity: Implications for rehabilitation after brain damage. *Journal of Speech, Language, and Hearing Research, 51*(1), S225–S239.

Koehler, R., Wilhelm, E. E., Shoulson, I., Institute of Medicine, & Committee on Cognitive Rehabilitation Therapy for Traumatic Brain Injury. (2012). *Cognitive rehabilitation therapy for traumatic brain injury: Evaluating the evidence*. Washington, DC: National Academies Press.

Kolb, B., & Muhammad, A. (2014). Harnessing the power of neuroplasticity for intervention. *Frontiers in Human Neuroscience, 8*(377).

Kranick, S. M., Gorrindo, T., & Hallett, M. (2011). Psychogenic movement disorders and motor conversion: A roadmap for collaboration between neurology and psychiatry. *Psychosomatics, 52*(2), 109–116.

Krasny-Pacini, A., Chevignard, M., & Evans, J. (2014). Goal management training for rehabilitation of executive functions: A systematic review of effectiveness in patients with acquired brain injury. *Disability and Rehabilitation, 36*(2), 105–116.

Krasny-Pacini, A., Evans, J., Sohlberg, M. M., & Chevignard, M. (2016). Proposed criteria for appraising goal attainment scales used as outcome measures in rehabilitation research. *Archives of Physical Medicine and Rehabilitation, 97*(1), 157–170.

Krasny-Pacini, A., Limond, J., Evans, J., Hiebel, J., Bendjelida, K., & Chevignard, M. (2014). Context-sensitive goal management training for everyday executive dysfunction in children after severe traumatic brain injury. *Journal of Head Trauma Rehabilitation, 29*(5), E49–E64.

Kreutzer, J. S., Kolakowsky-Hayner, S. A., Ripley, D., Cifu, D. X., Rosenthal, M., Bushnik, T., . . . High, W. (2001). Charges and lengths of stay for acute and inpatient rehabilitation treatment of traumatic brain injury 1990–1996. *Brain Injury, 15*(9), 763–774.

Kreutzer, J. S., Marwitz, J. H., Sima, A. P., Mills, A., Hsu, N. H., & Lukow, H. R. II (2018). Efficacy of the resilience and adjustment intervention after traumatic brain injury: A randomized controlled trial. *Brain Injury, 32*(8), 963–971.

Kreutzer, J. S., Serio, C. D., & Bergquist, S. (1994). Family needs after brain injury: A quantitative analysis. *Journal of Head Trauma Rehabilitation, 9*(3), 104–115.

Kucheria, P., Moore Sohlberg, M., Machalicek, W., Seeley, J., & DeGarmo, D. (2020). A single-case experimental design investigation of collaborative goal setting practices in hospital-based speech-language pathologists when provided supports to use motivational interviewing and goal attainment scaling. *Neuropsychological Rehabilitation, 32*(1), 1–32.

Kusec, A., Panday, J., Froese, A., Albright, H., & Harris, J. E. (2020). Getting motivated: Long-term perspectives on engaging in community-based programs after acquired brain injury. *Brain Injury, 34*(10), 1331–1338.

Kutlubaev, M. A., Xu, Y., Hackett, M. L., & Stone, J. (2018). Dual diagnosis of epilepsy and psychogenic nonepileptic seizures: Systematic review and meta-analysis of frequency, correlates, and outcomes. *Epilepsy & Behavior, 89*, 70–78.

Lahera, G., Ruiz, A., Branas, A., Vicens, M., & Orozco, A. (2017). Reaction time, processing speed and sustained attention in schizophrenia: Impact on social functioning. *Revista de Psiquiatr y Salud Mental, 10*(4), 197–205.

Lambez, B., & Vakil, E. (2021). The effectiveness of memory remediation strategies after traumatic brain injury: Systematic review and meta-analysis. *Annals of Physical and Rehabilitation Medicine, 64*(5), 101530.

Lamm, A. G., Goldstein, R., Giacino, J. T., Niewczyk, P., Schneider, J. C., & Zafonte, R. (2019). Changes in patient demographics and outcomes in the inpatient rehabilitation facility traumatic brain injury population from 2002 to 2016: Implications for patient care and clinical trials. *Journal of Neurotrauma, 36*(17), 2513–2520.

Lane, J. D., & Gast, D. L. (2014). Visual analysis in single case experimental design studies: Brief review and guidelines. *Neuropsychological Rehabilitation, 24*(3–4), 445–463.

Langer, K. G., & Padrone, F. J. (1992). Psychotherapeutic treatment of awareness in acute rehabilitation of traumatic brain injury. *Neuropsychological Rehabilitation, 2*(1), 59–70.

Langhorn, L., Holdgaard, D., Worning, L., Sørensen, J. C., & Pedersen, P. U. (2015). Testing a reality orientation program in patients with traumatic brain injury in a neurointensive care unit. *Journal of Neuroscience Nursing, 47*(1), E2–E10.

Larkins, B. M., Worrall, L. E., & Hickson, L. M. (2004). Stakeholder opinion of functional communication activities following traumatic brain injury. *Brain Injury, 18*(7), 691–706.

Lawson, M. J., & Rice, D. N. (1989). Effects of training in use of executive strategies on a verbal memory problem resulting from closed head injury. *Journal of Clinical and Experimental Neuropsychology, 11*(6), 842–854.

Ledbetter, A. K., Sohlberg, M. M., Fickas, S. F., Horney, M. A., & McIntosh, K. (2019). Evaluation of a computer-based prompting intervention to improve essay writing in undergraduates with cognitive impairment after acquired brain injury. *Neuropsychological Rehabilitation, 29*(8), 1226–1255.

Lemoncello, R., & Ness, B. (2013). Evidence-based practice & practice-based evidence applied to adult, medical speech-language pathology. *Perspectives on Gerontology, 18*(1), 14–26.

Leopold, A., Lourie, A., Petras, H., & Elias, E. (2015). The use of assistive technology for cognition to support the performance of daily activities for individuals with cognitive disabilities due to traumatic brain injury: The current state of the research. *NeuroRehabilitation, 37*(3), 359–378.

Lequerica, A. H., & Kortte, K. (2010). Therapeutic engagement: A proposed model of engagement in medical rehabilitation. *American Journal of Physical Medicine and Rehabilitation, 89*(5), 415–422.

Levin, H., O'Donnell, V., & Grossman, R. (1979). The Galveston Orientation Amnesia Test: A practical scale to assess cognition after head injury. *Journal of Nervous and Mental Disease, 167*, 675–684.

Levin, H. S. (1990). Memory deficit after closed-head injury. *Journal of Clinical and Experimental Neuropsychology, 12*(1), 129–153.

Levine, B., Robertson, I. H., Clare, L., Carter, G., Hong, J., Wilson, B., . . . Stuss, D. T. (2000). Rehabilitation of executive functioning: An experimental-clinical validation of goal management training. *Journal of the International Neuropsychological Society, 6*, 299–312.

Li, K., Alonso, J., Chadha, N., & Pulido, J. (2015). Does generalization occur following computer-based cognitive retraining?: An exploratory study. *Occupational Therapy in Health Care, 29*(3), 283–296.

Lidstone, S. C., Araújo, R., Stone, J., & Bloem, B. R. (2020). Ten myths about functional neurological disorder. *European Journal of Neurology, 27*(11), e62–e64.

Linscott, R. J., Knight, R. G., & Godfrey, H. P. (1996). The Profile of Functional Impairment in Communication (PFIC): A measure of communication impairment for clinical use. *Brain Injury, 10*(6), 397–412.

LoPresti, E. F., Mihailidis, A., & Kirsch, N. (2004). Assistive technology for cognitive rehabilitation: State of the art. *Neuropsychological Rehabilitation, 14*(1–2), 5–39.

The Lumosity Team. (2010). *Lumosity: Reclaim your brain*™. Dakim. www.lumosity.com.

Lumosity to Pay $2 Million to Settle FTC Deceptive Advertising Charges for Its "Brain Training" Program [Press release]. (2016). www.ftc.gov/news-events/press-releases/2016/01/lumosity-pay-2-million-settle-ftc-deceptive-advertising-charges.

Lundahl, B., Moleni, T., Burke, B. L., Butters, R., Tollefson, D., Butler, C., & Rollnick, S. (2013). Motivational interviewing in medical care settings: A systematic review and meta-analysis of randomized controlled trials. *Patient Education and Counseling, 93*(2), 157–168.

Lynch, B. (2002). Historical review of computer-assisted cognitive retraining. *Journal of Head Trauma Rehabilitation, 17*(5), 446–457.

MacArthur, C. A., Graham, S., Schwartz, S. S., & Schafer, W. D. (1995). Evaluation of a writing instruction model that integrated a process approach, strategy instruction, and word processing. *Learning Disability Quarterly, 18*(4), 278–291.

MacLennan, D., & Sohlberg, M. M. S. (2018). *Beyond workbooks: Functional cognitive rehabilitation following brain injury* [Webinar]. American Speech Language Hearing Association. https://apps.asha.org/eweb/olsdynamicpage.aspx?title=beyond+workbooks%3A+functional+cognitive+rehabilitation+for+traumatic+brain+injuries&webcode=olsdetails

Mahncke, H. W., DeGutis, J., Levin, H., Newsome, M. R., Bell, M. D., Grills, C., . . . Merzenich, M. M. (2021). A randomized clinical trial of plasticity-based cognitive training in mild traumatic brain injury. *Brain, 144*(7), 1994–2008.

Manasse, N. J., Hux, K., & Snell, J. (2005). Teaching face-name associations to survivors of traumatic brain injury: A sequential treatment approach. *Brain Injury, 19*(8), 633–641.

Manly, T., Fish, J., & Robertson, I. (2010). The rehabilitation of attention. In J. M. Gurd, U. Kischka, & J. C. Marshall (Eds.), *Handbook of clinical neuropsychology* (pp. 97–119). Oxford, UK: Oxford University Press.

Marchand-Martella, N. E., Slocum, T. A., & Martella, R. C. (2004). *Introduction to direct instruction.* Boston: Pearson/Allyn & Bacon.

Markowitsch, H. J. (1998). Editorial: Cognitive neuroscience of memory. *Neurocase, 4*(6), 429–435.

Martins, S., Guillery-Girard, B., Jambaque, I., Dulac, O., & Eustache, F. (2006). How children suffering severe amnesic syndrome acquire new concepts? *Neuropsychologia, 44*(14), 2792–2805.

Mashima, P. A., Waldron-Perrine, B., MacLennan, D., Sohlberg, M. M., Perla, L. Y., & Eapen, B. C. (2021). Interprofessional collaborative management of postconcussion cognitive symptoms. *American Journal of Speech-Language Pathology, 30*(4), 1598–1610.

Mashima, P., Waldron-Perrine, B., Seagly, K., Milman, L., Ashman, T., Mudar, R., & Paul, D. (2019). Looking beyond test results: Interprofessional collaborative management of persistent mild traumatic brain injury symptoms. *Topics in Language Disorders, 39*(3), 293–312.

Maslow, A. H. (1966). *The psychology of science: A reconnaissance.* New York: Harper & Row.

Mastropieri, M. A., Scruggs, T. E., Bakken, J. P., & Whedon, C. K. (1996). Reading comprehension: A synthesis of research in learning disabilities. *Advances in Learning and Behavioral Disabilities, 10*, 201–227.

Mateer, C. A., Sira, C. S., & O'Connell, M. E. (2005). Putting Humpty Dumpty together again: The importance of integrating cognitive and emotional interventions. *Journal of Head Trauma Rehabilitation, 20*(1), 62–75.

Matin, N., Young, S. S., Williams, B., LaFrance, W. C. Jr., King, J. N., Caplan, D., . . . Perez, D. L. (2017). Neuropsychiatric associations with gender, illness duration, work disability, and motor subtype in a U.S. functional neurological disorders clinic population. *Journal of Neuropsychiatry and Clinical Neuroscienc, 29*(4), 375–382.

McCauley, R. J., & Swisher, L. (1984). Psychometric review of language and articulation tests for preschool children. *Journal of Speech and Hearing Disorders, 49*(1), 34–42.

McDonald, S. (2013). Impairments in social cognition following severe traumatic brain injury. *Journal of the International Neuropsychological Society, 19*(3), 231–246.

McDonald, S., Flanagan, S., Rollins, J., & Kinch, J. (2003). TASIT: A new clinical tool for assessing social perception after traumatic brain injury. *Journal of Head Trauma Rehabilitation, 18*(3), 219–238.

McDougall, J., & King, G. (2007). *Goal attainment scaling: Description, utility, and applications in pediatric therapy services* (2nd ed.). London, ON, Canada: Thames Valley Children's Centre.

McGaugh, J. L. (2000). Memory—a century of consolidation. *Science, 287*(5451), 248–251.

McKenzie, K. J., Pierce, D., & Gunn, J. M. (2015). A systematic review of motivational interviewing in healthcare: The potential of motivational interviewing to address the lifestyle factors relevant to multimorbidity. *Journal of Comorbidity, 5*(1), 162–174.

McNally, K. A., Patrick, K. E., LaFleur, J. E., Dykstra, J. B., Monahan, K., & Hoskinson, K. R. (2018). Brief cognitive behavioral intervention for children and adolescents with persistent post-concussive symptoms: A pilot study. *Child Neuropsychology, 24*(3), 396–412.

McVicker, S., Parr, S., Pound, C., & Duchan, J. (2009). The communication partner scheme: A project to develop long-term, low-cost access to conversation for people living with aphasia. *Aphasiology, 23*(1), 52–71.

McWhirter, L., Ritchie, C., Stone, J., & Carson, A. (2020). Functional cognitive disorders: A systematic review. *Lancet Psychiatry, 7*(2), 191–207.

McWreath, M. (2005). *Picturing aphasia.* Retrieved from *www.aphasia.tv.*

Medley, A. R., & Powell, T. (2010). Motivational Interviewing to promote self-awareness and engagement in rehabilitation following acquired brain injury: A conceptual review. *Neuropsychological Rehabilitation, 20*(4), 481–508.

Merriam-Webster's Collegiate Dictionary. (1986). Springfield, MA: Merriam-Webster.

Meulenbroek, P., Bowers, B., & Turkstra, L. S. (2016). Characterizing common workplace communication skills for disorders associated with traumatic brain injury: A qualitative study. *Journal of Vocational Rehabilitation, 44*(1), 15–31.

Meulenbroek, P., Ness, B., Lemoncello, R., Byom, L., MacDonald, S., O'Neil-Pirozzi, T. M., & Moore Sohlberg, M. (2019). Social communication following traumatic brain injury part 2: Identifying effective treatment ingredients. *International Journal of Speech-Language Pathology, 21*(2), 128–142.

Michie, S., van Stralen, M. M., & West, R. (2011). The behaviour change wheel: A new method for characterising and designing behaviour change interventions. *Implementation Science, 6*, 42.

Millar, D. C., Light, J. C., & Schlosser, R. W. (2006). The impact of augmentative and alternative communication intervention on the speech production of individuals with developmental disabilities: A research review. *Journal of Speech, Language, and Hearing Research, 49*(2), 248–264.

Miller, E. M., Walton, G. M., Dweck, C. S., Job, V., Trzesniewski, K. H., & McClure, S. M. (2012). Theories of willpower affect sustained learning. *PLoS One, 7*(6), e38680.

Miller, W. R., & Rollnick, S. (1991). *Motivational interviewing: Preparing people to change addictive behavior.* New York: Guilford Press.

Miller, W. R., & Rollnick, S. (2012). *Motivational interviewing: Helping people change.* New York: Guilford Press.

Milman, L., Seagly, K., Waldron Perrine, B., Mudur, R., Mashima, P. A., Ashman, T., & Paul, D. (2019). *Interprofessional collaboration: Overcoming barriers to successful reintegration for working-age adults with acquired brain injury (ABI).* Paper presented at the annual convention of the American Speech–Language–Hearing Association, Orlando, FL.

Miotto, E. C., Evans, J. J., Souza de Lucia, M. C., & Scaff, M. (2009). Rehabilitation of executive dysfunction: A controlled trial of an attention and problem solving treatment group. *Neuropsychological Rehabilitation, 19*(4), 517–540.

Mirsky, A. F., Anthony, B. J., Duncan, C. C., Ahearn, M. B., & Kellam, S. G. (1991). Analysis of the elements of attention: A neuropsychological approach. *Neuropsychology Review, 2*(2), 109–145.

Mittenberg, W., Tremont, G., Zielinski, R. E., Fichera, S., & Rayls, K. R. (1996). Cognitive-behavioral prevention of postconcussion syndrome. *Archives of Clinical Neuropsychology, 11*(2), 139–145.

Montessori, M. (1912). *The Montessori method: Scientific pedagogy as applied child education in "The Children's Houses," with additions and revisions by the author.* New York: Frederick A. Stokes.

Moro, V., Pernigo, S., Zapparoli, P., Cordioli, Z., & Aglioti, S. M. (2011). Phenomenology and neural correlates of implicit and emergent motor awareness in patients with anosognosia for hemiplegia. *Behavioural Brain Research, 225*(1), 259–269.

Mortimer, D., Trevena-Peters, J., McKay, A., & Ponsford, J. (2019). Economic evaluation of activities of daily living retraining during posttraumatic amnesia for inpatient rehabilitation following severe traumatic brain injury. *Archives of Physical Medicine and Rehabilitation, 100*(4), 648–655.

Morton, K., Beauchamp, M., Prothero, A., Joyce, L., Saunders, L., Spencer-Bowdage, S., . . . Pedlar, C. (2015). The effectiveness of motivational interviewing for health behaviour change in primary care settings: A systematic review. *Health Psychology Review, 9*(2), 205–223.

Muraven, M., & Baumeister, R. F. (2000). Self-regulation and depletion of limited resources: Does self-control resemble a muscle? *Psychological Bulletin, 126*(2), 247–259.

Murray, L. L., & Clark, H. M. (2014). *Neurogenic disorders of language and cognition: Evidence-based clinical practice.* Austin, TX: Pro-Ed.

Nakase-Richardson, R., Sherer, M., Seel, R. T., Hart, T., Hanks, R., Arango-Lasprilla, J. C., . . . Hammond, F. (2011). Utility of post-traumatic amnesia in predicting 1-year productivity following traumatic brain injury: Comparison of the Russell and Mississippi PTA classification intervals. *Journal of Neurology, Neurosurgery, and Psychiatry, 82*(5), 494–499.

Nakase-Richardson, R., Yablon, S. A., & Sherer, M. (2007). Prospective comparison of acute confusion severity with duration of post-traumatic amnesia in predicting employment outcome after traumatic brain injury. *Journal of Neurology, Neurosurgery, and Psychiatry, 78*(8), 872–876.

Nazroo, J. Y. (1998). Genetic, cultural or socio-economic vulnerability?: Explaining ethnic inequalities in health. *Sociology of Health & Illness, 20*(5), 710–730.

Neils-Strunjas, J., Paul, D., Clark, A. N., Mudar, R., Duff, M. C., Waldron-Perrine, B., & Bechtold, K. T. (2017). Role of resilience in the rehabilitation of adults with acquired brain injury. *Brain Injury, 31*(2), 131–139.

Nelson, T. O., & Narens, L. (1990). Metamemory: A theoretical framework and new findings. *Psychology of Learning and Motivation, 26*, 125–173.

Neuhaus, M., Bagutti, S., Yaldizli, O., Zwahlen, D., Schaub, S., Frey, B., . . . Penner, I. K. (2018). Characterization of social cognition impairment in multiple sclerosis. *European Journal of Neurology, 25*(1), 90–96.

Nicholson, C., Edwards, M. J., Carson, A. J., Gardiner, P., Golder, D., Hayward, K., . . . Stone, J. (2020). Occupational therapy consensus recommendations for functional neurological disorder. *Journal of Neurology, Neurosurgery, and Psychiatry, 91*(10), 1037–1045.

Nielsen, G., Stone, J., Matthews, A., Brown, M., Sparkes, C., Farmer, R., . . . Edwards, M. (2015). Physiotherapy for functional motor disorders: A consensus recommendation. *Journal of Neurology, Neurosurgery, and Psychiatry, 86*(10), 1113–1119.

Niemeijer, M., Svaerke, K. W., & Christensen, H. K. (2020). The effects of computer based cognitive rehabilitation in stroke patients with working memory impairment: A systematic review. *Journal of Stroke and Cerebrovascular Diseases, 29*(12), 105265.

Nijsse, B., Spikman, J. M., Visser-Meily, J. M. A., de Kort, P. L. M., & van Heugten, C. M. (2019). Social cognition impairments are associated with behavioural changes in the long term after stroke. *PLoS One, 14*(3), e0213725.

Nobriga, C., & Clair, J. S. (2018). Training goal writing: A practical and systematic approach. *Perspectives of the ASHA Special Interest Groups, 3*(11), 36–47.

Novakovic-Agopian, T., Kornblith, E., Abrams, G., Burciaga-Rosales, J., Loya, F., D'Esposito, M., & Chen, A. J. (2018). Training in goal-oriented attention self-regulation improves executive functioning in veterans with chronic traumatic brain injury. *Journal of Neurotrauma, 35*(23), 2784–2795.

Novakovic-Agopian, T., Kornblith, E., Abrams, G., McQuaid, J. R., Posecion, L., Burciaga, J., . . . Chen, A. J. W. (2019). Long-term effects of executive function training among veterans with chronic TBI. *Brain Injury, 33*(12), 1513–1521.

O'Connell, N., Jones, A., Chalder, T., & David, A. S. (2020). Experiences and illness perceptions of patients with functional symptoms admitted to hyperacute stroke wards: A mixed-method study. *Neuropsychiatric Disease and Treatment, 16*, 1795–1805.

O'Neil-Pirozzi, T. M., Kennedy, M. R., & Sohlberg, M. M. (2016). Evidence-based practice for the use of internal strategies as a memory compensation technique after brain injury: A systematic review. *Journal of Head Trauma Rehabilitation, 31*(4), E1–E11.

O'Neil-Pirozzi, T. M., Strangman, G. E., Goldstein, R., Katz, D. I., Savage, C. R., Kelkar, K., . . . Glenn, M. B. (2010). A controlled treatment study of internal memory strategies (I-MEMS) following traumatic brain injury. *Journal of Head Trauma Rehabilitation, 25*(1), 43–51.

O'Rourke, A., Power, E., O'Halloran, R., & Rietdijk, R. (2018). Common and distinct components of communication partner training programmes in stroke, traumatic brain injury and dementia. *International Journal of Language Communication Disorders, 53*(6), 1150–1168.

Oaten, M., & Cheng, K. (2006). Improved self-control: The benefits of a regular program of academic study. *Basic and Applied Social Psychology, 28*(1), 1–16.

Oberg, L., & Turkstra, L. S. (1998). Use of elaborative encoding to facilitate verbal learning after adolescent traumatic brain injury. *Journal of Head Trauma Rehabilitation, 13*(3), 44–62.

Ochsner, K. N., & Lieberman, M. D. (2001, September). The emergence of social cognitive neuroscience. *American Psychologist, 56*(9),717–734.

Ownsworth, T., Fleming, J., Tate, R., Shum, D. H., Griffin, J., Schmidt, J., . . . Chevignard, M. (2013). Comparison of error-based and errorless learning for people with severe traumatic brain injury: Study protocol for a randomized control trial. *Trials, 14*, 369.

Ownsworth, T. L., & McFarland, K. (1999). Memory remediation in long-term acquired brain injury: Two approaches in diary training. *Brain Injury, 13*(8), 605–626.

Park, N. W., & Ingles, J. L. (2001). Effectiveness of attention rehabilitation after an acquired brain injury: A meta-analysis. *Neuropsychology, 15*(2), 199–210.

Paul, D., Frattali, C. M., Holland, A. L., Thompson, C. K., Caperton, C. J., & Slater, S. (2005). *Quality of Communication Life Scale*. Rockville, MD: American Speech–Language–Hearing Association.

Pegg, P. O. Jr., Auerbach, S. M., Seel, R. T., Buenaver, L. F., Kiesler, D. J., & Plybon, L. E. (2005). The impact of patient-centered information on patients' treatment satisfaction and outcomes in traumatic brain injury rehabilitation. *Rehabilitation Psychology, 50*(4), 366–374.

Pei, Y., & O'Brien, K. H. (2021). Reading abilities post traumatic brain injury in adolescents and adults: A systematic review and meta-analysis. *American Journal of Speech-Language Pathology, 30*(2), 789–816.

Pennington, C., Ball, H., & Swirski, M. (2019). Functional cognitive disorder: Diagnostic challenges and future directions. *Diagnostics (Basel), 9*(4), 131.

Pennington, C., Hayre, A., Newson, M., & Coulthard, E. (2015). Functional cognitive disorder: A common cause of subjective cognitive symptoms. *Journal of Alzheimer's Disease, 48*(1, Suppl.), S19–S24.

Perla, L., Jackson, P., Hopkins, S., Daggert, M., & VanHorn, L. (2013). Transitioning home: Comprehensive case management for America's heroes. *Rehabilitation Nursing, 38*, 231–239.

Pertz, M., Kowalski, T., Thoma, P., & Schlegel, U. (2021). What is on your mind?: Impaired social cognition in primary central nervous system lymphoma patients despite ongoing complete remission. *Cancers, 13*(5), 943.

Pick, S., Anderson, D. G., Asadi-Pooya, A. A., Aybek, S., Baslet, G., Bloem, B. R., . . . Nicholson, T. R. (2020). Outcome measurement in functional neurological disorder: A systematic review and recommendations. *Journal of Neurology, Neurosurgery, and Psychiatry, 91*(6), 638–649.

Pitel, A. L., Perruchet, P., Vabret, F., Desgranges, B., Eustache, F., & Beaunieux, H. (2010). The advantage of errorless learning for the acquisition of new concepts' labels in alcoholics. *Psychological Medicine, 40*(3), 497–502.

Ponsford, J., Janzen, S., McIntyre, A., Bayley, M., Velikonja, D., & Tate, R. (2014). INCOG recommendations for management of cognition following traumatic brain injury, part I: Posttraumatic amnesia/delirium. *Journal of Head Trauma Rehabilitation, 29*(4), 307–320.

Ponsford, J., Sloan, S., & Snow, P. (2012). *Traumatic brain injury: Rehabilitation for everyday adaptive living*. Hove, UK: Psychology Press.

Posner, M. I., & Petersen, S. E. (1990). The attention system of the human brain. *Annual Review of Neuroscience, 13*, 25–42.

Pottgen, J., Dziobek, I., Reh, S., Heesen, C., & Gold, S. M. (2013). Impaired social cognition in multiple sclerosis. *Journal of Neurology, Neurosurgery, and Psychiatry, 84*(5), 523–528.

Povlishock, J. T., & Katz, D. I. (2005). Update of neuropathology and neurological recovery after traumatic brain injury. *Journal of Head Trauma Rehabilitation, 20*(1), 76–94.

Powell, L. E., Gau, J., Glang, A., Corrigan, J. D., Ramirez, M., & Slocumb, J. (2021). Staff Traumatic Brain Injury Skill Builder: Evaluation of an online training program for paraprofessional staff serving adults with moderate-severe TBI. *Journal of Head Trauma Rehabilitation, 36*(5), E329–E336.

Powell, L. E., Glang, A., Ettel, D., Todis, B., Sohlberg, M. M., & Albin, R. (2012). Systematic instruction for individuals with acquired brain injury: Results of a randomised controlled trial. *Neuropsychological Rehabilitation, 22*(1), 85–112.

Powers, M., Vording, M., & Emmelkamp, P. (2009). Acceptance and commitment therapy: A meta-analytic review. *Psychotherapy and Psychosomatics, 78*, 73–80.

Premack, D., & Woodruff, G. (1978). Does the chimpanzee have a theory of mind? *Behavioral and Brain Sciences, 1*(4), 515–526.

Prescott, S., Fleming, J., & Doig, E. (2015). Goal setting approaches and principles used in rehabilitation for people with acquired brain injury: A systematic scoping review. *Brain Injury, 29*(13–14), 1515–1529.

Prideaux, G. D. (1991). Syntactic form and textural rhetoric: The cognitive basis for certain pragmatic principles. *Journal of Pragmatics, 16*(2), 113–129.

Prigatano, G. P., & Sherer, M. (2020). Impaired self-awareness and denial during the postacute phases after moderate to severe traumatic brain injury. *Frontiers in Psychology, 11*, 1569.

Prinsen, S., Evers, C., & de Ridder, D. (2016). "Oops, I did it again": Examining self-licensing effects in a subsequent self-regulation dilemma. *Applied Psychology: Health and Well-Being, 8*(1), 104–126.

Rakoczy, H., Harder-Kasten, A., & Sturm, L. (2012). The decline of theory of mind in old age is (partly) mediated by developmental changes in domain-general abilities. *British Journal of Psychology, 103*(1), 58–72.

Randolph, C. (2001). *Repeatable Battery for the Assessment of Neuropsychological Status.* San Antonio, TX: Psychological Corporation.

Rao, V., & Lyketsos, C. (2000). Neuropsychiatric sequelae of traumatic brain injury. *Psychosomatics, 41*(2), 95–103.

Raskin, N. J., & Rogers, C. R. (2005). Person-centered therapy. In *Current psychotherapies* (7th instructor's ed., pp. 130–165). Belmont, CA: Thomson Brooks/Cole.

Rath, J. F., Simon, D., Langenbahn, D. M., Sherr, R. L., & Diller, L. (2003). Group treatment of problem-solving deficits in outpatients with traumatic brain injury: A randomised outcome study. *Neuropsychological Rehabilitation, 13*, 461–488.

Raymer, A. M., Beeson, P., Holland, A., Kendall, D., Maher, L. M., Martin, N., . . . Gonzalez Rothi, L. J. (2008). Translational research in aphasia: from neuroscience to neurorehabilitation. *Journal of Speech, Language, and Hearing Research, 51*(1), S259–S275.

Ricker, T. J., Nieuwenstein, M. R., Bayliss, D. M., & Barrouillet, P. (2018). Working memory consolidation: Insights from studies on attention and working memory. *Annals of New York Academy of Sciences, 1424*(1), 8–18.

Rietdijk, R., Power, E., Brunner, M., & Togher, L. (2019). A single case experimental design study on improving social communication skills after traumatic brain injury using communication partner telehealth training. *Brain Injury, 33*(1), 94–104.

Roberts, C. M., Spitz, G., Mundy, M., & Ponsford, J. L. (2018). Retrograde personal semantic memory during post-traumatic amnesia and following emergence. *Journal of the International Neuropsychological Society, 24*(10), 1064–1072.

Robertson, I. H., Ward, T., Ridgeway, V., & Nimmo-Smith, I. (1994). *Test of everyday attention.* San Antonio, TX: Pearson.

Rollnick, S., & Miller, W. R. (1995). What is motivational interviewing? *Behavioural and Cognitive Psychotherapy, 23*(4), 325–334.

Rose-Krasnor, L. (1997). The nature of social competence: A theoretical review. *Social Development, 6*(1), 111–135.

Roth, R. M., Isquith, P. K., & Gioia, G. A. (2005). *Behavior Rating Inventory of Executive Function* (adult ed.). Lutz, FL: Par Inc.

Rothbart, A., & Sohlberg, M. M. (2021). Resilience as a mainstream clinical consideration for speech-language pathologists providing post–acquired brain injury neurorehabilitation. *Perspectives of the ASHA Special Interest Groups, 6*(5), 1026–1032.

Rowley, D. A., Rogish, M., Alexander, T., & Riggs, K. J. (2017). Cognitive correlates of pragmatic language comprehension in adult traumatic brain injury: A systematic review and meta-analyses. *Brain Injury, 31*(12), 1564–1574.

Ryan, N. P., Catroppa, C., Cooper, J. M., Beare, R., Ditchfield, M., Coleman, L., . . . Anderson, V. A. (2015). The emergence of age-dependent social cognitive deficits after generalized insult to the developing brain: A longitudinal prospective analysis using susceptibility-weighted imaging. *Human Brain Mapping, 36*(5), 1677–1691.

Sander, A. M., Clark, A. N., Atchison, T. B., & Rueda, M. (2009). A Web-based videoconferencing approach to training caregivers in rural areas to compensate for problems related to traumatic brain injury. *Journal of Head Trauma Rehabilitation, 24*(4), 248–261.

Scherer, M. J., & Craddock, G. (2005). Matching Person & Technology assessment process. *Technology & Disabilities, 14*(3), 125–132.

Scherer, M. J., & Federici, S. (2015). Why people use and don't use technologies: Introduction to the special issue on assistive technologies for cognition/cognitive support technologies. *NeuroRehabilitation, 37*(3), 315–319.

Schiehser, D. M., Delis, D. C., Filoteo, J. V., Delano-Wood, L., Han, S. D., Jak, A. J., . . . Bondi, M. W. (2011). Are self-reported symptoms of executive dysfunction associated with objective executive function performance following mild to moderate traumatic brain injury? *Journal of Clinical and Experimental Neuropsychology, 33*(6), 704–714.

Schilbach, L., Timmermans, B., Reddy, V., Costall, A., Bente, G., Schlicht, T., & Vogeley, K. (2013). Toward a second-person neuroscience. *Behavioral Brain Science, 36*(4), 393–414.

Schmidt, J., Fleming, J., Ownsworth, T., & Lannin, N. A. (2013). Video feedback on functional task performance improves self-awareness after traumatic brain injury: A randomized controlled trial. *Neurorehabilitation and Neural Repair, 27*(4), 316–324.

Schmidt, J., Lannin, N., Fleming, J., & Ownsworth, T. (2011). Feedback interventions for impaired self-awareness following brain injury: A systematic review. *Journal of Rehabilitation Medicine, 43*(8), 673–680.

Schmidtke, K., Pohlmann, S., & Metternich, B. (2008). The syndrome of functional memory disorder: Definition, etiology, and natural course. *American Journal of Geriatric Psychiatry, 16*(12), 981–988.

Schmitter-Edgecombe, M., Fahy, J. F., Whelan, J. P., & Long, C. J. (1995). Memory remediation after severe closed head injury: Notebook training vs. supportive therapy. *Journal of Consulting and Clinical Psychology, 63*(3), 484–489.

Schulkin, J. (2000). *Roots of social sensibility and neural function.* Cambridge, MA: MIT Press.

Selven, A., & Batts, B. (2021*). Implementation of the teach-back method of psychoeducation for management of individuals with persistent concussion symptoms.* Unpublished manuscript.

Serino, A., Ciaramelli, E., Di Santantonio, A., Malagu, S., Servadei, F., & Ladavas, E. (2006). Central executive system impairment in traumatic brain injury. *Brain Injury, 20*(1), 23–32.

Serino, A., Ciaramelli, E., Di Santantonio, A., Malagù, S., Servadei, F., & Làdavas, E. (2007). A pilot study for rehabilitation of central executive deficits after traumatic brain injury. *Brain Injury, 21*(1), 11–19.

Sharpe, M., Stone, J., Hibberd, C., Warlow, C., Duncan, R., Coleman, R., . . . Carson, A. (2010). Neurology out-patients with symptoms unexplained by disease: Illness beliefs and financial benefits predict 1-year outcome. *Psychological Medicine, 40*(4), 689–698.

Shelton, C., & Shryock, M. (2007). Effectiveness of communication/interaction strategies with patients who have neurological injuries in a rehabilitation setting. *Brain Injury, 21*(12), 1259–1266.

Shmueli, D., & Prochaska, J. J. (2009). Resisting tempting foods and smoking behavior: Implications from a self-control theory perspective. *Health Psychology, 28*(3), 300–306.

Siegal, M., & Varley, R. (2006). Aphasia, language, and theory of mind. *Society for Neuroscience, 1*(3–4), 167–174.

Sigmundsdottir, L., Longley, W. A., & Tate, R. L. (2016). Computerised cognitive training in acquired brain injury: A systematic review of outcomes using the International Classification of Functioning (ICF). *Neuropsychological Rehabilitation, 26*(5–6), 673–741.

Sit, J. W., Chair, S. Y., Choi, K. C., Chan, C. W., Lee, D. T., Chan, A. W., . . . Taylor-Piliae, R. E. (2016). Do empowered stroke patients perform better at self-management and functional recovery after a stroke?: A randomized controlled trial. *Clinical Interventions in Aging, 11*, 1441–1450.

Skidmore, E. R. (2015). Training to optimize learning after traumatic brain injury. *Current Physical Medicine and Rehabilitation Reports, 3*(2), 99–105.

Smith, M. S., & Testani-Dufour, L. (2002). Who's teaching whom?: A study of family education in brain injury. *Rehabilitation Nursing, 27*(6), 209–214.

Snow, P., & Ponsford, J. (1995). Assessing and managing changes in communication and interpersonal skills following TBI. In J. Ponsford (Ed.), *Traumatic brain injury: Rehabilitation for everyday adaptive living* (pp. 137–164). Hove, UK: Lawrence Erlbaum.

Sohlberg, M. M., Ehlhardt, L., & Kennedy, M. (2005). Instructional techniques in cognitive rehabilitation: A preliminary report. *Seminars in Speech and Language, 26*(4), 268–279.

Sohlberg, M. M., Harn, B., MacPherson, H., & Wade, S. L. (2014). A pilot study evaluating attention and strategy training following pediatric traumatic brain injury. *Clinical Practice in Pediatric Psychology, 2*(3), 263–280.

Sohlberg, M. M., Kennedy, M., Avery, J., Coehlo, C., Turkstra, L. S., Ylvisaker, M., & Yorkston, K. (2007). Evidence-based practice for the use of external memory aids as a memory compensation technique. *Journal of Medical Speech Language Pathology, 15*(1), xv–li.

Sohlberg, M. M., Kucheria, P., Fickas, S., & Wade, S. L. (2015). Developing brain injury interventions on both ends of the treatment continuum depends upon early research partnerships and feasibility studies. *Journal of Speech, Language, and Hearing Research, 58*(6), S1864–S1870.

Sohlberg, M. M., MacDonald, S., Byom, L., Iwashita, H., Lemoncello, R., Meulenbroek, P., . . . O'Neil-Pirozzi, T. M. (2019). Social communication following traumatic brain injury part I: State-of-the-art review of assessment tools. *International Journal of Speech-Language Pathology, 21*(2), 115–127.

Sohlberg, M. M., & Mateer, C. A. (1987). Effectiveness of an attention-training program. *Journal of Clinical and Experimental Neuropsychology, 9*(2), 117–130.

Sohlberg, M. M., & Mateer, C. A. (2001). *Cognitive rehabilitation: An integrative neuropsychological approach*. New York: Guilford Press.

Sohlberg, M. M., & Mateer, C. (2011). *Attention Process Training APT-3: A direct attention training program for persons with acquired brain injury*. Youngsville, NC: Lash & Associates Publishing/Training.

Sohlberg, M. M., & Turkstra, L. S. (2011). *Optimizing cognitive rehabilitation: Effective instructional methods*. New York: Guilford Press.

Speed, J., & Mooney, G. (1997). Rehabilitation of conversion disorders: An operant approach. *NeuroRehabilitation, 8*(3), 175–181.

Spikman, J. M., Boelen, D. H., Lamberts, K. F., Brouwer, W. H., & Fasotti, L. (2010). Effects of a multifaceted treatment program for executive dysfunction after acquired brain injury on indications of executive functioning in daily life. *Journal of the International Neuropsychological Society, 16*(1), 118–129.

Spikman, J. M., Timmerman, M. E., Milders, M. V., Veenstra, W. S., & van der Naalt, J. (2012).

Social cognition impairments in relation to general cognitive deficits, injury severity, and pre-frontal lesions in traumatic brain injury patients. *Journal of Neurotrauma, 29*(1), 101–111.

Stafslien, E. H. D., & Turkstra, L. S. (2020). Sex-based differences in expectations for social communication after TBI. *Brain Injury, 34*(13–14), 1756–1762.

Stagg, K., Douglas, J., & Iacono, T. (2019). A scoping review of the working alliance in acquired brain injury rehabilitation. *Disability and Rehabilitation, 41*(4), 489–497.

Stamenova, V., & Levine, B. (2019). Effectiveness of goal management training® in improving executive functions: A meta-analysis. *Neuropsychological Rehabilitation, 29*(10), 1569–1599.

Stark, C., Stark, S., & Gordon, B. (2005). New semantic learning and generalization in a patient with amnesia. *Neuropsychology, 19*(2), 139–151.

Stein, M., Carnine, D., & Dixon, R. (1998). Direct instruction: Integrating curriculum design and effective teaching practice. *Intervention in School and Clinic, 33*(4), 227–233.

Stojanoski, B., Wild, C. J., Battista, M. E., Nichols, E. S., & Owen, A. M. (2021). Brain training habits are not associated with generalized benefits to cognition: An online study of over 1000 "brain trainers." *Journal of Experimental Psychology: General, 150*(4), 729–738.

Stone, J., Carson, A., Aditya, H., Prescott, R., Zaubi, M., Warlow, C., & Sharpe, M. (2009). The role of physical injury in motor and sensory conversion symptoms: A systematic and narrative review. *Journal of Psychosomatic Research, 66*(5), 383–390.

Stone, J., Carson, A., & Hallett, M. (2016). Explanation as treatment for functional neurologic disorders. *Handbook of Clinical Neurology, 139*, 543–553.

Stone, J., Carson, A., & Sharpe, M. (2005). Functional symptoms in neurology: Management. *Journal of Neurology, Neurosurgery, and Psychiatry, 76*(1, Suppl.), i13–i21.

Stone, J., Pal, S., Blackburn, D., Reuber, M., Thekkumpurath, P., & Carson, A. (2015). Functional (psychogenic) cognitive disorders: A perspective from the neurology clinic. *Journal of Alzheimer's Disease, 48*(1, Suppl.), S5–S17.

Stone, J., Reuber, M., & Carson, A. (2013). Functional symptoms in neurology: Mimics and chameleons. *Practical Neurology, 13*(2), 104–113.

Sunderland, A., Harris, J. E., & Baddeley, A. D. (1983). Do laboratory tests predict everyday memory?: A neuropsychological study. *Journal of Verbal Learning & Verbal Behavior, 22*(3), 341–357.

Svoboda, E., & Richards, B. (2009). Compensating for anterograde amnesia: A new training method that capitalizes on emerging smartphone technologies. *Journal of the International Neuropsychological Society, 15*(4), 629–638.

Svoboda, E., Richards, B., Leach, L., & Mertens, V. (2012). PDA and smartphone use by individuals with moderate-to-severe memory impairment: Application of a theory-driven training programme. *Neuropsychological Rehabilitation, 22*(3), 408–427.

Swan, K., Hopper, M., Wenke, R., Jackson, C., Till, T., & Conway, E. (2018). Speech-language pathologist interventions for communication in moderate-severe dementia: A systematic review. *American Journal of Speech-Language Pathology, 27*(2), 836–852.

Swanson, H. L. (1999). Reading research for students with LD: A meta-analysis of intervention outcomes. *Journal of Learning Disabilities, 32*(6), 504–532.

Swanson, H. (2001). Searching for the best model for instructing students with learning disabilities. *Focus on Exceptional Children, 34*(2), 1–15.

Swanson, H. L., Carson, C., & Saches-Lee, C. M. (1996). A selective synthesis of intervention research for students with learning disabilities. *School Psychology Review, 25*(3), 370–391.

Swanson, H. L., & Hoskyn, M. (1998). Experimental intervention research on students with learning disabilities: A meta-analysis of treatment outcomes. *Review of Educational Research, 68*(3), 277–321.

Talevski, J., Wong Shee, A., Rasmussen, B., Kemp, G., & Beauchamp, A. (2020). Teach-back: A systematic review of implementation and impacts. *PLoS One, 15*(4), e0231350.

Tate, R., Kennedy, M., Ponsford, J., Douglas, J., Velikonja, D., Bayley, M., & Stergiou-Kita, M.

(2014). INCOG recommendations for management of cognition following traumatic brain injury, part III: Executive function and self-awareness. *Journal of Head Trauma Rehabilitation, 29*(4), 338–352.

Thoene, A. I., & Glisky, E. L. (1995). Learning of name-face associations in memory impaired patients: A comparison of different training procedures. *Journal of the International Neuropsychological Society, 1*(1), 29–38.

Togher, L., Hand, L., & Code, C. (1996). A new perspective on the relationship between communication impairment and disempowerment following head injury in information exchanges. *Disability and Rehabilitation, 18*(11), 559–566.

Togher, L., McDonald, S., Tate, R., Power, E., & Rietdijk, R. (2013). Training communication partners of people with severe traumatic brain injury improves everyday conversations: A multicenter single blind clinical trial. *Journal of Rehabilitation Medicine, 45*(7), 637–645.

Togher, L., McDonald, S., Tate, R., Power, E., Ylviskaker, M., & Rietdijk, R. (2010). *TBI Express: A social communication training manual for people with traumatic brain injury (TBI) and their communication partners.* Sydney: Australian Society for the Study of Brain Impairment.

Togher, L., Power, E., Tate, R., McDonald, S., & Rietdijk, R. (2010). Measuring the social interactions of people with traumatic brain injury and their communication partners: The adapted Kagan scales. *Aphasiology, 24*(6–8), 914–927.

Togher, L., Wiseman-Hakes, C., Douglas, J., Stergiou-Kita, M., Ponsford, J., Teasell, R., . . . Panel, I. E. (2014). INCOG recommendations for management of cognition following traumatic brain injury, part IV: Cognitive communication. *Journal of Head Trauma Rehabilitation, 29*(4), 353–368.

Toglia, J., Johnston, M. V., Goverover, Y., & Dain, B. (2010). A multicontext approach to promoting transfer of strategy use and self regulation after brain injury: An exploratory study. *Brain Injury, 24*(4), 664–677.

Toglia, J., & Kirk, U. (2000). Understanding awareness deficits following brain injury. *Neurorehabilitation, 15*(1), 57–70.

Tomasello, M., Carpenter, M., Call, J., Behne, T., & Moll, H. (2005). Understanding and sharing intentions: The origins of cultural cognition. *Behavioral and Brain Sciences, 28*(5), 675–691; see discussion 691–735.

Tornas, S., Lovstad, M., Solbakk, A. K., Evans, J., Endestad, T., Hol, P. K., . . . Stubberud, J. (2016). Rehabilitation of executive functions in patients with chronic acquired brain injury with goal management training, external cuing, and emotional regulation: A randomized controlled trial. *Journal of the International Neuropsychological Society, 22*(4), 436–452.

Traumatic Brain Injury Model Systems National Data and Statistical Center. (2020). Annual Traumatic Brain Injury Model Systems Presentation.

Trevena-Peters, J., McKay, A., Spitz, G., Suda, R., Renison, B., & Ponsford, J. (2018). Efficacy of activities of daily living retraining during posttraumatic amnesia: A randomized controlled trial. *Archives of Physical Medicine and Rehabilitation, 99*(2), 329–337.

Trevena-Peters, J., Ponsford, J., & McKay, A. (2018). Agitated behavior and activities of daily living retraining during posttraumatic amnesia. *Journal of Head Trauma Rehabilitation, 33*(5), 317–325.

Tschopp, M. K., Frain, M. P., & Bishop, M. (2009). Empowerment variables for rehabilitation clients on perceived beliefs concerning work quality of life domains. *Work, 33*(1), 59–65.

Tulsky, D. S., Kisala, P. A., Victorson, D., Carlozzi, N., Bushnik, T., Sherer, M., . . . Cella, D. (2016). TBI-QOL: Development and calibration of item banks to measure patient reported outcomes following traumatic brain injury. *Journal of Head Trauma Rehabilitation, 31*(1), 40–51.

Tulving, E., & Markowitsch, H. J. (1998). Episodic and declarative memory: Role of the hippocampus. *Hippocampus, 8*(3), 198–204.

Turkstra, L. S. (2001). Partner effects in adolescent conversations. *Journal of Communication Disorders, 34*(1–2), 151–162.

Turkstra, L. S. (2013). Inpatient cognitive rehabilitation: Is it time for a change? *Journal of Head Trauma Rehabilitation, 28*(4), 332–336.

Turkstra, L. S., Clark, A., Burgess, S., Hengst, J. A., Wertheimer, J. C., & Paul, D. (2017). Pragmatic communication abilities in children and adults: Implications for rehabilitation professionals. *Disability and Rehabilitation, 39*(18), 1872–1885.

Turkstra, L. S., Coelho, C. A., & Ylvisaker, M. (2005). The use of standardized tests for individuals with cognitive-communication disorders. *Seminars in Speech and Language, 26*(4), 215–222.

Turkstra, L. S., McDonald, S., & Kaufmann, P. M. (1996). Assessment of pragmatic communication skills in adolescents after traumatic brain injury. *Brain Injury, 10*(5), 329–345.

Turkstra, L. S., Mutlu, B., Ryan, C. W., Despins Stafslien, E. H., Richmond, E. K., Hosokawa, E., & Duff, M. C. (2020). Sex and gender differences in emotion recognition and theory of mind after TBI: A narrative review and directions for future research. *Frontiers in Neurology, 11*, 59.

Turkstra, L. S., Norman, R. S., Mutlu, B., & Duff, M. C. (2018). Impaired theory of mind in adults with traumatic brain injury: A replication and extension of findings. *Neuropsychologia, 111*, 117–122.

Turner, S., & Whitworth, A. (2006). Conversational partner training programmes in aphasia: A review of key themes and participants' roles. *Aphasiology, 20*(6), 483–510.

Valitchka, L., & Turkstra, L. S. (2013). Communicating with inpatients with memory impairments. *Seminars in Speech and Language, 34*(3), 142–153.

van Heugten, C. M., Ponds, R. W., & Kessels, R. P. (2016). Brain training: Hype or hope? *Neuropsychological Rehabilitation, 26*(5–6), 639–644.

van Hout, M. S., Wekking, E. M., Berg, I. J., & Deelman, B. G. (2008). Psychosocial and cognitive rehabilitation of patients with solvent-induced chronic toxic encephalopathy: A randomised controlled study. *Psychotherapy and Psychosomatics, 77*(5), 289–297.

Vanderploeg, R. D., Belanger, H. G., Curtiss, G., Bowles, A. O., & Cooper, D. B. (2019). Reconceptualizing rehabilitation of individuals with chronic symptoms following mild traumatic brain injury. *Rehabilitation Psychology, 64*(1), 1.

Vargha-Khadem, F., Gadian, D. G., Watkins, K. E., Connelly, A., Van Paesschen, W., & Mishkin, M. (1997). Differential effects of early hippocampal pathology on episodic and semantic memory. *Science, 277*(5324), 376–380.

Varni, J. W., Seid, M., & Rode, C. A. (1999). The PedsQL: Measurement model for the pediatric quality of life inventory. *Medical Care, 37*(2), 126–139.

Vas, A. K., Chapman, S. B., Cook, L. G., Elliott, A. C., & Keebler, M. (2011). Higher-order reasoning training years after traumatic brain injury in adults. *Journal of Head Trauma Rehabilitation, 26*(3), 224–239.

Vasquez, B. P., Lloyd-Kuzik, A., & Moscovitch, M. (2021). Mobile app learning in memory intervention for acquired brain injury: Neuropsychological associations of training duration. *Neuropsychological Rehabilitation*, 1–27.

Velikonja, D., Tate, R., Ponsford, J., McIntyre, A., Janzen, S., Bayley, M., & Panel, I. E. (2014). INCOG recommendations for management of cognition following traumatic brain injury, part V: Memory. *Journal of Head Trauma Rehabilitation, 29*(4), 369–386.

Vereijken, B., & Whiting, H. (1990). In defence of discovery learning. *Canadian Journal of Sport Sciences, 15*(2), 99–106.

Verhaeghe, S., Defloor, T., & Grypdonck, M. (2005). Stress and coping among families of patients with traumatic brain injury: A review of the literature. *Journal of Clinical Nursing, 14*(8), 1004–1012.

Vermeij, A., Kessels, R. P. C., Heskamp, L., Simons, E. M. F., Dautzenberg, P. L. J., & Claassen, J. A. H. R. (2017). Prefrontal activation may predict working-memory training gain in normal aging and mild cognitive impairment. *Brain Imaging and Behavior, 11*(1), 141–154.

Vinney, L. A., van Mersbergen, M., Connor, N. P., & Turkstra, L. S. (2016). Vocal control: Is it susceptible to the negative effects of self-regulatory depletion? *Journal of Voice, 30*(5).

von Cramon, D. Y., Cramon, G. M.-v., & Mai, N. (1991). Problem-solving deficits in brain-injured patients: A therapeutic approach. *Neuropsychological Rehabilitation, 1*(1), 45–64.

Wade, S. L., Carey, J., & Wolfe, C. R. (2006). An online family intervention to reduce parental distress following pediatric brain injury. *Journal of Consulting and Clinical Psychology, 74*(3), 445–454.

Wade, T. K., & Troy, J. C. (2001). Mobile phones as a new memory aid: A preliminary investigation using case studies. *Brain Injury, 15*(4), 305–320.

Wakefield, S. J., Blackburn, D. J., Harkness, K., Khan, A., Reuber, M., & Venneri, A. (2018). Distinctive neuropsychological profiles differentiate patients with functional memory disorder from patients with amnestic-mild cognitive impairment. *Acta Neuropsychiatrica, 30*(2), 90–96.

Waldron-Perrine, B., Mudar, R., Mashima, P., Seagly, K., Sohlberg, M., Bechtold, K. T., . . . & Dunn, R. (2022). Interprofessional collaboration and communication to facilitate implementation of cognitive rehabilitation in persons with brain injury. *Journal of Interprofessional Care.* [Epub ahead of print]

Walker, H. M., Irvin, L. K., Noell, J., & Singer, G. H. S. (1992). A construct score approach to the assessment of social competence. *Behavior Modification, 16*(4), 448–474.

Walker, V. L., Douglas, S. N., Douglas, K. H., & D'Agostino, S. R. (2020). Paraprofessional-implemented systematic instruction for students with disabilities: A systematic literature review. *Education and Training in Autism and Developmental Disabilities, 55*(3), 303–317.

Ware, J., Jr., Kosinski, M., & Keller, S. D. (1996). A 12-item Short-Form Health Survey: Construction of scales and preliminary tests of reliability and validity. *Medical Care, 34*(3), 220–233.

Watanabe, T. K., Black, K. L., Zafonte, R. D., Millis, S. R., & Mann, N. R. (1998). Do calendars enhance posttraumatic temporal orientation?: A pilot study. *Brain Injury, 12*(1), 81–86.

Webb, P. M., & Glueckauf, R. L. (1994). The effects of direct involvement in goal setting on rehabilitation outcome for persons with traumatic brain injuries. *Rehabilitation Psychology, 39*(3), 179.

Weinman, J., Petrie, K. J., Moss-Morris, R., & Horne, R. (1996). The Illness Perception Questionnaire: A new method for assessing the cognitive representation of illness. *Psychology & Health, 11*(3), 431–445.

West, R. L. (1995). Compensatory strategies for age-associated memory impairment. In A. W. Baddeley, B. A. Wilson, & F. N. Watts (Eds.), *Handbook of memory disorders* (pp. 481–500). Oxford, UK: Wiley.

Westby, C., Burda, A., & Mehta, Z. (2003). Asking the right questions in the right ways: Strategies for ethnographic interviewing. *ASHA Leader, 8*, 4.

White, A. A. III, Logghe, H. J., Goodenough, D. A., Barnes, L. L., Hallward, A., Allen, I. M., . . . Llerena-Quinn, R. (2018). Self-awareness and cultural identity as an effort to reduce bias in medicine. *Journal of Racial and Ethnic Health Disparities, 5*(1), 34–49.

White-Chu, E. F., Graves, W. J., Godfrey, S. M., Bonner, A., & Sloane, P. (2009). Beyond the medical model: The culture change revolution in long-term care. *Journal of the American Medical Directors Association, 10*(6), 370–378.

Whiteneck, G. G., Charlifue, S. W., Gerhart, K. A., Overholser, J. D., & Richardson, G. N. (1992). Quantifying handicap: A new measure of long-term rehabilitation outcomes. *Archives of Physical Medicine and Rehabilitation, 73*(6), 519–526.

Whyte, J. (2014). Contributions of treatment theory and enablement theory to rehabilitation research and practice. *Archives of Physical Medicine and Rehabilitation, 95*(1, Suppl.), S17–S23.

Whyte, J., Dijkers, M. P., Hart, T., Van Stan, J. H., Packel, A., Turkstra, L. S., . . . Ferraro, M. (2019). The importance of voluntary behavior in rehabilitation treatment and outcomes. *Archives of Physical Medicine and Rehabilitation, 100*(1), 156–163.

Whyte, J., & Turkstra, L. S. (2021). Building a theoretical foundation for cognitive rehabilitation. *Brain, 144*(7), 1933–1935.

Williams, K. N., Perkhounkova, Y., Herman, R., & Bossen, A. (2017). A communication intervention to reduce resistiveness in dementia care: A cluster randomized controlled trial. *Gerontologist, 57*(4), 707–718.

Willmott, C., & Ponsford, J. (2009). Efficacy of methylphenidate in the rehabilitation of attention following traumatic brain injury: A randomised, crossover, double blind, placebo controlled inpatient trial. *Journal of Neurology, Neurosurgery, and Psychiatry, 80*(5), 552–557.

Wilson, B. A. (1995). Management and remediation of memory problems in brain-injured adults. In A. D. Baddeley, B. A. Wilson, & F. N. Watts (Eds.), *Handbook of memory disorders* (pp. 451–479). Oxford: John Wiley & Sons.

Wong, D., Sinclair, K., Seabrook, E., McKay, A., & Ponsford, J. (2017). Smartphones as assistive technology following traumatic brain injury: A preliminary study of what helps and what hinders. *Disability and Rehabilitation, 39*(23), 2387–2394.

Working Group to Develop a Clinician's Guide to Cognitive Rehabilitation in Mild Traumatic Brain Injury: Application for Military Service Members and Veterans. (2016). *Clinician's guide to cognitive rehabilitation in mild traumatic brain injury: Application for military service members and veterans.* American Speech–Language–Hearing Association. www.asha.org/siteassets/practice-portal/traumatic-brain-injury-adult/clinicians-guide-to-cognitive-rehabilitation-in-mild-traumatic-brain-injury.pdf.

World Health Organization. (2021). *International classification of functioning, disability and health.* www.who.int/standards/classifications/international-classification-of-functioning-disability-and-health.

Worthington, A., & Wood, R. L. (2018). Apathy following traumatic brain injury: A review. *Neuropsychologia, 118*(Part B), 40–47.

Wright, J., & Sohlberg, M. M. (2021). The implementation of a personalized dynamic approach for the management of prolonged concussion symptoms. *American Journal of Speech-Language Pathology, 30*(4), 1611–1624.

Wright, J., Sohlberg, M. M., McIntosh, K., Seeley, J., Hadley, W., Blitz, D., & Lowham, E. (2022). What is the effect of personalized cognitive strategy instruction on facilitating return-to-learn for individuals experiencing prolonged concussion symptoms? *Neuropsychological Rehabilitation.* [Epub ahead of print]

Wright, P., Rogers, N., Hall, C., Wilson, B., Evans, J., Emslie, H., & Bartram, C. (2001). Comparison of pocket-computer memory aids for people with brain injury. *Brain Injury, 15*(9), 787–800.

Ylvisaker, M., & Feeney, T. J. (2000). Reconstruction of identity after brain injury. *Brain Impairment, 1*(1), 12–28.

Ylvisaker, M., & Gioia, G. (1998). Cognitive assessment. In M. Ylvisaker (Ed.), *Traumatic brain injury rehabilitation* (2nd ed., pp. 159–179). Boston: Butterworth-Heinemann.

Ylvisaker, M., Mcpherson, K., Kayes, N., & Pellett, E. (2008). Metaphoric identity mapping: Facilitating goal setting and engagement in rehabilitation after traumatic brain injury. *Neuropsychological Rehabilitation, 18*(5–6), 713–741.

Ylvisaker, M., Turkstra, L. S., & Coelho, C. A. (2005). Behavioral and social interventions for individuals with traumatic brain injury: A summary of the research with clinical implications. *Seminars in Speech and Language, 26*(4), 256–267.

Yuan, W., Treble-Barna, A., Sohlberg, M. M., Harn, B., & Wade, S. L. (2017). Changes in structural connectivity following a cognitive intervention in children with traumatic brain injury. *Neurorehabilitation and Neural Repair, 31*(2), 190–201.

Yves Von Cramon, D., & Cramon, G. M. V. (1994). Back to work with a chronic dysexecutive syndrome?: A case report. *Neuropsychological Rehabilitation, 4*(4), 399–417.

Zelazo, P. D., Forston, J. L., Masten, A. S., & Carlson, S. M. (2018). Mindfulness plus reflection training: Effects on executive function in early childhood. *Frontiers in Psychology, 9*, 208.

Zickefoose, S., Hux, K., Brown, J., & Wulf, K. (2013). Let the games begin: A preliminary study using Attention Process Training-3 and Lumosity brain games to remediate attention deficits following traumatic brain injury. *Brain Injury, 27*(6), 707–716.

Index